Spa Bodywork
A Guide for Massage Therapists

Spa Bodywork
A Guide for
Massage Therapists

Anne Williams

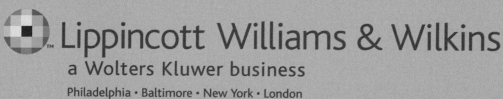 Lippincott Williams & Wilkins
a Wolters Kluwer business

Philadelphia · Baltimore · New York · London
Buenos Aires · Hong Kong · Sydney · Tokyo

Acquisitions Editor: John Goucher
Managing Editor: David R. Payne
Marketing Manager: Hilary Henderson
Signing Publisher Representative: Susan Schlosstein
Production Editor: Paula C. Williams
Designer: Doug Smock
Artwork: Dragonfly Media
Photography: Mel Curtis
Compositor: Maryland Composition, Inc.
Printer: R.R. Donnelley & Sons—Willard

Printed in the United States of America

Library of Congress Cataloging-in-Publication Data

Williams, Anne, BFA.
    Spa bodywork : a guide for massage therapists / Anne Williams
        p. ; cm.
    Includes bibliographical references and index.
    ISBN 13: 978-0-7817-5578-8
    ISBN 10: 0-7817-5578-6 (alk. paper)
1. Massage therapy. I. Title.
    [DNLM: 1. Massage—methods. 2. Health Resorts. WB 537 W721s 2007]
RM721.W55 2007
615.8'22—dc22

                                                                                    2006009315

*The publishers have made every effort to trace the copyright holders for borrowed material. If they have inadvertently
overlooked any, they will be pleased to make the necessary arrangements at the first opportunity.*

To purchase additional copies of this book, call our customer service department at **(800) 638-3030** or fax
orders to **(301) 223-2320**. International customers should call **(301) 223-2300**.

Visit Lippincott Williams & Wilkins on the Internet: http://www.LWW.com. Lippincott Williams & Wilkins
customer service representatives are available from 8:30 am to 6:00 pm, EST.

06 07 08 09 10
2 3 4 5 6 7 8 9 10

For my parents, Marsha and Lloyd; for my sister, Cindy; for my husband, Keith; for my cousin, Natalie; and for my dear friend, Erin, who support me, cheer when it works, and pick up the pieces when it doesn't.

Preface

Spa Bodywork: A Guide for Massage Therapists is primarily a textbook for massage students enrolled in spa programs. It is also a guide for practicing massage therapists who wish to add spa treatments to a private practice or work in the spa industry. To some extent, the text can be used by estheticians to improve their product knowledge and develop new skills for "full-body" skin care.

As the title implies, *Spa Bodywork* aims to illuminate the powerful links between massage and spa treatments. By providing the background on common treatments, I am able to show that many of the spa products often used just for beauty have the same physiological effects as massage or act in synergy with massage techniques. Seaweed, for example, stimulates circulation and lymph flow and supports the detoxification process of the body. Many useful minerals in seaweed can be absorbed through the skin. Seaweed treatments can have a pronounced effect on the thyroid, so they must be used carefully. This requires a good knowledge of the products and application methods being used. Similarly, therapeutic mud such as Dead Sea mud and Moor mud have proven anti-inflammatory properties, so they are used in Europe to treat arthritis and other musculoskeletal disorders. Such products can be used to support relaxation and stress reduction or as part of a treatment plan for injury rehabilitation.

Spa Bodywork breaks down each spa treatment into an easy-to-understand sequence of steps carefully designed to provide an efficient routine for practitioners and a satisfying experience for clients. The book provides instructions for standard methods of delivery as well as for some creative options that make sense when the service is provided by a massage therapist. In these cases, the service is designed to incorporate a natural healing substance such as mud, seaweed, shea butter, or essential oils into the massage. Clients do not have to give up their massage to enjoy a spa treatment.

The basic concepts and application methods covered earlier in the book lay the foundation for more advanced techniques that are described in later chapters. All aspects of a treatment are addressed, including indications and contraindications for the treatment, equipment needs, product choices, promotion, combining one service with another, and client management during the treatment.

Although wet room treatments (i.e., treatments that depend on expensive hydrotherapy equipment such as Vichy showers) are discussed in Chapters 3 and 4, the emphasis is on the delivery of spa treatments in a dry room setting (i.e., no shower). This makes the book usable in a wide range of surroundings because it shows how spa services that are usually thought to be too difficult to deliver in a dry room (e.g., seaweed, mud) can be used in both day spas and small private practices without the need for expensive equipment.

Organization and Structure

Spa Bodywork is practical and comprehensive in its approach. For example, spa instructors will find that the materials are presented in a format that can be easily referenced and that is flexible enough to allow them to use as little or as much of the information as they choose. Students can be directed to the treatment considerations and procedure section, and advanced therapists will find the detailed background on spa products useful. The topics have been divided into three main areas.

Part 1: Spa Foundations, provides a framework for massage therapists venturing into the world of spa. Chapter 1, "Overview of the Spa Industry," gives a history of the spa industry and defines the types of spas that are common in America. Chapter 2, **"Preparation for Spa Treatment Delivery"** describes the equipment needed to deliver spa treatments, sanitation protocols, the documentation process, and contraindications to spa treatments. Although skin care is out of the scope of practice for massage therapists in most states, every therapist working in a spa should have a basic understanding of the skin. This information is provided in Chapter 2 along with an introduction to product types and important product terms.

Chapter 3, "Foundation Skills for Spa Treatment Delivery," teaches core techniques that are used in the treatment chapters of the book. These techniques include spa draping, positioning the client for product application, removal techniques for the dry room and wet room, spa massage, and treatment enhancers such as firming face massages and paraffin dips. In Chapter 4, "Water Therapies," the basic principles of hydrotherapy are discussed together with wet room equipment such as Vichy showers and hydrotherapy tubs.

It is important to have a solid understanding of aromatherapy when working in the spa industry. Chapter 5, "Introduction to Spa Aromatherapy," introduces aromatherapy, provides an overview of the physiological and psychological effects of essential oils, describes basic methods of application, and presents some simple ways to add essential oils to any treatment. Smell-scapes refer to the aroma landscape that a therapist creates to enhance a spa treatment. This concept is defined, and readers are given practical advice about creating smell-scapes and blending essential oils safely.

In **Part 2: Spa Treatments**, the lessons learned in Part 1 become a stepping stone for more advanced techniques. Common treatments delivered routinely at most spas are described in step-by-step detail in Chapter 6, "Exfoliation Treatments," and Chapter 7, "Body Wraps." In Chapter 8, "Spa Foot Treatments," reflexology, satisfying massage techniques, and various products such as clay and seaweed are combined for pain-relieving and revitalizing foot services. The sample treatments described under each section heading show how basic treatments can be combined with different treatment concepts and promotional descriptions to create many "ready-to-use" services.

Fangotherapy, the use of clay, mud, and peat for healing purposes, is discussed in Chapter 9, "Fangotherapy." This chapter looks at the traditional use of fango in Europe as well as its evolution in the United States. Popular relaxation treatments used before the application of fango for acute, subacute, and chronic muscular conditions are described.

In Chapter 10, "Thalassotherapy," the therapeutic benefits of seaweed are explored in relationship to a number of popular services. In each of these chapters, traditional approaches are described along with variations in techniques and creative departures that suit the special skills of a massage therapist.

The final chapters of Part 2 are Chapter 11, "Ayurveda" and Chapter 12, "Stone Massage." The techniques described in these chapters require an attention to detail and a willingness to embrace new ideas. Ayurveda, the 5000-year-old Indian medical system, incorporates spiritual as well as practical methods for addressing wellness. Readers learn about core concepts in ayurveda that support unique body treatments, including abhyanga massage, marma point massage, Indian head massage, shirodhara (a treatment in which a thin stream of oil is played over the forehead), and udvartana (massage with herbal paste).

Stone massage is a popular massage modality at spas and clinics across the country. It requires focus and commitment to the treatment, attention to detail, and good massage skills. The routine taught in Chapter 12 walks readers through the basic elements of a stone massage before teaching more advanced techniques that require practice. The goal is to move beyond effleurage with stones to a more satisfying form of bodywork that includes a variety of techniques, including deep tissue and range of motion.

Part 3: Putting It All Together begins with an in-depth look at treatment design and the signature spa treatment in Chapter 13, "Treatment Design and the Signature Spa Treatment." Readers learn how to develop their own original services and to view spa treatments as works of art. In Chapter 14, "Careers in Spa," readers are encouraged to define their own spa philosophies and use those philosophies to identify a good spa job or write a spa program for their massage practice or spa. Practical issues such as the creation of a spa menu are addressed as well as marketing activities, retail sales, and budget considerations.

Pedagogical Features

To facilitate learning, each chapter in the book begins with an outline and a list of key terms with definitions. The treatment chapters have the same internal structure so that information can be found quickly. Each of these chapters has the following components:

- **Introduction:** At the beginning of each chapter, the topic is introduced and the framework for the treatment is set up. If the treatment has a unique history, as is the case with thalassotherapy, it is briefly described. If the chapter is broad in scope, as it is in Chapter 11 on ayurveda, the introduction is used to provide an overview and organize the topic. Product details are also described in this section when appropriate. For example, a number of different types of fango are used in spa treatments, and each has a different set of therapeutic benefits. When developing a spa service, the therapist needs to have enough information to be able to choose the fango most likely to achieve the desired therapeutic goal.

- **General Treatment Considerations:** These sections discuss the indications, contraindications, and any other special considerations for the delivery of each service. For example, in a body wrap, claustrophobia is always a concern. Even clients who have no previous history of claustrophobia may become panic stricken when wrapped. This section gives practical advice about how to avoid or deal with such situations.

- **Treatment Snapshots:** The snapshots allow therapists to get a speedy overview of the indications, contraindications, supplies, and treatment steps involved in each service. These snapshots are of benefit to therapists who like a concise list and want to find information quickly.

- **Treatment Procedures:** Each Treatment Procedure describes how to prepare for the treatment and position the client at the beginning of the service. The treatment is broken down into easy-to-follow steps accompanied by photographs that illustrate how to position the client and how to apply the products. When appropriate, variations in treatment delivery methods are discussed, taking into account the available equipment, positioning of the client, timing limitations, and implications of combining a treatment with enhancers or other treatments. Although wet room options are stated briefly, when appropriate, all of the treatment steps are based on dry room delivery.

- **Sanitation Boxes:** Sanitation Boxes appear in the Procedure sections to remind therapists about cleanliness and hygiene. Methods for cleaning specific equipment used in the treatments are described.

- **Broaden Your Understanding Boxes:** Some chapters contain a box that helps to provide an understanding of the broader application of spa therapies. Some of these boxes focus on the use of a unique product in other countries (e.g., the use of fango in Europe), and others focus on treatments or techniques used by estheticians (e.g., What is a facial?).

- **Sample Treatments:** The basic treatment procedure, or a variation of it, is described within the context of an overall treatment concept. Promotional descriptions and ready-to-use recipes provide valuable resources for planning how to add spa services to an existing massage practice. By using the main treatment as a starting point and adding other therapeutic elements to it, the therapist can learn to develop highly original spa services.

- **Review Questions:** Review questions at the end of each chapter allow spa students to test their knowledge and comprehension.

In the Appendix section, a master list of essential oils with botanical names and a list of sources for products and equipment are given to help therapists find the necessary materials for the delivery of the treatments described in the book. A helpful list of spa associations is also provided.

Final Note

In the past 10 years, complementary therapies such as massage, traditional Chinese medicine, acupuncture, aromatherapy, meditation, yoga, and hydrotherapy have gained a wider acceptance with the general public. At the same time, stress in the workplace has increased, resulting in a higher incidence of diseases such as repetitive musculoskeletal injury, heart disease, high blood pressure, and panic attacks. There has never been a better time for therapists to promote the use of spa therapies, and the continuing expansion of the spa industry is evidence for the strong demand that exists. From spa's origins in ancient cultures and from its established use in Europe, it is plain that spa assimilates many forms of therapy into a comprehensive system that leads to wellness. The spa experience can be life changing. Far from being just a luxury, spa therapy represents the bold first step toward a better form of health care. Its future is in the hands of dedicated therapists and visionary spa owners who have the ability to provide a space where clients can experience balance and celebrate life while receiving exceptional care.

I hope that this book inspires massage therapists to include spa therapies in their practices or to find jobs in the spa industry that are challenging and rewarding. I believe that the use of the products and treatments described in these chapters will support better health and wellness. I am grateful for the opportunity to share spa with all of the talented therapists and students who populate this wonderful profession, and I invite therapists to share their spa experiences, best practices, and suggestions. These can be sent by email to anne@spabodywork.com

Sincerely,
Anne Williams

User's Guide

Spa Bodywork: A Guide for Massage Therapists will guide you through each step of delivering a treatment—from a consideration of the indications and contraindications to scope of practice issues, the supplies needed, how to set-up the room and practical tips on the specific steps involved. It also provides ideas for massage therapists on integrating massage techniques, spa products and enhancing accents, so you can create and deliver unique services.

You'll find these great features in the text:

More than 350 striking full-color photographs clearly illustrate each spa technique and treatment. ▶

◀ Each chapter begins with a **chapter outline** and list of **key terms** to orient you to the content in the chapter.

Broaden Your Understanding boxes provide you with additional information and alternative methods. ▶

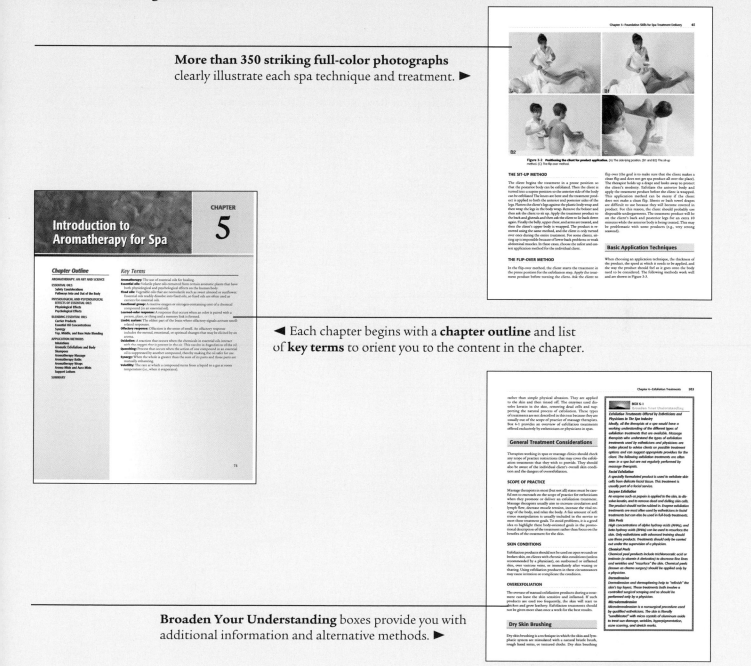

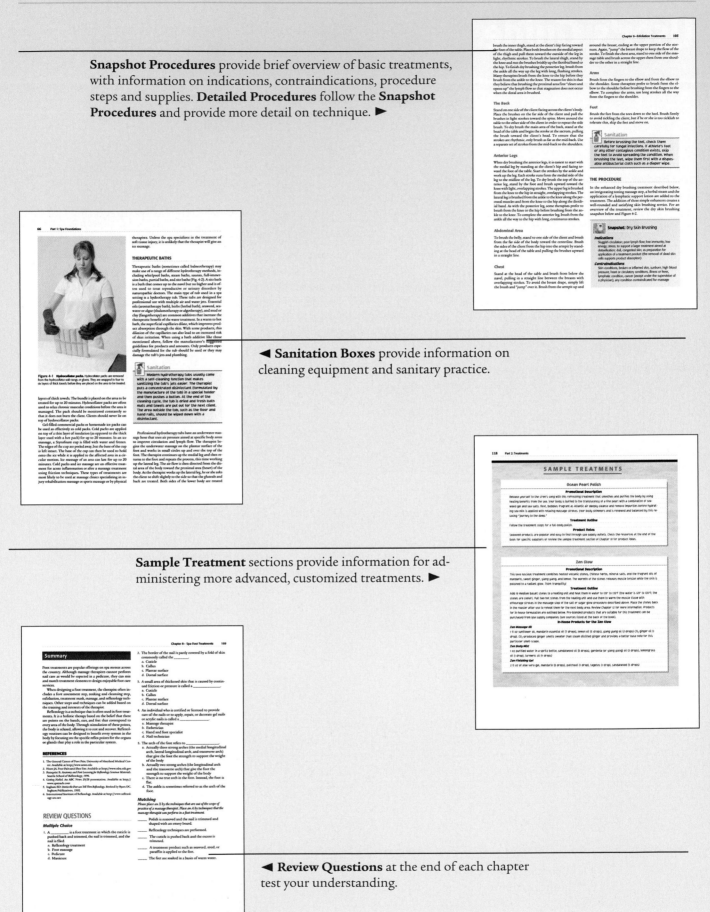

Snapshot Procedures provide brief overview of basic treatments, with information on indications, contraindications, procedure steps and supplies. **Detailed Procedures** follow the **Snapshot Procedures** and provide more detail on technique. ▶

◀ **Sanitation Boxes** provide information on cleaning equipment and sanitary practice.

Sample Treatment sections provide information for administering more advanced, customized treatments. ▶

◀ **Review Questions** at the end of each chapter test your understanding.

Acknowledgments

Writing and producing *Spa Bodywork* has involved the contributions of many people, some of whom are unknown. I am thankful to all of them and would like to acknowledge those who stand out here.

I am grateful to have had the opportunity to work with the team at Lippincott Williams & Wilkins, and I am thankful for their tireless enthusiasm and hard work. I would particularly like to thank Pete Darcy for his creativity, vision, and insight; David Payne for always being sensible and practical (while remaining flexible); and Susan Schlosstein for her continued support and interest.

During its development, *Spa Bodywork* has been reviewed by a number of professionals in the massage industry, each of whom have given thoughtful and helpful input, so I would like to thank them for their time and contribution.

Thanks to the photographer Mel Curtis and his team, Connie and Doug, for their visual contribution to the book and for being such lovely people. Thank you also to June Pendleton of Universal Companies and Professor Jim Simon of Rutgers University for help with some of the images. Thank you to the team at Savi Day Spa for allowing us to use their facility for the location shots, especially Kelly Wilson and Mary Wilson. Thank you to the models that gave up their weekends and did their best with body mechanics on the slippery floor! The models were Debbie Bates, Destiny Harrison, Catharine Jakeman, Sunny Kim, Melody Lickert, Natalie Mayer-Yeager, Faithann McVeigh, Erin Murphy, Earl Nabritt, Jason Priest, Keith Shawe, Jenni Shires, Jill Wells, Tiffany Williams, and Gloria Mayer.

The material for this book was originally developed for four different spa programs, and so I am deeply grateful to the individuals who believed in spa and aromatherapy training for massage therapists and were willing to invest in the equipment and training necessary to launch these programs. These individuals include Feliz Rodriguez for the original program at Ashmead College; Meredyth Given, Kim Lothian, Lorine Hill, Siri McElliott, and Eric Rasmussen for the second program at Ashmead College (Washington and Oregon); Chris Froelich and the team at Somerset School of Massage Therapy (New Jersey); Jill Standard and the team at Oregon School of Massage Therapy (Oregon); and Lisa Hensel at Seattle School of Reflexology for the Reflexology Foot Spa Workshops. Thank you to both Randy Rogers and John Smith at Corinthian Colleges for their interest and support.

I extend my sincere appreciation to my family and friends for understanding when I couldn't be there because of the book and for their unwavering support and encouragement during the time that I was writing.

I would also like to thank the amazing spa instructors, aromatherapists, administrative staff, workshop participants, and individuals that I have had the privilege of working with and learning from, especially Kim Virant, Anthony Knoll, Melody Lickert, Jacki Borde, Katharine Appleyard, Judy Scheller, Kitty Lawrence, Alla Kammers, Ingrid Martin, Erin Murphy, Deby Giske, Anita Harper, Lincoln Heartsong, Mary Bryan, Andrea McClelland, Cindy Babb, Margie Miller, Jack Elias, Geraldine Thompson, Tani Bigalli, Kate Bromley, Faithann McVeigh, Alicia Chapman, Meghan Lawrence, Christy Cael, Gemini Sanford, Jade Shutes, Julie Carico, Andrea Niemeyar, Veronica McHugh, Marsha Elston, Shannon Alyea, Kim Marshal, Roz Burnet, Amanda Flynn, Cheryl Young, Chris Damalas, Terri Zelepuza, Suzanne Smith, Taffie Lewis, Jolie Griffin, Bill Fee, Edna Ciallella, Jenni Shires, Patty Glen, Carrie Ebling, Angie Coxon, David Christian, and Angie Schneider. A special thank you to my friend and business partner Bill Langford of Aromatic Body Stone Therapy for teaching me stone massage, being so much fun, and putting so much care into every set of stones for the workshops.

Reviewers

Kimberly Coleman, MEd
Massage Therapist
O'Fallon, Missouri

Linda Derrick, MA
Director of Education
CT Center for Massage Therapy
Andover, Connecticut

Susan Pomfret, MA
Lead Instructor, Massage Therapy Program
East Valley Institute of Technology
Mesa, Arizona

Timothy Starkey, LPN, LMT, CPT, CHT
Director of Education and Massage Department Head
Headhunter SpaTech Institute
Worcester, Massachusetts

Kelli Lene Yearwood
Department Head, Massage Therapy
Community Care College
Coweta, Oklahoma

Brief Contents

Expanded Contents

CHAPTER **3**

Foundation Skills for Spa Treatment Delivery

39

CHAPTER 4   **Water Therapies**   **61**

CHAPTER *7*   **Body Wraps**   **121**

CHAPTER *8*   **Spa Foot Treatments**   **145**

CHAPTER **9**   **Fangotherapy**   **171**

CHAPTER **10**   **Thalassotherapy**   **193**

CHAPTER **11**   **Introduction to Ayurveda for Spa**   **209**

CHAPTER 12   Stone Massage   243

PART three PUTTING IT ALL TOGETHER 263

Appendix   309

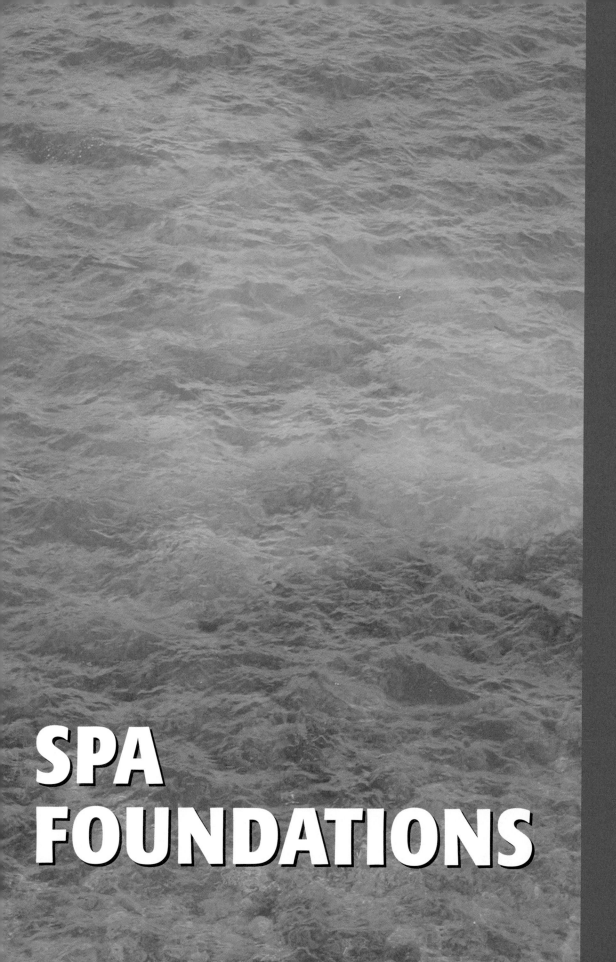

SPA
FOUNDATIONS

Overview of the Spa Industry

Chapter Outline

Key Terms

Esthetician: This word is a variant of the word *aesthetician*, which is derived from *aesthetic*, a branch of philosophy dealing with the nature of beauty. Estheticians are beauty specialists with around 300 to 750 hours of training. Their scope of practice includes skin care, hair removal, and makeup application.

Hamam: An Islamic bath characterized by a vaulted ceiling and a raised, heated marble platform called a *hararat*, which is used for massage or exfoliation.

Hydrotherapy: The use of water in one of its three forms (liquid, solid, or vapor) at specific temperatures for therapeutic purposes.

The Kur system: A German medical system that includes spa treatments as part of a wider system for health and wellness. Kur treatments are medically prescribed and paid for by the national health care system.

Luxury spa: A spa with exceptional accommodations, a full range of treatments, the latest advances in spa technology, a full array of wet-room equipment, and well-trained staff.

Radon: A naturally occurring atmospheric gas that is radioactive and is released as uranium in rock and soil as it breaks down. It is used in trace amounts in Europe for the treatment of arthritis and asthma.

Spa: A commercial establishment that provides health and wellness treatments.

Spa therapy: A general term for a wide range of spa treatment methods or techniques used by various professionals in different settings to support health and wellness.

Spa treatment: A general term for a treatment that uses water, specialized products, and various techniques to bring about relaxation, address a specific pathology, or support overall health and wellness.

Terme: Thermal bath. From the Greek *therme* meaning heat, and *thermai* meaning of or related to hot springs.

Thermal mud: Mud that comes from the areas around hot springs. It can be applied at the site while still hot from the spring water, or it can be extracted and heated for later application elsewhere.

The spa industry is dynamic, changeable, and difficult to define or categorize. It uses a variety of professionals that may include physicians, chiropractors, ayurvedic doctors, massage therapists, **estheticians**, life coaches, counselors, dietitians, yoga instructors, spiritual leaders, cosmetologists, dermatologists, cosmetic surgeons, naturopathic doctors, hypnotherapists, fitness trainers, and others. A wide range of therapies may be offered in an array of different settings under the heading of "**spa**." This chapter aims to briefly describe the historical roots of the spa industry and its evolution in the United States and to define broad categories of spas and the types of individuals that frequent them. It also looks at the future of spas and the potential role that spas play in a broader system of health care.

A Brief History of Spas

It is hard to pin down the origin of spa therapy. Mineral springs and **thermal muds** were probably used long before the first civilizations developed. In Finland, for example, nomadic people heated holes in the ground with hot rocks and covered them with a tarpaulin to have a warm place for bathing.[1] These saunas were also holy places where births and deaths took place. In much the same way, North American Indian tribes used a separate hut or a covered sweat lodge built partly into the ground. Large stones were heated in a fire and taken inside the hut, where they were sprinkled with water. Many early civilizations had a version of the spa bath that combined some form of social interaction with cleanliness. Russian steam baths, which can still be found in Europe, combine hot air and steam piped from a boiler. The atmosphere is humid, and the aim is to get the body to perspire continuously for a period after the bath has finished.

Traditionally, Arabs would bathe, only in cold water and would never use a tub, which would subject the bather to his or her own filth.[2] Cleanliness is intertwined with Islamic spirituality. The *hamam* (bath) became popular around 600 AD after Muhammed recommended sweat baths. They gained religious significance after this and began to be built close to mosques. When the Arabs conquered Syria, they quickly adopted Roman and Greek forms of bathing with hot water and steam, and cold water bathing fell out of fashion. The *hamam* became central to the community, serving as both a place of spiritual retreat and for socializing with friends. The beautiful vaulted ceilings, which were cut through to allow disks of natural light to shine down on the bathers, were more modest than those of their Roman counterparts. Bathers would stop first at the *camekan*, a small court of changing cubicles surrounding a fountain, before entering the *hararat* (hot marble baths). Bathers would receive a vigorous massage or *kese* (exfoliation with a rough cloth) on a raised marble platform above the wood or coal furnaces that are used to heat the *hararat*.

Although the use of public *hamam* is on the decline, travelers to Istanbul can still experience a Turkish bath complete with an exfoliating scrub and a brief, invigorating massage. Historical *hamams* such as the Galatasaray *Hamam* in Beyoglu give visitors a glimpse of the lasting splendor of the Ottoman Empire.

Perhaps the most famous ancient spas were those of the Roman Empire, where public baths were a part of the culture that served an important social function as well as providing a means of hygiene. The central role of spas in Roman culture led to a well-developed use of **hydrotherapy** (healing with water), and garrisons were often built around hot springs so that the soldiers could heal their battle wounds. By 43 AD, the Roman public viewed the baths as a way to relax and maintain health, and by the early fifth century AD, there were 900 baths in Rome alone. Although not everyone could afford a massage, all classes used the baths. Apart from the bath itself, there was usually an area that served as a community center, a restaurant, fitness center, bar, and a performance center where a juggler, a musician, or even a philosopher might entertain.

EUROPEAN SPAS IN THE 18TH AND 19TH CENTURIES

In the 18th and 19th centuries, Europeans would "take the waters" for common ailments such as rheumatism and respiratory disorders. Spas were often built in secluded mountain towns, providing visitors with spectacular views; fresh, clean air; and exercise on nature walks. A trend in spas at the time was to use medical professionals who carefully monitored each visitor's treatment. Eventually, spas expanded to include restaurants, casinos, theaters, racetracks, and other forms of entertainment. One such mineral spring town is Spa in Belgium (Fig. 1-1). The rich, royal, and famous have been visiting the mineral springs of Spa since the 16th century. The writer Victor Hugo was an advocate of Spa's curative waters and visited it often. The town, situated in a wooded valley surrounded by undulating hills and mineral-rich springs and rivers, is still a favored destination for those seeking rest and relaxation. Some speculate that the word "spa" can be traced to the name of the town, but it is more likely that it comes from the Latin words *espa* (fountain) and *sparsa* (from *spargere*, or "to bubble up"). *Sanus per aquam* (SPA) is Latin for "health through or by water," and *solus per aqua* (SPA) means "by water alone."

The use of water has long been central to **spa therapy** because bathing in mineral-rich water has some positive effects on the body. The medical benefits of "taking the waters" were advanced in Europe by two natural healers who developed their ideas in the early 1800s. The first was the Austrian Vincent Priessnitz (1799–1852), who promoted "the cold water cure." The "cure" consisted of drinking large amounts of cold water, bathing in cold water, following a simple diet, and participating in physical activity in the open air. Priessnitz was able to use the cold water cure

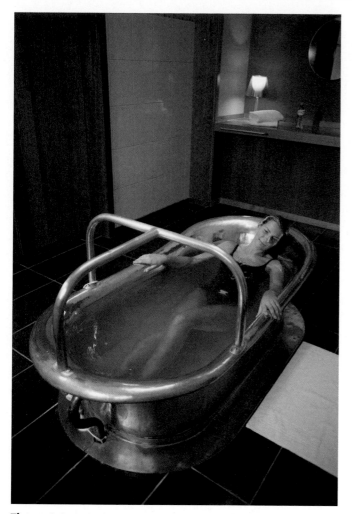

Figure 1-1   Spa, Belgium. The copper tubs used at Termes de Spa in Belgium date back to the 1800s. (Courtesy of Termes de Spa, Belgium.)

to care for a personal injury that doctors of the time thought untreatable. In 1826, Priessnitz opened a water cure establishment at Grafenberg in the mountains of Silesia, where his ideas were adopted by many prominent physicians.[3]

The second natural healer was Father Sebastian Kneipp (1824–1897), a German priest who cured himself of pulmonary tuberculosis by bathing in the icy Danube River and "shocking" his body into health. In one of his many books, *My Water-Cure* (1894), Kneipp writes, "Being a priest, the salvation of immortal souls is the first object for which I wish to live and die. During the last 30 or 40 years, however, the care for mortal bodies has absorbed a considerable portion of my time and strength."[4] Instead of administering last rites to gravely ill people, Kneipp used water and herbs to cure them. Kneipp's healing system, which combined physical exercise, simple food, hydrotherapy, and herbs, forms the basis of modern naturopathy. He is well known for the "wet nightshirt" treatment in which the remedy was to wear a shirt that had been dipped into water with salt or hay flower.

MODERN EUROPEAN SPAS

The modern spas of Europe are still based on the hydrotherapy principles developed by Priessnitz and Kneipp. For example, visitors to Bad Hofgastein Spa in Austria stay at a comfortable hotel with an indoor thermal pool fed by the mountain's waters. The spa also offers a whirlpool, sauna, Turkish bath, fango (mud) treatments, massage, radon baths, and a bar with a fireplace. Arthritic patients at the spa are given the "Gastein cure," which consists of visits to the **radon** caves of the Radhausberg Mountain and seems to be effective for arthritis, sinusitis, and chronic asthma sufferers (Fig. 1-2). Radon is a naturally occurring radioactive gas released by rock, soil, and water from the breakdown of uranium. It is absorbed by the body in very small doses through inhalation and through the skin in the 70% to 80% humidity that is found deep in the mountain caves. The use of environments with trace amounts of radon is not unique in Europe. In fact, some research appears to support the use of radon inhalation and radon baths for individuals with asthma, hypertension, osteoarthritis, and diabetes.[5–8]

Visitors to the little spa town of le-Mont-Dore in Auvergne, France, can take the radon-rich air in the form of a nasal irrigation with a tube inserted up one nostril. They breathe in a gas drawn from a nearby natural hot spring. Although this gas is mostly carbon dioxide, it also contains a

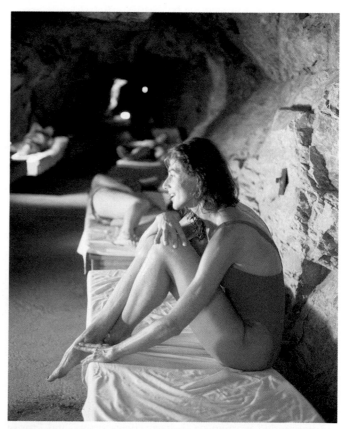

Figure 1-2   Bad Hofgastein Radon Cave at Bad Hofgastein Spa in Austria. (Courtesy of Bad Hofgastein Spa, Austria.)

radon concentration that is well above average. The radon is supposed to activate the blood, combat allergies, improve digestion, and stimulate the immune system.[9]

The Italian towns of Abano, Montegrotto, Galzignano, and Battaglia, which lie in a broad, green plain northeast of the Euganaean Hills in the Veneto of Italy, are famous for their ancient thermal baths. The spa at Montegrotto dates from the Roman times, and the remains of Roman spas in the area can still be seen. Abano Terme (*terme* means thermal bath) is considered one of the oldest spa centers in the world. According to legend, the Abano waters were warmed when Phaeton, the offspring of the sun, fell and landed in the mineral springs. It is likely that the inactive volcano there feeds the 130 hot springs in the area that still flow at a constant temperature of 188°F (86°C). Guests enjoy thermal treatments under the supervision of medical staff, and the Euganian Hills mud found in the area is used for arthritis, fibrosis, neuritis, gout, and metabolic problems.

It is common in Italy, as in many European spas, for guests to stay up to 3 weeks and receive daily treatments. In Germany, for example, spa therapies are regarded as medical treatments and as a general preventative against poor health. More than 9 million Germans enjoy the benefits of **"the Kur"** each year. In the Kur (cure) system, people spend 2 to 4 weeks in a climate chosen for their condition. They receive a wide range of treatments, including massage, mud, herbal and seaweed applications, inhalation therapy, and the use of mineral and thermal water. Part of the treatment is enjoying leisure time in a beautiful, efficiently run natural setting. Long-term studies show that the number of sick days taken by German workers who received Kur treatments dropped by an average of 60%.[10] Medical drug consumption and other health care costs also decreased. The long-term effects of the Kur system include a decrease in the number of early retirements and an increase in productivity throughout the patient's working life.

SPAS IN THE UNITED STATES

After the Industrial Revolution, **spa treatments** were seen as less scientifically viable than fast-acting, medically measurable drugs. As a result, the European concept of spas did not cross the Atlantic intact. Even though hydrotherapy cures quickly gained popularity in mid-1800s America, spa and "complementary" therapies developed in different directions.

In the early 1900s, water-cure centers became rallying points for new medical ideas, including meat-free diets and drugless healing, which were among the forerunners of alternative medicine as we know it today. Dr. John Harvey Kellogg pioneered many of the practices that have been proven in modern medicine at the Battle Creek Sanitarium (the San) in Michigan. Kellogg recommended a good vegetarian diet, regular exercise, correct posture, fresh air, and proper rest. He persuaded women to discard their corsets and ignore fashion to improve their breathing. Kellogg also practiced some questionable medicine, including electropathy and radium cures. Many regarded him as a quack even though he was one of the nation's leading surgeons. Kellogg's program was offered in a luxurious, restful, and elegant setting that was often attended by the rich and famous.[11]

In 1934, Elizabeth Arden turned her Maine summer home into a beauty and health spa called the Maine Chance. She targeted two groups of women: those who were middle-aged and trying to recapture youth and plain women looking for a means to achieve "beauty in a jar."[12] With cosmetics as her primary product, Arden pioneered the integration of diet, exercise, sports, yoga, facials, massage, beauty training, and pampering into a focused spa program. She used science and technology to develop her concept of beauty and to turn that concept into a $20 million industry. Today, Arden's signature Red Door Salons are recognized worldwide.

Spas in the early 1960s developed the stigma of "fat farms" for wealthy women who wanted to lose weight and detoxify (sometimes from drug and alcohol addictions).[13] The "fat farm" stigma may have slowed the growth of the spa industry for some time, but the concept of an integrated program of fitness, diet, and healthy lifestyle training, balanced with pampering treatments and beauty, became established. This comprehensive approach differentiates the American spa from its European counterpart, where the focus is usually on treating a recognized medical condition.

In the 1970s, hair salons seeking to expand their businesses started to offer *à la carte* spa treatments as well as regular salon services. This transformation of the salon into the day spa was the idea of Noel De Caprio.[14] She regularly attended spas in Europe and wanted to offer her clients a mini-spa experience in the convenience of her salon. She also recognized that Americans rarely had the time or the money to travel for 3 or 4 weeks to experience spa treatments in Europe. Making these services available locally, in easy-to-manage half- or full-day packages, added to their popularity. Other salon owners quickly followed De Caprio's lead. By 2004, there were an estimated 12,100 spas in the United States, and seven of every 10 of these establishments is a day spa.[15]

Over the past 10 years, complementary therapies such as massage, traditional Chinese medicine, acupuncture, aromatherapy, meditation, yoga, and hydrotherapy have gained acceptance with the public, especially for illnesses and injuries that are not effectively treated using conventional medical approaches.[16] At the same time, Americans now have greater access to information about health care options. This has led to the birth of integrative approaches in which alternative and conventional medicine are practiced side by side in many spas to improve health and fight disease.[17] Other factors in the growth of the spa industry are the general increase in the level of stress experienced by Americans and a decrease in the amount of leisure time.[18] Spas offer guests a way to decrease stress while improving their health at the same time.

According to a survey conducted by the International Spa Association (ISPA), 136 million visits were made to U.S.

spas in 2003, producing $11.2 billion in revenue. Spas have grown at an annual rate of 19% in the past 5 years. Shopping malls, cruise ships, and fitness clubs are adding spas, and they have also become a feature or focus of large hotels and resorts. At one time, spas were only for wealthy and privileged individuals, but today a spa experience is available for every budget. American spa owners are a vibrant and creative bunch and draw inspiration from a range of healing modalities, spiritual systems, and cultural influences to create a unique experience for their guests.

Basic Spa Categories

Because of the diversity that currently exists within the industry, spas are difficult to place into clear categories. For example, spas might be grouped on the length of the client's stay or on the focus of the spa program. A destination spa might be a weight loss spa, or it might be a spiritual retreat. A resort spa might be an adventure spa focusing on healthy athletes or a family spa with programs for both adults and children. Spas might be **luxury spas** with expensive treatments and high-tech equipment or "budget" spas with moderately priced services and a relaxed décor. The following list of spa types will help the reader begin to understand the general differences between basic spa categories.

DESTINATION SPAS

Guests visit destination spas for a weekend, a 4-day program, or longer to make significant lifestyle changes or to relax completely. Spa programs focus on fitness, healthy diet, detoxification, and lifestyle education. Some destination spas offer classes and services geared toward spiritual as well as physical renewal. Many destination spas offer a full menu of beauty services in addition to the spa program. A good example is the New Age Health Spa in New York

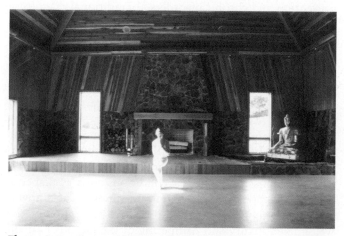

Figure 1-3   New Age Health Spa, New York. (Courtesy of New Age Health Spa, Neversink, NY.)

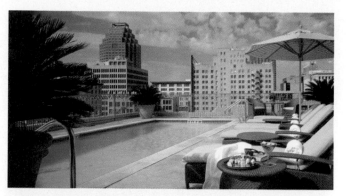

Figure 1-4   The Watermark Hotel and Spa in San Antonio, TX. (Courtesy of the Watermark Hotel and Spa, San Antonio, TX.)

(Fig. 1-3). This is a destination spa with a philosophy of mindful living, a calm mind, and a strong body. The spa offers guests a program that is spiritual while promoting fitness, good nutrition, and enjoyment of the outdoors. A typical day includes a morning meditation, a 3-mile hike, and yoga classes. For those who wish to detoxify, a juice fast replaces regular meals. Body treatments include a full range of services, such as a Shirodhara spiritual treatment, aromatherapy body wrap, and a maple sugar body scrub. As the name suggests, this type of spa targets clients who are looking for a spiritual as well as physical experience.[19]

RESORT SPAS

A resort spa offers different recreational opportunities such as hiking, rock climbing, water sports, shopping, tennis, golf, and horseback riding, as well as spa services. Often, the beautiful natural landscape around a resort is the primary reason for the visit, and the spa is just one of many activities offered to the resort or hotel guest. Some resort spas are a cross between a destination and hotel spa, where health programs are offered and guests can choose from low-fat spa cuisine or more traditional fare. For example, the Watermark Hotel and Spa in San Antonio, Texas, is a resort spa that sits right on San Antonio's famous River Walk (Fig. 1-4). Guests can explore the 2.5 miles of trails that follow the San Antonio River, shop in boutiques, or make an excursion to the Alamo. The spa, which occupies the entire second floor of the hotel, offers various beauty services, massage, and hydrotherapy *à la carte*.[20]

AMENITY SPAS

At one time, amenity spas, which are usually found in hotels, offered basic services only and were really afterthoughts, even in large hotels. A massage room, a simple fitness center containing little more than a treadmill, and a basic salon were usually all that was offered to guests. Many hotels now view spa services as an important contributor to

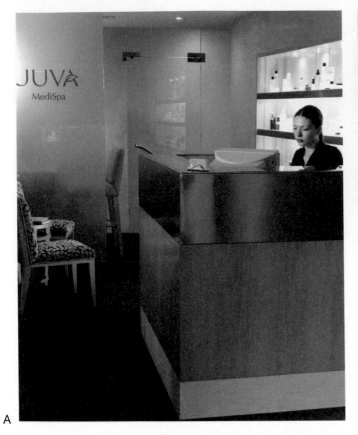

A

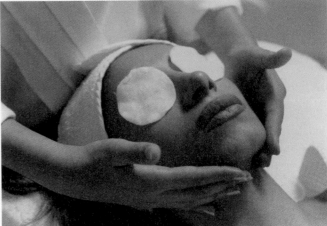

B

Figure 1-5 **Juva MediSpa, New York.** (Courtesy of Dr. Bruce Katz. MediSpa is a registered trademark owned by Dr. Bruce Katz.)

the bottom line,[21] so they have started to offer full-service facilities. Keeping pace with this trend, smaller hotels, bed and breakfast establishments, and even some time shares have moved toward offering in-room massages or mobile spa services if they do not have room for a full-service spa.

MEDICAL SPAS

In many ways, medical spas are a direct counterpart of European spas at which guests receive health care services in a relaxing and beautiful natural setting. Some hospitals are adding spas to ease the discomfort of terminally ill individuals and to help with pain management. Three different types of medical spas (sometimes called "medi-spas" or "medspas") are listed by SpaFinder.[22]

The first type is the esthetics-oriented medical spa, which includes services such as Botox or collagen injections, chemical skin peels, laser hair removal, laser skin treatments, liposuction, plastic surgery, and sclerotherapy (spider vein elimination). In this type of spa, medical cosmetic and clinical esthetics procedures are offered together with revitalizing treatments (e.g., massage) to support the recovery process. A good example is the Juva MediSpa, which is linked to the Juva Health and Wellness Center.[23] Skin health and beauty are addressed with anti-aging and skin damage treatments, Botox injections, liposuction, and breast augmentation. The mind–body connection and its

effect on health are treated using hypnotherapy, psychotherapy, fitness training, and nutritional consultations (Fig. 1-5).

The second type of medical spa is the complementary or alternative medicine spa, where the program designed for each guest is based on one of the alternative medicine systems such as ayurveda or Chinese Traditional Medicine. Naturopathic medicine, nutrition therapy, Western herbal medicine, and acupuncture all fall into this category. The Maharishi Vedic Health Center in Lancaster, Massachusetts, uses authentic ayurveda treatments for disease prevention and chronic disorders.[24] Traditional diagnostic procedures such as Vedic pulse diagnosis are used in designing the treatment and spa regimen. Guests can also take part in yoga classes, healthy cooking instruction, and evening lectures on Maharishi Vedic medicine.

The third type of medical spa is the preventative health care spa, in which medical staff members carry out a number of tests (e.g., blood tests, bone density screening) before designing the treatment program. Some of these spas specialize in general areas such as weight loss, pain management, or pre- or postnatal care. They may also offer specific programs for particular conditions such as diabetes, high blood pressure, or chronic insomnia. The Canyon Ranch Health Resort in Tucson, Arizona, combines the well-known luxury and pampering of the famous Canyon Ranch Spas with a health and healing center (Fig 1-6). The Executive Wellness Program is a 4-day health program that

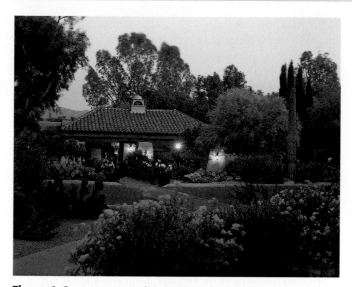

Figure 1-6   Canyon Ranch Spa Executive Health Program.
(Courtesy of Canyon Ranch Spa, Tucson, AZ.)

includes a complete physical examination as well as lifestyle assessment. The general approach of Canyon Ranch is to encourage guests to make long-term commitments to healthy living so as to decrease the occurrence of disease.[25]

At the time of writing (2004), medical spas comprised only 3% of the U.S. spa industry, but between 2002 and 2004, this was the segment of the industry that had grown the fastest.[26]

DAY SPAS

Day spas are mini retreats with services delivered *à la carte* or in half- to full-day packages. The Day Spa Association defines a day spa as a spa that offers a full range of treatments, including massage, body treatments, hydrotherapy treatments, esthetic services, weight management, yoga, or meditation, with hair care, manicures, and pedicures. Many business owners use the term "day spa" loosely to indicate an establishment that focuses on beauty, wellness, or both. An example of a creative day spa concept is Embodywork, a day spa in Decatur, Georgia, which offers daily retreats based on the principle that "a good life begins with being good to ourselves" (Fig. 1-7). Clients can choose a half- or full-day retreat that begins with a conversation about health, diet, relationships, and exercise goals. Conscious breathing exercises progress to a full-body massage and body polish. After lunch, the client can choose between a facial, reflexology, hand and foot treatment, or body wrap for their final service.[27]

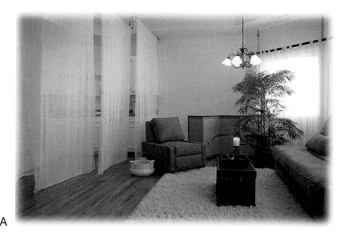

A

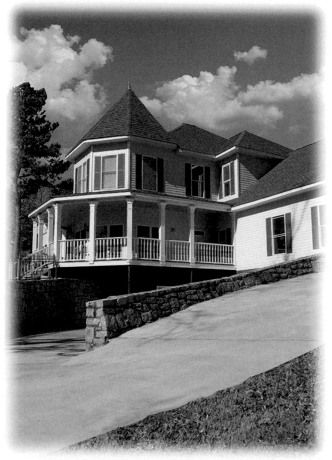

B

Figure 1-7   Embodywork, a creative day spa concept in Decatur, GA. (Courtesy of Embodywork, Decatur, GA.)

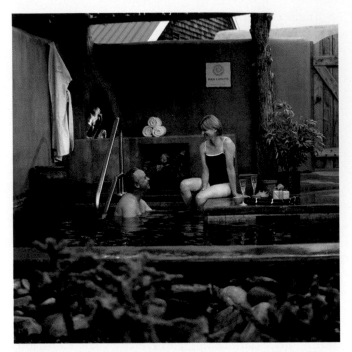

Figure 1-8 Ojo Caliente Hot Spring. Photo courtesy of Ojo Caliente Hot Spring, NM.

HOT SPRING SPAS

Hot springs spas use the natural thermal waters from hot springs in their spa regimen or treatments. The Ojo Caliente Spa surrounds the Ojo Caliente hot springs in New Mexico (Fig. 1-8). This spring was sacred to the ancestors of the Tewa tribes that still live in the region.[28] The mineral pools are open to the public for an entry fee, or spa guests can opt for a private pool and spa treatments that include facials, massage, and body wraps.

MOBILE SPAS

Mobile spas bring day spa services directly to clients at their home, office, hotel room, or at a party. The treatments are designed to be set up and delivered on site and are popular as a feature at bachelorette parties, prom parties, and corporate retreats. Treatments include seated massages, manicures, pedicures, reflexology, facials, and diet consultations.

Spa Clients

In Roman times, the local spa was a focal point of the community and enjoyed by all social classes. This is still the case in some parts of Europe, where spas are a part of the mainstream health care system. Although the American spa industry encourages the idea that spas are for everyone and should be a regular part of a healthy lifestyle, there is still a bias in the social status of individuals who attend spas.

In the 1960s and the 1970s, the average American spa client was most likely to be wealthy, female, and overweight. Her goals for visiting the spa probably included weight loss, exercise, and pampering in the form of beauty treatments. She expected the best possible service and was a discriminating customer.[13] Although spas in the United States go out of their way to attract a more diverse clientele, the ISPA Spa-Goer Survey for 2003 shows that the primary spa client is still female but has a middle to upper middle class income ($72,200 annual household income).[30] This client is most likely to be white (87%), with African Americans and those of Asian decent making up only 9% of the spa-going population. To promote greater diversity, spas are branching out, and spa owners are targeting various income backgrounds and age groups. The number of men attending spas is growing rapidly, and men currently comprise 29% of the market. Products and services for teenagers are also on the rise.

Although massage remains the most accepted treatment at spas, facials, manicures, and pedicures are also popular. Clients report that they want to focus on health, fitness, anti-aging, increased energy, and stress reduction.[31] Many clients visit spas simply to revitalize themselves and give themselves a break from work stresses. Cultural elements that include Ayuvedic medicine, Native American wisdom, and Asian influences are used to inspire treatments and create links to the environment and the global community.

In general terms, spas attract clients by adopting a philosophy and creating a menu of services that appeal to a specific group of clients. The facility, its visual appearance, the equipment available, and the price of its services also play roles in attracting these target clients to the spa. Clients are as diverse and difficult to define as the spas they attend, so it is helpful to look at the different ways that spas design their programs to attract a particular type of client.

SPAS FOR WOMEN

Spas for women can take many forms. A spa for women might offer expensive high-tech skin care or detoxification, vegetarian cuisine, and yoga. Anything and everything is possible. A spa might cater to brides, to mothers and babies, to athletes, or to grandmothers. For example, the target client of the Body Shop Spa in Utah, close to Zion National Park, is a woman on a budget (services are moderately priced), between the ages of 18 and 65, who wants to lose weight and enjoy the outdoors. The program at the spa is based on a seven-point philosophy that addresses nutrition, endurance, strength, flexibility, self-awareness, education, and relaxation. Manicures, pedicures, and massage are available, but rock climbing lessons and hiking replace other normal spa services.[32]

The Olympus Health Spa in Washington is a women-only spa because clothing throughout the spa is optional. Body scrubs and massage are offered in a Roman bath setting while other guests lounge nearby in the hot pools or converse in the sauna. It is a communal experience that caters to groups of women enjoying each other's company while they relax and renew. This spa has built its business by selling the "just for women" experience.[33]

SPAS FOR MEN

Research carried out using Spa Finder shows that nearly 29% of men book their own appointments, and the number of men attending spas has tripled since 1987. The International Spa and Fitness Association suggests that spas can target men by linking spa treatments to health and fitness, by offering discount treatments for men, and by using spa treatments as interesting giveaways at business meetings and conventions. The Nickel Spa in New York City, which has cobalt and sliver décor, was designed specifically for men. It has a menu of massage and facials that meet the special needs of men, including a Love Handle Wrap, a full-body wax called the Bodybuilder's Special, and 15 different skin care lines.[34]

SPAS FOR FAMILIES

Spas that target families offer services that fit every member's needs. There may be a full spa offering services for men and women as well as programs geared toward teens. Child care facilities for the younger members of the family might be offered with programs designed to get everyone together, such as horseback riding or hiking. The Point Hilton in Phoenix, Arizona, is a good example of this. This hotel offers a full-service spa, coyote camp for the kids, a family pool, and a golf course.[35]

SPA PROGRAMS FOR TEENS

Some day spas focus on the needs of teenagers, with treatments that address oily skin, acne, and sports injuries. Spa prom parties are a clever way to introduce young women and men to the benefits of spa treatments. Teens enjoy the chance of preparing for the big event surrounded by a group of friends getting manicures, pedicures, facials, and body wraps.

Spas in the Future

By their very nature, spas are indefinable, ever changing, diverse, and evolving. Therapists and clients alike are embracing spa treatments as a means of promoting health and wellness. This seems likely to continue as the public understanding of spa treatments develops. The rate of growth in the industry is expected to become steadier as the dramatic boom of recent years slows down. It is likely that spas will continue to drive a movement toward a more integrated form of medicine. Currently, one third of all Americans are

in favor of complementary medicine's becoming more widely available within the conventional medical system. This is the trend in Europe, where 60% of the public in Belgium and 74% of the public in the United Kingdom use alternative forms of medicine for wellness. Spas provide a place where conventional medicine and exceptional client care have become integrated. Taking care of oneself by being willing to receive care and pampering is an important aspect of healing in a spa environment. Although spas are still often considered just luxuries, it is likely that spa services will come to be viewed as necessary for thriving in a fast-paced contemporary lifestyle.

The ISPA Education Committee developed the Ten Elements of the Spa Experience image shown in Figure 1-9.[36] ISPA's goal was "to help define the elusive and ever changing nature of the spa experience" and to "create a foundation, a common language and career path for the emerging spa professional." Many concepts important to the practice of spa emerge from the ISPA's dialog around the Ten Elements image. The most important perhaps is the idea of integration. Everything is connected: Feeling beautiful, feeling joyous, feeling healthy and energetic are signs of a balanced life. A balanced life requires both reflection and action. Spas provide a space where clients can experience each element represented in the image and reflect on its presence or absence in their lives. Movement, touch, an appreciation of beauty, a connection to the environment, cultural expression, social contribution, the healing quality of water, and nourishment of both the body and the soul are the essential concepts upon which spa therapy is founded. The spa experience can be life changing. Far from being just a luxury, spa therapy represents the bold first step toward a better form of health care. Its future is in the hands of dedicated therapists and visionary spa owners who have the ability to provide a space where clients can experience balance and celebrate life while receiving exceptional care.

Summary

It is difficult to pin down the origin of spa therapy because mineral springs and thermal mud were probably used long before civilizations evolved and history was first recorded. Many early civilizations had a version of the spa bath that combined some form of social interaction with cleanliness.

Spas emerged in America in the 1960s as expensive retreats for wealthy women who wanted to lose weight, detoxify, and relax. Since then, American spas have evolved to include a wide range of complementary therapies that embrace concepts in preventative health, wellness, spirituality, fitness, rehabilitation, and beauty. Although the primary spa client is still a middle upper class woman, spas are now reaching out to other demographics, including men and teenagers.

THE TEN ELEMENTS OF THE SPA EXPERIENCE

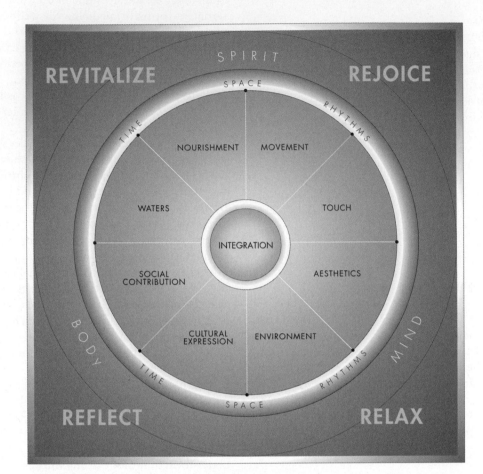

Waters: The internal and external use of water in its many forms.

Nourishment: What we feed ourselves: food, herbals, supplements, and medicines.

Movement: Vitality and energy through movement, exercise, stretching and fitness.

Touch: Connectivity and communication embraced through touch, massage and bodywork.

Integration: The personal and social relationship between mind, body, spirit and environment.

Aesthetics: Our concept of beauty and how botanical agents relate to the biochemical components of the body.

Environment: Location, placement, weather patterns, water constitution, natural agents and social responsibility.

Cultural Expression: The spiritual belief systems, the value of art and the scientific and political view of the time.

Social Contribution: Commerce, volunteer efforts, and intention as they relate to well-being.

Time, Space Rhythms: The perception of space and time and its relationship to natural cycles and rhythms.

Circle concept created by R. Zill for ISPA 2001

ISPA would like to thank the ISPA education committees past and present.

Figure 1-9 International SPA Association 10 elements image. (Reprinted with permission from the International SPA Association. Circle concept created by R. Zill for ISPA 2001.)

Spas provide a space for clients to rest, reflect, and make positive life changes that lead to a more balanced life. As integrative approaches to health continue to develop, spas are likely to play a larger role in meeting people's health care needs.

REFERENCES

1. Aaland M: *Finnish sauna: History of the Nordic bath.* Available at http://www.cyberbohemia.com
2. Aaland M: Sweat: *The Illustrated History and Description of the Finnish Sauna, Russian Bania, Islamic Hamam, Japanese Mushi-Buro, Mexican Temescal, and Americ.* Santa Barbara: CAPRA Press, 1978.
3. Buchman DD: *The Complete Book of Water Healing.* New York: McGraw-Hill, 2002.
4. Kneipp S: *My Water-Cure,* 3rd ed. Kempten, Bavaria: Jos. Koesel Publishers, 1894.
5. Mitsunobu F, et al. Elevation of antioxidant enzymes in the clinical effects of radon and thermal therapy for bronchial asthma. *J Radiation Res* 2003;44:95–99.
6. Marshalik BE, Fen'ko AN: The use of air-radon baths for rehabilitating the immune system of patients with bronchial asthma [translated from Russian]. *Vopr Kurortol Fizioter Lech fiz Kult* 1991;6:6–10.
7. Yamaoka K, et al: Basic study on radon effects and thermal effects on humans in radon therapy. *Physiol Chem Phys Med NMR* 2001;33:133–138.
8. Yamoka K, et al: Effects of radon inhalation on biological function-lipid peroxide level, superoxide dismutase activity, and membrane fluidity. *Arch Biochem Biophys* 1993;302:37–41.
9. Emsley J: *Nature's Building Blocks: An A-Z Guide to the Elements.* Oxford, UK: Oxford University Press, 2001.
10. Hyde F: *The German Way.* New York: McGraw-Hill, 1996.
11. Great American Quacks: The Museum of Questionable Medical Devices. Available at http://www.mtn.org/quack/amquack/kellogg.html
12. Elizabeth Arden. Available at http://www.enterprisingwomanexhibit.org/beauty/adreu.html
13. Miller ET: *Salon Ovations: Day Spa Techniques.* Albany, NY: Milady Publishing, 1996.
14. Noelle Spa, Stamford, CT. Available at http://www.noelle.com
15. *The ISPA 2004 Spa Industry Executive Summary.* Available at http://www.experienceispa.com/media/industrystudy-o11805.html
16. Peeke PM: *The Birth of Integrative Medicine.* Available at http://www.experienceispa.com/confrenses/articles/birth.html
17. Peeke PM: *The American Spa: A Renaissance of Ancient Wisdom and Modern Medicine.* Available at http://www.experienceispa.com/articles/renaissance.html
18. *Americans and Stress.* Available at http://www.stress.org
19. The New Age Health Spa, Neversink, NY. Available at http://www.newagehealthspa.com
20. The Watermark Hotel and Spa, San Antonio, TX. Available at http://www.watermarkhotel.com
21. Wylie J: *Today's Spas are More Than an Amenity at Hotels and Resorts.* Available at http://www.e-hospitality.com
22. *Medical spas.* Available at http://www.spafinder.com/spas/medical/procedures.is
23. *The Juva Medi Spa in New York.* Available at http://www.juvaskin.com
24. *Maharishi Vedic Health Center, Lancaster, MA.* Available at http://www.landcasterhealth.com
25. The Canyon Ranch Health Resort in Tucson, Arizona, accessed 03.02.05. Available at http://www.canyonranch.com/tucson/index.asp
26. The ISPA 2004 Spa Industry Study. Available at http://www.experienceispa.com/learn/resources.html
27. Embodywork Spa, Decatur, GA. Available at http://www.embody.com
28. The Ojo Caliente Hot Spring Spa, New Mexico. Available at http://www.ojocalientespa.com
29. Brown MT: *Spa and Medicine: Mindful of the Past, Movement of the Future.* Available at http://www.spamangament.com/les%20cadres/medi/introduction.html
30. *Key Findings of the 2003 ISPA Spa Goer Survey.* Available at http://www.discoverspas.com
31. Monteson P, Singer J: What today's spa client seeks. *ISHC Lodging Hospitality* 1998 (November).
32. The Body Shop Spa, St. George, UT. Available at http://www.bodyshopspa.com
33. The Olympus Spa, Tacoma, WA. Available at http://www.olympusspa.com
34. The Nickel Spa in New York, NY. Available at http://www.nickelformen.com
35. The Point Hilton Resort, Phoenix, AZ. Available at http://www.pointhilton.com
36. *Pulse Magazine.* January/February 2002. Available at http://www.experienceISPA.com

REVIEW QUESTIONS

Multiple Choice

1. Many early civilizations had a version of a:
   a. Spa shower
   b. Exfoliation treatment
   c. Meditation center
   d. Spa bath

2. Roman baths may have originally been built to treat soldiers' battle injuries. By 43 AD, they were used by:
   a. Field soldiers only
   b. Emperors only
   c. All classes of the Roman Empire
   d. Men only

3. The Turkish bath is also called a:
   a. Sweat lodge
   b. Garrison
   c. *Hamam*
   d. *Camekan*

4. In the 18th and 19th centuries, Europeans would go to spa towns to heal common ailments such as rheumatism and respiratory disorders. This practice was know as
   a. "Take the mud"
   b. "Take the waters"
   c. "Take the cure"
   d. "Take the air"

5. The word *spa* originated from:
   a. A mineral spring town in Belgium named Spa
   b. The Latin words for *fountain* (*espa*)
   c. The Latin words for *by water alone* (*solus per aqua*)
   d. No one is really sure, although more than likely it is from a Latin source.

Fill in the Blank

6. In Germany, there is widespread acceptance of spa therapies as a viable form of treatment for individuals who have not responded to conventional medicine. This system is called the _____ system.

7. An Austrian healer named Vincent Priessnitz was an advocate of the _____ cure.

8. Naturopathic medicine is rooted in the healing methods of a German priest named _____.

9. At Bad Hofgastein, patients with arthritis, sinusitis, and chronic asthma take part in the "Gastein cure." This cure consists of visits to caves where _____ is absorbed and inhaled in small amounts.

10. The International Spa Association Spa-Goer Survey for 2003 indicates that the primary spa client will be of middle to upper class income and _____.

Preparation for Spa Treatment Delivery

Chapter Outline

Key Terms

Antiseptic: An agent that prevents or arrests the growth of microorganisms.

Barrier function: The ability of the skin to prevent penetration by microorganisms and chemicals that might otherwise damage tissues or enter the circulation. The skin also reduces water loss.

Disinfectant: A chemical that destroys harmful microorganisms; usually used on inanimate objects such as floors, walls, and countertops.

Sanitation protocol: The spa or clinic's procedure for keeping the facility clean and disinfected during operation.

Stratum corneum: The outermost layer of the epidermis of the skin that provides the skin with its barrier function.

Universal Precautions: The policy of the Centers for Disease Control on blood and body fluids, which are potentially infectious sources of human immunodeficiency virus (HIV), hepatitis B virus (HBV), and other bloodborne pathogens.

This chapter aims to introduce new spa therapists to areas that need attention and careful planning before a particular spa treatment is offered at the spa or clinic. First, it is helpful to explore the different equipment choices that are available for dry room treatments (see Chapter 4 for descriptions of wet room equipment). The therapist must also evaluate and, if necessary, modify any **sanitation protocols** used to ensure proper disinfection of the spa equipment and to prevent contamination of spa products. Forms are needed to document the client's overall condition and to keep a record of the spa treatment. Understanding how spa treatments might affect a client's condition adversely and when to postpone a treatment or suggest a different service are also important. Finally, it is useful to have a basic understanding of the skin and the effects of different spa product ingredients. This knowledge helps therapists decide when it is appropriate to refer clients to skin care professionals and enables them to ensure that clients are comfortable and that treatments are carried out safely.

Basic Dry Room Equipment and Setup

There is no doubt that the luxurious surroundings of an upscale spa enhance the mood and character of the spa experience. But with attention to detail and with an eye toward functional ambiance, spa treatments can also be delivered satisfactorily in small spas and massage clinics without inordinate expense.

Soothing color combinations set the tone for a room. Color combinations should be determined by the type of spa or the type of treatments offered at the facility. For example, some spas located at fitness centers have a high-tech look with shiny surfaces of glass and metal. This styling suits a purposeful, streamlined, urban concept. Earth tones with accents of natural texture (woven baskets, rattan mats, bamboo, and stone) are presently in style. These organic backgrounds set the stage for the culturally inspired treatments that are the current trend in the industry. Multiple pools of soft light are more relaxing than one bright light in a corner or even a treatment room that is too dark. Although candles define a reflective atmosphere, open flames are often against the fire codes. Candles look beautiful the first time they are lit, but as they start to melt and become misshapen, they appear messy. Tea lights are a neater option.

The centerpiece of the room will be the treatment table and the manner in which it is made up with linens. For a spa on a budget, plain sheets and a large bath towel might be used. Beige or cream sheets and an earth-toned towel seem to make a more elegant impression than stark white sheets and a colorful beach towel. Multi-tonal colors in slightly varying shades give an impression of texture and depth. An upscale spa might opt for Egyptian cotton and a matching coverlet with a multitude of throw pillows. Spa suppliers provide everything from the basics to very expensive linens.

Added touches such as fleece table covers that provide softness and warmth, and gel-filled face cradle covers are important touches that indicate that care has been taken to make clients welcome and comfortable.

Whenever possible, keep larger pieces of equipment out of the treatment room or hide them behind a screen until they are needed. It is helpful to have a movable cart available to hold any spa products used in the treatment. Arrange the cart with care. Dirty bottles that are half full of spa products look messy, and even worse, may not be clean. Use only sanitized, clean, new-looking product bottles or remove the products from the used bottles and put them onto elegant Japanese platters, colorful glass bowls, spotless stainless steel, or pure white porcelain. The local import store is a good place to look for attractive containers that will improve the ambience of a treatment room. Avoid glass containers on hardwood, tile, or slate floors in case they break when dropped. It is often the simple touches that make the most difference. A flower tucked inside the fold of the coverlet or a platter with fruit placed on a sideboard suggests a place for rest, reflection, and renewal.

In upcoming chapters, individual treatments are described. Each of these treatments will be preceded by a "snapshot" that helps the reader get an overview of the service. A supply list is included as part of the snapshot. For therapists new to spa treatment, it is helpful to discuss equipment and equipment options in detail so that these snapshots will not be confusing (Fig. 2-1). Spa suppliers and equipment resources are listed in Appendix B.

HOT TOWEL HEATING UNIT

Hot towels are required throughout a spa body treatment, even when a shower is available. Therapists have a number of options in the way they heat and maintain their towels. These include a hot towel cabinet, hydroculator, roaster oven, or a simple soda cooler (see Fig. 2-1A).

Hot Towel Cabinet (Cabbi)

Hot towel cabinets (often called a cabbi) range in size from small six-towel units to much larger 72-towel units. They look like small refrigerators and are placed somewhere convenient close to the treatment table.

Hydrocollator

Hydrocollators are most often used to heat hydrocollator packs (see Chapter 4), but they also heat towels and hot sheets for body wraps. They keep water at a constant 165°F, and in busy spas, are useful as a source of hot water for filling foot soak containers.

Roaster Oven

For spas that are on a budget, a roaster oven filled with water is a cheap and efficient alternative to the more expensive

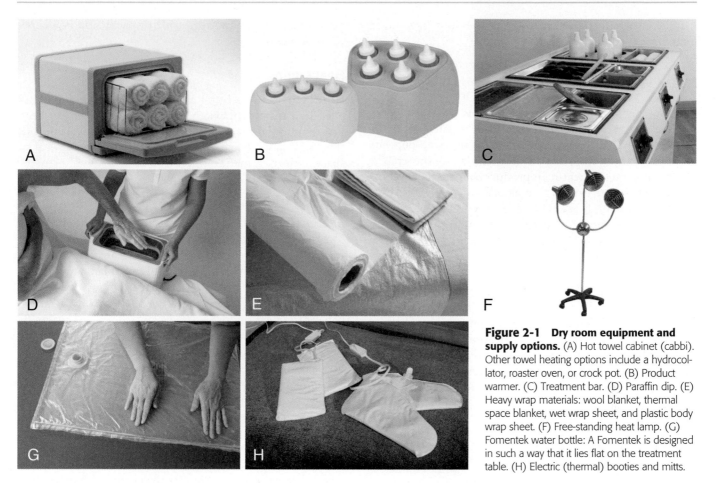

Figure 2-1   Dry room equipment and supply options. (A) Hot towel cabinet (cabbi). Other towel heating options include a hydrocollator, roaster oven, or crock pot. (B) Product warmer. (C) Treatment bar. (D) Paraffin dip. (E) Heavy wrap materials: wool blanket, thermal space blanket, wet wrap sheet, and plastic body wrap sheet. (F) Free-standing heat lamp. (G) Fomentek water bottle: A Fomentek is designed in such a way that it lies flat on the treatment table. (H) Electric (thermal) booties and mitts.

cabbi. A roaster oven can hold up to 20 towels and is also a useful heater for hot sheet wraps, spa products, and the stones used in a hot stone massage. Remove the towels from the roaster oven and ring out the excess water before putting them into an insulated soda cooler to keep them hot until use. If only a few towels are needed for the treatment, a crock pot serves the same purpose.

Soda Cooler

When the therapist removes products with hot towels, the towels must be close at hand to keep the process quick and efficient. Walking back and forth to a hot towel cabbi disrupts the flow of the treatment and is time consuming. Instead, transfer the towels from the heating unit to a small soda cooler (9- to 12-quart size) and place it near the treatment table for convenience.

PRODUCT WARMERS

There are some situations in which the product is meant to be applied cold, but in most cases, products are warmed before they are applied to the body. There are many different types of spa product warmers. Some are effectively double boilers with two pots so that the spa product can warm inside a small pot placed inside a second larger water-filled heating pot or an electrically heated outer pot. Lotion warmers heat spa products to around 122°F with a thermostat to control the temperature (see Fig. 2-1B). A roaster oven can hold towels on one side and a metal or Pyrex container full of spa product on the other. To avoid contamination, cover the container with a lid while it is in the oven. Metal warmers contaminate seaweed and mud, so these products are usually heated in a Pyrex glass container in a water bath and then placed in a plastic container before the treatment (glass may break and so is dangerous). Never use a microwave oven to heat spa products because microwaves are likely to affect many of the products' therapeutic properties. Lastly, many products break down if they are left in a warmer for too long.

Treatment bars are an expensive but handy way to heat several products at the same time. These bars are usually built into the treatment room and have a number of inlaid pans on a large heater, similar to the food heaters used in buffets at restaurants. The heater pans can hold such varied items as towels; hot stones; products; hot, soapy water for hand washing; hot wrap sheets; and product application brushes (see Fig. 2-1C).

PARAFFIN DIPS

Paraffin dips for the hands and feet are used to treat arthritis and sore joints and to enhance other spa services (see Fig. 2-1D). It is best to use a high-quality professional unit on a rolling stand rather than an ordinary home care unit, which usually heats up more slowly and does not have good temperature control.

BODY WRAP MATERIALS

In many spa body treatments, the client is "wrapped" to allow the treatment product to absorb or to encourage perspiration. The type of material used for the wrap depends on the amount of trapped body heat needed for the wrap to be effective and the treatment product being used. Layers of heavy material are needed to make the client perspire during the treatment. If the client does not need to perspire, a cotton blanket should be used instead. When using messy products such as mud or honey, the client is wrapped in plastic or Mylar (almost like tinfoil) first (see Fig. 2-1E).

Heavy Wool Blanket

A heavy wool blanket is ideal for trapping enough heat to make the client perspire in detoxification wraps. The blanket must be large enough to wrap up and around a large person (80 to 90 inches long works well). A washable wool is best because the blanket will need to be washed between clients.

Thermal "Space" Blanket

A thermal "space" blanket is a heavy emergency blanket. It is plastic on the outside and has foil on the inside to prevent loss of body heat.

Wrap Sheets

Hot (or cold) wet wrap sheets (for wet wraps such as herbal, coffee, or milk and honey) are made of 100% cotton, heavy muslin, or a combination of linen and either cotton or fleece. Flannel is never used with hot wet sheet wraps because it is difficult to wring out completely, so it may burn the client.

Body Wrap Plastic and Mylar

Plastic and Mylar sheeting are used with messy products such as seaweed and mud. If the body were wrapped in a fabric, the fabric rather than the body would absorb the product. Plastic and Mylar come on large rolls that are cut to about 6 feet per client. Mylar tends to keep the body warmer, but is a bit more expensive.

BODY-WARMING EQUIPMENT

In a spa body treatment, the client may only be draped with one hand towel across the breasts and one hand towel across the genitals. There are many ways to keep the client warm, including the use of heat lamps; electric table warmers; corn, rice, or flax seed packs; hydrocollator packs; and Fomentek water bottles.

Heat Lamps

Heat lamps can be hung above the treatment table and placed on a dimmer switch to allow for more or less heat. Free-standing units with flexible "necks" are available, but they have large, heavy bases that take up a good deal of space in the treatment room (Fig. 2-1F).

Table Warmers

Electric table warmers can be used to heat up the sheets before the client gets onto the treatment table. For body wrap treatments, the client will often be lying on a piece of plastic sheeting that sits on top of a thermal blanket and wool wrap blanket. Electric table warmers cannot warm the client sufficiently through all of these layers, and many therapists believe the heating elements disrupt the electromagnetic fields of their clients. If this is a problem, use a Fomentek instead to keep the client warm. A Fomentek is a large water bottle designed to sit flat on the treatment table (see Fig. 2-1G). Put the bottle under a pillowcase and place it directly beneath the plastic layer or the wet sheet. This provides warmth and comfort during a body wrap. Corn, rice, or flax packs heated in a microwave are a good alternative. Do not use a hydrocollator pack because the client may get burned if he or she lies down on top of the pack. Instead, hydrocollator packs can be placed under the client's feet to increase core body temperature.

Electric (Thermal) Booties and Mitts

Electric booties and mitts are good for keeping spa products warm on the feet or hands (see Fig. 2-1H). They can be used at any time to keep the client warm, but if used for too long, the client's limbs may start to feel heavy and swollen. Because thermal booties and mitts cause increased vasodilatation in the distal limb, it is important to use flushing strokes toward the heart after removing them.

SPA CLOTHING

Disposable undergarments are highly recommended because many clients are modest about the degree of exposure in a spa treatment, even when draped. Small-, medium-, and large-sized women's briefs, thongs, and bras and men's briefs or boxers need to be available. For wet room treatments, dark blue or black disposable undergarments are much better than white ones, which become transparent when wet. Spa products can be applied on top of some types of disposable undergarments because they are porous, so the product will still be able to reach the skin. A fluffy terry robe, washable spa slippers, terry hair protectors, and terry body wraps allow clients to move about in the spa and to move from one treatment room to another in comfort.

Sanitation Protocols

Whether the therapist is practicing spa treatments in an expensive spa or at a small private clinic, strict sanitation protocols should be used. The state board of massage, state board of cosmetology, state department of health, and Centers for Disease Control and Prevention (CDC) are useful sources for information on suitable sanitation protocols. The protocols should include therapist hygiene; sanitation of the treatment room, equipment, and product containers; and general cleanness of the facility.

THERAPIST HYGIENE

Practitioners working in a health care environment should shower daily and wash their hair regularly. Hair should be tied back so that it does not touch clients during treatments. For better hygiene and client comfort, keep the nails short, natural, and filed to smooth edges. Avoid long nails, nail polish, and artificial nails. Launder uniforms and clothing worn by therapists at the end of each working day. Short sleeves are preferable to long sleeves, which may touch clients' skin and become contaminated. Remove jewelry, including rings, wristwatches, bracelets, and necklaces. These items contain small crevices and sharp edges that can harbor bacteria or potentially scratch a client. Proper sanitation of the hands is probably the single most important part of the sanitation protocol for therapists.

The CDC recommends that health care workers wash their hands with either a non-antimicrobial soap or an antimicrobial soap for 15 to 30 seconds using friction and lather to lift contaminants off the skin's surface. Clean the nails before the hands using a personal nailbrush that has not been used by anybody else. Cleaning should include the area between the fingers and from the forearms to the elbows. Rinse the arms and hands thoroughly with running water and dry them with a disposable towel. Use the same towel to turn off the water tap and to open any doors on the way to the treatment room. An alcohol-based hand rub is recommended for decontaminating the hands before the treatment, before or after some steps of the treatment, and at the end of a treatment. Non–alcohol-based hand rubs have not been adequately evaluated by the CDC and, therefore, are not recommended. Wash the hands and decontaminate them before putting on gloves and right away after removing the gloves. Decontaminate the hands with an alcohol rub before moving from a potentially contaminated body area (e.g., the feet), to a clean body area (e.g., the face) during the treatment. Do the same when moving from contact with an unsanitized inanimate object (e.g., a product container) to the client. Last, wash and decontaminate the hands before and after eating and after using the rest room.[1]

Every client potentially has a bacterial, fungal, or viral infection that he or she may spread to the therapist or to other clients at the same facility. This may be as minor as a foot fungus that spreads easily if clients walk around on the floor barefoot or as serious as hepatitis. To avoid infection, therapists should always practice **Universal Precautions** for their own safety.

Universal Precautions are the policy of the CDC on blood and body fluids.[2] The purpose of the policy is to remind workers to protect themselves from bloodborne diseases transmitted through broken skin or mucous membranes. If the therapist's hands have scratches or cuts, the therapist should wear gloves. Therapists should also wear gloves if the client has any areas of skin that are not intact or if the client says that he or she has a bloodborne condition such as hepatitis or HIV, even if the skin appears to be intact. Latex gloves break down when exposed to oil, lotion, or cream products. Polyvinyl chloride (PVC), nitrile, and neoprene gloves are suitable alternatives to latex. Gloves serve a second purpose by protecting the therapist's hands from overexposure to spa products, which may cause sensitivity.

If the therapist is suffering from allergies or coughing, a face mask should be used. If clothing or linen is contaminated with blood or body fluid droplets, use chlorine bleach in the wash cycle. Handle such articles with gloves and launder them as soon as possible.

SANITATION OF THE TREATMENT ROOM, EQUIPMENT, AND PRODUCT CONTAINERS

In preparation for the session, the therapist should decontaminate his or her hands and then decontaminate the treatment area, equipment, and implements. Sanitation consists of a cleaning step that removes visible contaminants and a disinfection step that removes most pathogenic organisms from inanimate objects. Wipe down countertops, equipment, treatment chairs and tables, the floor, and any other hard surface (e.g., doorknobs, handles, cabinets) with an approved **disinfectant** between clients. Most approved disinfectants are EPA approved and eliminate HIV, hepatitis, and tuberculosis. Consult the board of health in your state because certain states require specific types of disinfectants in health care settings.

Remove all spa products from their original closed containers with a sanitized spoon or spatula and place them into presanitized holders for later use during the treatment. Cover the spa product with plastic wrap to avoid contamination before use. Spa products become contaminated when therapists use their hands to remove the products or dip into original containers during treatments. Discard any unused spa products rather than returning them to their original containers. Some products are dispensed directly into the client's hand using a pump top or flip lid. In this case, take care to decontaminate the product container both before and after the treatment.

During a body or a facial treatment, proper waste disposal procedures are important. Some items used in treatments are one-time-use products such as gauze, sponges, and plastic body wrap. These items should be deposited in a closed trash can immediately after use. Put all used towels, sheets, smocks, and hair wraps in a closed, ventilated container until they are moved to the laundry area. At the end of the treatment, wash them in hot water, dry them with heat, and store them in a closed cabinet. Wash all reusable equipment (e.g., metal or plastic bowls, spatulas, application brushes, and the cooler) in hot, soapy water and disinfect them with alcohol. Even surfaces that do not come into direct contact with clients should be sanitized after treatments. These surfaces include the treatment table and the thermal space blanket, which is often forgotten in the clean-up process. Spray the thermal space blanket with alcohol and allow it to air dry before folding it and placing it in a closed cabinet.

Clients wear washable robes and washable or disposable slippers when moving about the spa. Clean, disinfect, and dry the shower after use by each client. The shower curtain and the floor outside the shower should also be disinfected.

Change all towels and the mat outside the shower for each client. Only use liquid soaps or shower gels. Bars of soap that have been used by more than one person are unsanitary and should not be left in the shower or where hands are washed. Clean, disinfect, and dry the hydrotherapy tub between clients. If the tub has jets, they must be flushed with bleach or a specialized **antiseptic** product (follow the manufacturer's directions) between clients. The same applies to pedicure or foot soak tubs with jets.

Spa supply outlets stock a variety of disinfectant products. The manufacturer's instructions often specify the best sort of disinfectant to use with the equipment. Table 2-1 lists some examples of common cleaning products used in spas, but this is just a sample of what is available. The Occupational Safety and Health Administration (OSHA)[3] requires spas to alert employees to the dangers of the chemicals that they use in the workplace. Material Safety Data Sheets (MSDS) must be available for all hazardous chemicals that are on site. Spa employees should always wear heavy cleaning gloves and eye protection when handling cleaning products.

Table 2-1 — Common Cleaning Products Used in Spas

NAME	DESCRIPTION
Quaternary ammonium compounds (quats)	A disinfectant that is formulated to kill pathogens on a variety of non-living surfaces. Accepted by OSHA's Bloodborne Pathogens Standard for cleanup of blood or body fluids. Effective against *Pseudomonas*, *Staphylococcus*, and *Salmonella*, spp.; certain bacteria; HIV-1; and hepatitis B and C. Low in toxicity for cleaning personnel.[14]
Phenolics (also called cresols)	Disinfectants that are effective against tuberculosis and accepted by OSHA's Bloodborne Pathogens Standard for cleanup of blood or body fluids. Higher toxicity for cleaning personnel than quats.[14]
Alcohols	Ethyl and isopropyl alcohol are used as antimicrobial agents against bacteria and fungi but do not have an effect on bacterial spores.
EPA-approved disinfectant	The EPA monitors disinfectant products and requires manufacturers to provide test data verifying claims about effectiveness as antimicrobial agents.[15]
CaviCide	A hospital-grade, EPA-approved disinfectant with a broad spectrum of action on viral, bacterial, and fungal pathogens. It is noted as effective against tuberculosis.
Mar-V-Cide	An EPA-approved disinfectant and germicidal effective against HIV-1, athlete's foot fungus, mold, mildew, and herpes simplex types 1 and 2.
Citrus II	A nontoxic, natural cleaning product made with citrus essential oils. Used for its general disinfectant properties on noncritical surfaces. This product is safe for the environment.
MadaCide-FD germicidal solution	An infection control spray that is alcohol based and kills HIV and tuberculosis.
Aerocide foam cleanser	A hospital-grade germicidal foam that cleans and disinfects hard surfaces to control infection and kill germs.

EPA = Environmental Protection Agency; OSHA = Occupational Safety and Health Administration.

CLEANLINESS OF THE FACILITY

A checklist of daily cleaning duties is helpful for ensuring that the spa or clinic is properly maintained. A cleaning checklist might include the following items:

1. Wash all bowls, implements, application brushes, trays, and other equipment with hot, soapy water and wipe them with alcohol before storing them in closed containers.
2. Wash cloth products such as robes, slippers, hand towels, bath towels, and shower mats in hot water with an appropriate detergent and dry them using heat before storing them in a closed container.
3. Wipe the countertops, treatment tables, mirrors, floors, equipment, doorknobs, sinks, and, in some cases, walls with a disinfectant.
4. Disinfect showers, hydrotherapy tubs, and all wet room equipment and then put fresh towels and mats in place between clients.
5. Clean and disinfect all bathrooms.
6. Wipe all product bottles and containers with alcohol and store them properly.
7. Empty all trash bins and disinfect them at the end of each day.

Because new information about communicable diseases is constantly emerging, it is important to keep up to date with the most recent standards and guidelines by visiting the CDC's website (http://www.cdc.gov). Throughout the treatment chapters, there are sanitation boxes, which have quick hints on how to clean up properly.

Basic Documentation

The client intake process is just as important for a spa treatment as it is for massage, and before being treated, all clients need an evaluation of their physical condition. To set a relaxing tone, the therapist can provide a cup of herbal tea and soak the client's feet in a decorative tub. This is a good time for the therapist to introduce himself or herself and to describe the benefits of the treatment the client is about to receive. If it is appropriate, the therapist can help the client to develop long-term health goals and identify how the spa or clinic can play a role in achieving those goals. The information obtained during the intake process helps the therapist to recommend other beneficial services or home care products for the client.

The type of information included on the health form depends on the scope of the spa, the services offered at the spa, and the needs of the therapist for that particular session. A nutritionist may ask some questions about the client's diet, an esthetician may focus on the condition of the skin, and a massage therapist may ask about muscular conditions. Spas can plan to have one intake form or several different forms that suit individual therapists or services. All therapists should plan some time at the beginning of every treatment, even for returning clients, to discuss the client's current condition. The primary purpose of the health form and treatment record is to check on the client's state of health, identify appropriate treatments, and make sure that there are no contraindications for the treatments selected (Figs. 2-2 and 2-3).

Contraindications

Massage and spa treatments may be contraindicated completely, contraindicated without a doctor's release, contraindicated for a specific body area, or require adaptive measures and increased vigilance.

Usually, if massage is contraindicated, spa treatments are also contraindicated; sometimes the opposite is true. A bruise is a good example. Although a therapist would never massage over a new bruise (< 72 hours old), applying seaweed, certain essential oils (e.g., *Helichrysum*, lemon), or a therapeutic mud would help the bruise to clear up. The same is true with sunburn. Massage is contraindicated, but a soothing aloe vera and German chamomile essential oil wrap are not.

The spa product chosen for a particular treatment, the surface area of the body that it is to cover, and the overall condition of the client all need careful consideration. A spot treatment may be safe when a full-body application is contraindicated. If the product or some of its ingredients can penetrate the skin and enter the circulation (e.g., essential oils), it must be used with more caution. In such a situation, a full-body application allows substantially more of the product to penetrate than a spot application.

Seaweed applications can affect thyroid medications, so they should be avoided in cases of hypo- or hyperthyroidism (except when used under the direction of a physician). Peppermint, eucalyptus, and rosemary essential oils counteract the effects of many homeopathic remedies, so they should not be applied to clients who are using such remedies to treat a condition. If a client is taking a prescription or over-the-counter medication that distorts his or her perception of hot, cold, pain, or pressure, the treatment should be postponed. For the same reason, clients under the influence of drugs or alcohol should not receive treatments. Also, offering wine, champagne, or other alcoholic drinks as part of the treatment or spa package endangers the client and may affect the legal liability of the clinic or spa.

Clients who are pregnant, in a weakened condition, have neurological or heart conditions, or uncontrolled high or low blood pressure (BP) should not receive hydrotherapy treatments except when under the care of a physician. Similarly, such clients need a doctor's release for full-body spa treatments, including mud, herbal hot sheet wraps, and seaweed wraps.

SPA HEALTH INFORMATION

Patient's Name _____ Date _____

Address _____ State _____ Zip _____

Phone_____ Occupation _____

Emergency Contact _____ Phone _____

Primary Health Care Provider

Name _____ Phone _____

Address _____ State _____ Zip _____

Current Health Information

Please list all conditions currently monitored by a health care provider.

_____

_____

Please list all the medications you took today (include pain relievers and herbal remedies).

_____

_____

Please list the medications you took in the past 3 months.

_____

_____

Please list and briefly explain (including dates and the treatment received) the following:

Surgeries_____

_____

Accidents _____

_____

Major
Illnesses _____

_____

Tobacco Use: ☐ Current   ☐ Past   ☐ Never   Comments _____

Alcohol Use: ☐ Current   ☐ Past   ☐ Never   Comments _____

Drug use: ☐ Current   ☐ Past   ☐ Never   Comments _____

Are you currently menstruating?   ☐ Yes   ☐ No

Have you received a spa treatment before?   ☐ Yes   ☐ No

If yes, what types of spa treatment have you received?   _____

_____

Figure 2-2   Spa health form.

Current and Previous Conditions

Please check all current and previous conditions and give a brief explanation, if appropriate, in the comments section at the end of this form.

Current	Past		Current	Past	
☐	☐	Headache	☐	☐	Lymphedema
☐	☐	Pain	☐	☐	High blood pressure
☐	☐	Sleep disorders	☐	☐	Low blood pressure
☐	☐	Fatigue	☐	☐	Poor circulation
☐	☐	Infections	☐	☐	Swollen ankles
☐	☐	Fever	☐	☐	Varicose veins
☐	☐	Sinus condition	☐	☐	Asthma
☐	☐	Skin conditions	☐	☐	Bowel dysfunction
☐	☐	Athlete's foot	☐	☐	Bladder dysfunction
☐	☐	Warts	☐	☐	Abdominal pain
☐	☐	Skin sensitivities	☐	☐	Thyroid dysfunction
☐	☐	Sunburn	☐	☐	Diabetes
☐	☐	Burns	☐	☐	Pregnancy
☐	☐	Bruises	☐	☐	Fibrotic cysts
☐	☐	Aversions to scent	☐	☐	Pacemaker
☐	☐	Aversion to oils	☐	☐	Phlebitis
☐	☐	Allergies	☐	☐	Raynaud's syndrome
☐	☐	Sensitivity to detergents			
☐	☐	Aversion to cold			
☐	☐	Claustrophobia			
☐	☐	Rheumatoid arthritis			
☐	☐	Osteoarthritis			
☐	☐	Spinal problems			
☐	☐	Disc problems			
☐	☐	Lupus			
☐	☐	Tendonitis, bursitis			
☐	☐	Fibromyalgia			
☐	☐	Dizziness, ringing in the ears			
☐	☐	Mental confusion			
☐	☐	Numbness, tingling			
☐	☐	Neuritis			
☐	☐	Neuralgia			
☐	☐	Sciatica, shooting pain			
☐	☐	Depression			
☐	☐	Anxiety, panic attacks			
☐	☐	Heart disease			
☐	☐	Blood clots			
☐	☐	Stroke			

Other Conditions:

_____

_____

_____

_____

_____

Comments:

_____

_____

_____

_____

_____

_____

Therapist's Name: _____

Signature: _____

Date: _____

SPA TREATMENT RECORD

Patient's Name _____ Date _____

Date: Treatment received:	Therapist:	Comments:	Retail items purchased:
Date: Treatment received:	Therapist:	Comments:	Retail items purchased:
Date: Treatment received:	Therapist:	Comments:	Retail items purchased:
Date: Treatment received:	Therapist:	Comments:	Retail items purchased:
Date: Treatment received:	Therapist:	Comments:	Retail items purchased:
Date: Treatment received:	Therapist:	Comments:	Retail items purchased:

Figure 2-3 Spa treatment record.

The term *hypertension* refers to a prolonged elevation of BP. It can lead to an increased risk of stroke and heart attack. Spa treatments that result in rapid detoxification or that are stimulating for the circulation may be dangerous for individuals with hypertension. If a client has risk factors for hypertension or has a known history of hypertension, the therapist should check the client's BP before and after the treatment just as is done before a massage. The risk factors for hypertension include pregnancy, history of heart disease, myocardial infarction, angina pectoris, arteriosclerosis, kidney disorders, diabetes, metabolic disorders such as hyperthyroidism, smoking, high stress, high sodium intake, and obesity. If the client has moderate to severe hypertension (systolic BP > 159, diastolic BP > 99), a doctor's release is required, and the temperature and duration of the treatment should be modified. Temperatures closer to natural body temperature are safer, and shorter treatments rather than longer treatments should be used.

With any client, the therapist should watch for increased pain, any discomfort, agitation, nausea, headache, and dizziness. If any of these symptoms occur during a treatment, the therapist should stop the session and allow the client to relax in a quiet environment at a normal temperature. Monitor the client at all times and do not allow them to go home until their symptoms have disappeared. Most often, symptoms such as nausea and headache are the result of accelerated detoxification. If the symptoms persist after the session has ended, a physician should be consulted. If the symptoms increase rapidly after the session has ended, the client could be in danger, and the therapist should call emergency services.

Sometimes massage or spa treatments are not contraindicated but need adaptation to make them safer or more comfortable for the client. This may mean that the way the client is positioned needs to be changed or the treatment needs to be shortened. The therapist may also need to work with less depth or allow a particular spa product to absorb for less time. In a hydrotherapy treatment, for example, the therapist can decrease the cardiovascular load on the client by using warm and cool applications rather than hot and cold ones. The closer the temperature of the application to the client's body temperature, the less intense the response will be. Hydrotherapy principles are covered in Chapter 4.

Each chapter of this book deals with a different type of treatment. Specific contraindications are listed in the treatment snapshots for common pathologies. Table 2-2 provides an overview of conditions for quick reference, but such lists should not be relied on completely. Each client and each situation is different, and therapists need to learn to reason clinically so they can make appropriate decisions for each client. Novice therapists may shy away from conditions that the experienced therapist can work with safely. An up-to-date medical dictionary, drug reference, and pathology reference book should be readily available to research unfamiliar conditions and medications. If there is

any doubt about the suitability of a given treatment for a particular client, be cautious and either suggest a different treatment to the client or postpone the treatment until he or she has a doctor's release.

What Every Therapist Should Know about Skin and Spa Products

A basic understanding of the skin and spa product ingredients is vital to every therapist working in a spa regardless of the scope of practice. When therapists understand something about the skin, they can direct the client to suitable treatments and appropriate home care retail items. In high-end spas, the clients tend to be well versed in different skin care treatments. A knowledgeable therapist sets the tone for the spa treatment and inspires confidence in the client. Massage is often the first treatment that a novice spa client will choose because other services may seem mysterious or intimidating. The massage therapist often becomes the client's personal guide to other treatments. Through interaction with the client during the massage, the therapist helps the client make treatment choices and encourages the client to try something new and different. For this reason, the massage therapist needs to have a basic understanding of every treatment that is offered at a spa and its benefits for the client.

Massage and body treatments products affect the skin, so they must be chosen with care. For example, although a product might be indicated for a client's muscular condition, it may be contraindicated for the client's skin condition. Therefore, massage therapists need a good knowledge of skin types and skin problems so that they know when to direct the client to an esthetician or dermatologist for professional skin care.

The essential oils used in aromatherapy are often misused in skin care because the word *oil* is misleading. Essential oils do not directly address dry skin conditions by adding oil or moisture to the skin. In fact, most essential oils are quite drying for the skin and can cause irritation if used inappropriately on a particular skin type. Essential oils are useful as antiseptics and for helping the body to relax.

Stress plays a role in many skin disorders, so massage therapists and estheticians can work together for clients' benefit. A full-body massage using spa products that are appropriate for a client's skin condition can significantly reduce stress and have a significant impact on skin health.

Improvements in the condition of the skin take a while and require patience. At least a month is required before a significant improvement can be seen in most conditions. Often skin conditions require many months to resolve. When estheticians and massage therapists recognize the potential synergy of the work they do, they can provide integrative and supportive treatment plans for clients.

Table 2-2 Contraindications Chart

CONDITION[a]	CONTRAINDICATED	DR. RELEASE	EXFOLIATION	HYDROTHERAPY	SEAWEED	MUD	CLAY	PEAT	MASSAGE	STONE MASSAGE	PARAFANGO	HOT WRAPS	WARM WRAPS	COOL WRAPS	SHIRODHARA	UDVARTANA	FOOT TREATMENTS	REFER TO SKIN CARE SPECIALIST
Abortion, recent			UC	AU	UC	UC	UC	UC	UC	C	UC	C	UC	UC	▲	UC	▲	
Acne vulgaris			C	UC	SC	SC	SC	SC	SC	SC	SC	UC	UC	UC	SC	SC	▲	X
Acromegaly		X	UC	UC	UC	UC	UC	UC	UC	UC	UC	C[b]	UC	UC	▲	UC	UC	
Addison's disease		X	UC	UC	UC	UC	UC	UC	UC	UC	UC	C	UC	UC	▲	UC	UC	
AIDS (client condition good)		X	UC	UC	UC	UC	UC	UC	UC	UC	UC	UC	UC	UC	▲	UC	UC	
Allergies: Shellfish, iodine, seafood			▲	▲	C	▲	▲	▲	▲	▲	▲	▲	▲	▲	▲	▲	▲	
Alzheimer's disease		X	UC	UC	UC	UC	UC	UC	UC	UC	▲	C	C	C	UC	UC	UC	
Amenorrhea			▲	▲	▲	▲	▲	▲	▲	▲	▲	▲	▲	UC	▲	▲	▲	
Angina pectoris		X	UC	C	UC	UC	UC	UC	C	C	C	C	UC	C	UC	UC	UC	
Anorexia nervosa appendicitis		X	UC	UC	C	▲	▲	▲	▲	▲	UC	▲	▲	C	▲	UC	▲	
Anxiety disorder		X	▲	UC	▲	▲	▲	▲	▲	▲	▲	C	C	C	▲	UC	▲	
Asthma			▲	UC	▲	▲	▲	▲	▲	▲	▲	C	▲	UC	▲	▲	UC	
Arteriosclerosis		X	UC	C[b]	UC	UC	UC	UC	UC	UC	UC	C	UC	C	▲	UC	UC	
Atherosclerosis		X	UC	C[b]	UC	UC	UC	UC	UC	UC	UC	C	UC	C	▲	UC	UC	
Athlete's foot			C	SC	▲	SC	SC	SC	SC	SC	SC	▲	UC	▲	▲	SC	SC	
Bed sore or pressure sore		X	SC	AU	SC	SC	SC	SC	SC	SC	SC	C	UC	UC	SC	SC	SC	
Bipolar disorder		X	UC	UC	UC	UC	UC	UC	UC	UC	UC	C	C	C	UC	UC	UC	
Boil			SC	UC	SC	SC	SC	▲	SC	SC	SC	▲	▲	UC	SC	SC	SC	
Bronchitis			▲	UC	▲	▲	▲	▲	▲	▲	▲	UC	▲	UC	▲	▲	▲	X
Bruise			SC	SC	▲	▲	▲	▲	▲	SC	SC	SC	▲	▲	▲	SC	SC	

[a] For a description of the conditions, please refer to a pathology textbook.
[b] Except under medical supervision or with advanced training or specialized understanding.
▲ = indicated/safe; AU = advanced understanding; C = contraindicated; SC = site contraindicated; UC = use caution.

Condition																	
Burns, recent	X		SC	C	UC	SC	SC	SC	SC	SC	SC	SC	SC	SC	SC	SC	SC
			UC	UC	SC	UC	UC	UC	UC	UC	UC	UC	UC	UC	UC		
Common cold (2 to 3 days after acute)	X		UC	UC	SC	UC	UC	UC	UC	UC	UC	UC	▲	UC	▲	▲	UC
Cardiac arrest, history of	X		UC	C	UC	UC	UC	UC	UC	UC	UC	C	UC	UC	UC	UC	UC
Cellulitis	X		SC	C	SC	SC	SC	SC	SC	SC	SC	SC	SC	SC	SC	SC	SC
Cerebral palsy		Xb															
Chickenpox		X															
Cholecystitis		Xb															
Cirrhosis of the liver		X															
Colitis		UC	UC	UC	UC	UC	UC	UC	UC	UC	C	UC	UC	▲	C	UC	UC
Constipation		▲	▲	▲	▲	▲	▲	▲	▲	▲	UC	▲	▲	▲	UC	▲	▲
Crohn's disease	X		UC	UC	UC	UC	UC	UC	UC	UC	C	UC	UC	UC	C	UC	UC
Chronic fatigue syndrome		UC	▲	▲	UC	▲	UC	▲	▲	▲	C	UC	▲	▲	C	UC	▲
Congestive heart failure		Xb															
Conjunctivitis (pinkeye)		X															
Contact dermatitis		SC	SC	SC	SC	SC	SC	SC	SC	SC	C	SC	C	SC	C	SC	SC
Contusion or concussion, recent		X															
Coronary artery disease	X		UC	Cb	UC	UC	UC	UC	UC	UC	C	UC	UC	▲	C	UC	UC
Cushing's disease	X		UC	UC	UC	UC	UC	UC	UC	C	C	UC	UC	UC	C	UC	UC
Cystic fibrosis	X		UC	AU	UC	UC	UC	UC	UC	UC	C	UC	▲	▲	C	UC	UC
Cystitis (chronic; acute C)		UC	▲	UC	▲	▲	▲	▲	▲	▲	C	▲	▲	▲	C	▲	▲
Depression	X		UC	UC	UC	UC	UC	UC	UC	UC	UC	UC	▲	UC	UC	UC	UC
Diabetes insipidus	X		UC	Cb	UC	UC	UC	UC	UC	UC	C	UC	UC	UC	C	UC	UC
Diabetes mellitus	X		UC	C	C	UC	UC	UC	UC	UC	C	C	▲	C	C	UC	C
Diarrhea		Xb															
Diverticulitis	X		UC	UC	UC	UC	UC	UC	UC	UC	C	UC	▲	UC	C	UC	UC
Diverticulosis	X		▲	UC	▲	▲	▲	▲	▲	▲	UC	▲	▲	▲	C	▲	▲
Dysmenorrhea		UC	▲	UC	UC	SC	UC	UC	UC	SC	UC	SC	UC	▲	UC	SC	UC
Eczema	X		SC	UC	UC	UC	SC	UC	SC	UC	UC	UC	▲	UC	UC	SC	UC
Embolism		UC	▲	Cb	C	C	C	C	C	C	C	C	C	C	C	C	C
Emphysema		UC	UC	UC	UC	UC	UC	UC	UC	UC	C	UC	UC	UC	UC	UC	UC
Endocarditis	X																
Endometriosis		▲	▲	▲	▲	▲	▲	▲	▲	▲	▲	▲	▲	▲	▲	▲	▲
Epilepsy	X		UC	UC	C	UC	UC	UC	UC	UC	C	C	C	C	C	UC	UC
Fever		X															

(continued)

Table 2-2 (continued)

CONDITION[a]	CONTRAINDICATED	DR. RELEASE	EXFOLIATION	HYDROTHERAPY	SEAWEED	MUD	CLAY	PEAT	MASSAGE	STONE MASSAGE	PARAFANGO	HOT WRAPS	WARM WRAPS	COOL WRAPS	SHIRODHARA	UBVARTANA	FOOT TREATMENTS	REFER TO SKIN CARE SPECIALIST
Fibrocystic breast disease			▲	▲	▲	▲	▲	▲	▲	▲	▲	▲	▲	▲	▲	▲	▲	
Fibroids			▲	▲	▲	▲	▲	▲	▲	▲	▲	▲	▲	▲	▲	▲	▲	
Fibromyalgia			▲	AU	▲	▲	▲	▲	▲	UC	▲	UC	UC	UC	▲	UC	UC	
Flaccid muscles			▲	AU	▲	▲	▲	▲	▲	UC	▲	UC	UC	UC	▲	▲	UC	
Folliculitis			SC	UC	UC	SC	UC	SC	SC	SC	SC	UC	UC	UC	SC	SC	▲	X
Gastritis (chronic; acute C)			UC	UC	UC	UC	UC	UC	UC	UC	UC	C	UC	UC	▲	UC	UC	
Gastroenteritis	X																	
Gastroesophageal reflux disease			UC	UC	UC	UC	UC	UC	UC	UC	UC	C	UC	UC	▲	UC	UC	
Goiter			UC	UC	C	▲	▲	▲	▲	SC	▲	UC	▲	▲	▲	UC	UC	
Gout			C	AU	AU	AU	AU	AU	SC	SC	SC	C	UC	UC	▲	SC	C	
Graves' disease		X	UC	UC	C	UC	UC	UC	UC	UC	UC	UC	UC	UC	▲	UC	UC	
Heart murmur		X	UC	UC	UC	UC	UC	UC	SC	SC	UC	UC	UC	UC	▲	UC	UC	
Hemangioma			SC	C[b]	SC	SC	SC	SC	SC	SC	SC	UC	UC	UC	▲	SC	SC	
Hematoma			SC	C	SC	SC	SC	SC	SC	SC	SC	C	UC	C	▲	SC	SC	
Hemophilia		X	C	C[b]	UC	UC	UC	UC	UC	C	C	C	C	C	▲	UC	UC	
Hemorrhage	X																	
Hepatitis (chronic; acute C)		X	UC	C[b]	UC	UC	UC	UC	UC	C	C	C	UC	UC	▲	UC	UC	
Hernia		X	SC	UC	SC	SC	SC	SC	SC	UC	SC	C	SC	SC	▲	SC	▲	
Herniated disk		X	SC	AU	SC	SC	SC	SC	SC	SC	SC	C	SC	UC	▲	SC	▲	
Herpes simplex			SC	SC	SC	SC	SC	SC	SC	SC	SC	SC	SC	SC	UC	SC	▲	
Hypercholesterolemia		X	UC	C[b]	UC	UC	UC	UC	UC	C	C	C	UC	C	▲	UC	UC	
Hypertension		X	UC	C[b]	UC	UC	UC	UC	UC	UC	UC	C	UC	C	▲	UC	UC	
Hyperthyroidism		X	UC	UC	C	UC	UC	UC	UC	UC	C	C	UC	UC	▲	UC	UC	

Condition															
Hypotension	X	UC	C^b	UC	UC	UC	UC	UC	UC	C	C	C	C	UC	UC
Hypothyroidism	X	UC	UC	C	UC	UC	UC	UC	UC	C	C	▲	UC	UC	UC
Ichthyosis vulgaris		UC	UC	UC	UC	UC	UC	UC	UC	C	UC	UC	UC	UC	UC
Impetigo														X	
Inflammation, acute	C	AU	AU	AU	AU	SC	SC	C	SC	C	AU	C	AU	AU	SC
Inflammation, chronic	▲	▲	▲	▲	▲	▲	▲	▲	▲	▲	▲	▲	▲	▲	▲
Inflammation, subacute	C	AU	AU	AU	AU	UC	UC	C	UC	UC	AU	UC	UC	SC	UC
Influenza	X														
Insomnia	▲	▲	▲	▲	▲	▲	▲	▲	▲	▲	▲	▲	▲	▲	▲
Intestinal obstruction	X														
Irritable bowel syndrome	UC	UC	UC	UC	UC	UC	UC	UC	UC	UC	UC	UC	UC	UC	UC
Jaundice	X														
Kidney stones (acute C)	X	UC	UC	▲	▲	▲	▲	▲	▲	SC	▲	▲	UC	UC	▲
Lice	X														
Lou Gehrig's disease (ALS)	X^b														
Lupus (in remission)	X	C	C	UC	UC	UC	C	C	C	C	C	C	I	UC	UC
Lyme disease		UC	UC	UC	UC	UC	UC	UC	UC	UC	UC	UC	▲	UC	UC
Lymphangitis	X														
Lymphedema	X^b														
Meningitis	X														
Menopause		UC	▲	▲	▲	UC	UC	UC	UC	C	UC	▲	▲	▲	▲
Mononucleosis	X^b														
Multiple sclerosis	X^b														
Muscular dystrophy	X	UC	UC	UC	UC	UC	C	C	UC	C	UC	C	▲	UC	UC
Myocardial infarction (history of)	X	C^b	UC	UC	UC	C	UC	C	C	UC	UC	UC	UC	C	UC
Myocarditis	X														
Neuropathy	X	C	SC	SC	SC	SC	SC	C	C	SC	C	UC	SC	SC	SC
Obesity		AU	UC	▲	▲	▲	C	▲	▲	UC	▲	C	▲	UC	▲
Osteoarthritis	X	UC	UC	UC	UC	UC	UC	UC	▲	C	▲	C	UC	UC	UC
Ovarian cysts	X	▲	▲	▲	▲	▲	▲	▲	▲	▲	▲	▲	▲	▲	▲
Pancreatitis (chronic; acute C)	X	UC	UC	UC	UC	UC	UC	UC	UC	UC	UC	UC	UC	UC	▲
Paralysis	X^b														
Parkinson's disease	X	UC	UC	UC	UC	UC	UC	UC	UC	C	C	UC	UC	UC	UC

(continued)

Table 2-2 *(continued)*

CONDITION[a]	CONTRAINDICATED	DR. RELEASE	EXFOLIATION	HYDROTHERAPY	SEAWEED	MUD	CLAY	PEAT	MASSAGE	STONE MASSAGE	PARAFANGO	HOT WRAPS	WARM WRAPS	COOL WRAPS	SHIRODHARA	UBVARTANA	FOOT TREATMENTS	REFER TO SKIN CARE SPECIALIST
Pelvic inflammatory disease	X																	
Pericarditis	X																	
Peripheral vascular disease, mild		X	SC	C	SC	SC	SC	SC	SC	C	C	C	UC	C	▲	SC	SC	
Peritonitis	X[b]																	
Phlebitis		X	SC	C	SC	SC	SC	SC	SC	C	C	C	UC	C	▲	SC	SC	
Pleurisy, nonbacterial		X	UC	C[b]	UC	UC	UC	UC	UC	UC	UC	C	UC	UC	▲	UC	UC	
Polycystic kidney disease		X	▲	UC	▲	▲	▲	▲	▲	UC	▲	C	▲	▲	▲	▲	▲	
Preeclampsia	X																	
Pregnancy			UC	AU	C	UC	UC	UC	UC	UC	UC	C	UC	C	C	C	UC	
Pregnancy, high risk		X	UC	C	C	C	C	C	UC	C	C	C	UC	C	C	C	UC	
Premenstrual syndrome			▲	▲	▲	▲	▲	▲	▲	▲	▲	▲	▲	▲	▲	▲	▲	
Prostatitis			▲	▲	▲	▲	▲	▲	▲	▲	▲	UC	▲	▲	▲	▲	▲	
Pseudo sciatica			UC	UC	UC	▲	▲	▲	▲	UC	▲	UC	▲	▲	▲	▲	▲	
Psoriasis		X	SC	AU	UC	UC	UC	UC	UC	UC	▲	UC	UC	UC	▲	UC	UC	X
Pulmonary edema	X[b]																	
Pyelonephritis	X																	
Raynaud's syndrome			UC	C[b]	UC	UC	UC	UC	UC	UC	UC	C	UC	C	▲	UC	UC	
Rheumatoid arthritis		X	UC	AU	UC	UC	UC	UC	UC	C	SC	C	UC	UC	▲	UC	UC	
Ringworm	X																	
Scabies	X																	
Scars, old			UC	▲	▲	▲	▲	▲	▲	▲	▲	▲	▲	▲	▲	▲	▲	
Scars, recent		X	SC	AU	UC	UC	UC	UC	UC	UC	UC	UC	UC	UC	UC	UC	UC	

Condition																
Scleroderma	X	UC	AU	UC	▲	▲	▲	UC	▲	C	UC	UC	UC	▲	▲	▲
Sebaceous cyst		UC	UC	UC	UC	UC	UC	UC	UC	SC	UC	▲	C	UC	UC	UC
Skin tabs		UC	▲	▲	▲	▲	▲	▲	▲	UC	UC	▲	UC	UC	UC	X
Sickle cell disease	X	UC	C	UC	C	UC	C	C	UC	UC	C	▲	C	UC	UC	X
Sinusitis (no fever present)		▲	▲	▲	▲	▲	▲	▲	▲	▲	▲	▲	▲	C	▲	
Site infection or fungus		SC	SC	SC	SC	SC	SC	SC	SC	SC	SC	SC	SC	SC	SC	SC
Stroke	X	UC	Cᵇ	UC	UC	UC	UC	UC	UC	C	C	UC	UC	UC	UC	
Substance abuse, recovery from	X	▲	UC	▲	▲	▲	▲	▲	▲	C	UC	UC	▲			
Sunburn		C	AU	C	C	C	C	C	C	C	SC	C	SC	SC		
Thromboangiitis obliterans	X	SC	C	SC	SC	SC	SC	SC	C	SC	C	SC	SC	SC		
Thrombophlebitis	X	SC	C	SC	SC	SC	C	UC	C	SC	C	UC	SC	SC		
Tonsillitis	X															
Tuberculosis (no longer infective)	X	UC	UC	▲	▲	▲	▲	▲	▲	UC	▲	UC	▲	▲		
Ulcers		▲	▲	▲	▲	▲	▲	▲	▲	UC	▲	▲	▲	▲		
Urethritis	X															
Varicose veins		SC	UC	UC	UC	UC	SC	SC	SC	UC	▲	UC	UC	UC	UC	UC

Table 2-3 provides an overview of skin types and conditions of which massage therapists should be aware. Some essential oils appropriate for each condition are included in the table. This information is useful for massage therapists making blends for a safe full-body massage and for estheticians using essential oils in skin care treatments. In addition, recommendations are given for products that should be avoided. The chapters on aromatherapy, body wraps, fangotherapy, and thalassotherapy provide detailed information.

THE SKIN

The skin is the largest organ of the body and has many important functions (Fig. 2-4). Color and texture changes, such as paleness, redness, bumpiness, or yellowing, reflect the overall health of the body and may indicate internal disease. Rashes and skin eruptions illustrate poor nutritional habits, stress, allergies, and sensitivities.

The outer layer of the skin is called the epidermis. It contains no blood vessels but has many nerve endings. The epidermis has multiple sublayers called strata. The bottom layer of the epidermis is the stratum basale layer, which produces a constant supply of new cells. Keratinocytes make up 80% to 90% of the epidermis and produce keratin. As the keratinocytes mature, they lose water and flatten out. They are shed when they reach the outermost layer of the epidermis, called the **stratum corneum**. The stratum corneum provides the **barrier function** of the skin, protecting the body from microbial invasion and injury. It also protects the body from water loss. In fact, this layer is 1000 times more impermeable to water than most other membranes of living organisms.[4]

A healthy stratum corneum is compact with an orderly arrangement of cells in what is often referred to as the "brick and mortar" of the skin. The bricks are dead cells filled with keratin. The mortar is the lipids between the cells that "cement" them together. When the corneum layer is damaged, the cells are thin and arranged in an uneven pattern. Damage allows preparations applied to the skin to penetrate more readily. This is why dry or scaly skin may give a burning sensation when products are applied to it.

On the stratum corneum, sebum, perspiration, and other water-soluble acids produce a pH of 4.4 to 5.6. This is the skin's acid mantle, which acts as a defense mechanism against invading microbes. Research indicates that the low pH in the stratum corneum also plays a role in corneocyte maturation (the maturation of the keratin-filled cells that make up the stratum corneum).[5]

The inner layer of the skin, the dermis, is thicker than the epidermis and is composed of connective tissue that contains collagen and elastin. Collagen makes up a large part of the dermis (70%) and gives the skin structural support for cells and blood vessels. It forms a network of microscopic interwoven fibers that allows for stretching and contraction of the skin. It also aids in the healing of wounds. Moisture is important for keeping the collagen network supple.

The follicles, sweat glands, sebaceous glands, most of the sensory receptors, and nerve endings are all found in the reticular layer of the dermis. The sebaceous glands secrete sebum, an oily, waxy substance composed of various kinds of lipids that lubricate the skin. Normally, it flows through the oil ducts leading to hair follicles. When sebum becomes hardened the follicle becomes blocked. This is what causes blackheads (comedones). Excessive flow of oil from the oil glands may produce seborrhea and problem skin. Emotional stress increases the flow of sebum.

The skin was thought to be impervious to most chemicals until, in the 1960s, dimethylsulfoxide (DMSO) was shown to transport other substances through the skin barrier and into the bloodstream. It is important to understand that some of the ingredients of spa products do pass through the skin into the bloodstream, where they may affect the body on a physiological level. Many factors contribute to the passage of these ingredients through the skin. Lipophilic (literally, "lipid-loving" or "fat-loving") ingredients penetrate better than hydrophilic ("water-loving") ingredients. Essential oils pass rapidly through the skin because of their lipophilic nature. The polysaccharides (mucilaginous, slimy substances) in seaweed also pass readily through the skin. It is not surprising that small-sized molecules penetrate faster than larger molecules or that a viscous formulation passes through more slowly than more fluid preparations. Dead cells and lipid accumulation in the stratum corneum, as well as sebum pH and skin thickness affect the rate at which a substance passes through the skin.[6] Some natural components increase skin penetration. These include linoleic acid (found in evening primrose oil and some other seed oils),[7] oleic acid (found in almond, cod liver oil, and others),[8] menthol (found in some essential oils such as peppermint),[9,10] and squalene (found in olives, wheat germ oil, and shark liver oil).[11]

SPA PRODUCT BASICS

Spa products fall into basic categories, including cleansers, toners or astringents, exfoliation products, masks (treatment products), and moisturizers.

Cleansers

Cleansers rid the skin of dead cells, excess sebum, dirt, and other impurities. An effective cleanser removes impurities from both the skin's surface and the pores. Soaps are alkaline and strip the skin of its acid mantle, upsetting the proper pH of the skin and leaving it dry. Soaps also leave a dulling film on the surface of the skin. It is important to find a gentle body cleanser that rinses off completely. A cleanser is often used at the beginning of a treatment to pu-

Table 2-3	Important Skin Types and Conditions	
BASIC SKIN TYPE OR SKIN CONDITION	**DESCRIPTION**	**GENERAL RECOMMENDATIONS**
Normal	The skin is clear, with an even tone and texture, and good color and is blemish free.	Full-body massage blends with essential oils of lavender, neroli, Roman or German chamomile, geranium, jasmine, frankincense, or rose. Citrus oils can also be used in moderation. Seaweed, clay, mud, and peat can be used at full strength.
Oily	Characterized by the overproduction of sebum. Enlarged pores (follicles) may be filled with visible grease and debris. Blemishes may be present on the face or back.	Full-body massage blends with essential oils of bergamot, tea tree, lemon, grapefruit, lavender, geranium, German chamomile, or cedarwood in a jojoba base. If inflammatory acne is present, products should be diluted or the client should be referred to an esthetician before the treatment progresses. Seaweed mixed with aloe vera and clay is appropriate. Mud and peat should be avoided.
Oil dry	Sebaceous output has slowed and the skin is not receiving enough natural oil. The skin appears dry and dehydrated.	Full-body massage blends with essential oils of lavender, German chamomile, geranium, rose, carrot seed oil, frankincense, myrrh, and Roman chamomile in shea butter or a heavy carrier oil such as sweet almond. Keep products covered and moist while on the skin and do not allow clay, peat, or seaweed to dry out. Refer the client to an esthetician for a professional skin care evaluation.
Water dry	Skin that is "water dry" has sufficient oil but lacks moisture. The skin is thin in texture, with small capillaries showing in certain areas. This type of skin is prone to fine lines, early wrinkles, and a flaky appearance.	Full-body massage blends with essential oils of carrot seed, seaweed essential oil, frankincense, myrrh, German chamomile, Roman chamomile, yarrow, *Helichrysum*, rose, or geranium. Avoid citrus oils in high concentrations. Avoid the use of clay and direct the client to mud, peat, seaweed, shea butter, or honey applications instead. Refer the client to an esthetician for a professional skin care evaluation.
Sensitive	The texture of the skin tends to be fine with redness, heat, broken capillaries, and itching patches. Sensitive skin reacts to strong chemicals, cleaning products, dyes, and fragrances.	Full-body massage blends with essential oils of *Helichrysum*, carrot seed, lavender, rose, frankincense, geranium in sweet almond oil, or expeller pressed sunflower oil (12 drops maximum of essential oil in 2 oz of oil). Avoid products with dyes and synthetic fragrances. Avoid hot treatments such as sheet wraps or Parafango. Dilute seaweeds to half strength with aloe vera gel or wheat germ oil. It is a good idea to keep hydrocortisone cream on hand in case of skin irritation.
Acne on the back	Blackheads, whiteheads, pimples, redness, and irritation may be present. If the condition is inflamed and hot, do not apply product to the area.	If the condition is mild, then the massage therapist can proceed with massage or a body treatment. Full-body massage blends that benefit oily skin and acne include tea tree, lavender, German chamomile, Roman chamomile, yarrow, grapefruit, bergamot, and lemon mixed in jojoba or hemp oil. Avoid the use of peat, paraffin, parafango, and mud and direct the client toward clay or seaweed instead.

Table 2-3	(continued)	

BASIC SKIN TYPE OR SKIN CONDITION	DESCRIPTION	GENERAL RECOMMENDATIONS
Psoriasis	Skin cells divide much faster than normal, resulting in round, reddish patches with silvery scales. Psoriasis usually affects the elbows, knees, lower back, ears, and scalp.	A wide range of essential oils is indicated because psoriasis is considered by many to be a stress-related disorder. Nurturing oils that are unlikely to cause irritation include neroli, ylang ylang, rose, lavender, cypress, *Helichrysum*, yarrow, and frankincense. A combination of these oils can be mixed in hemp seed oil, apricot kernel oil, or expeller pressed sunflower oil. Although mild cases of psoriasis do not seem to be irritated by spa products, mud and peat should be avoided. Direct the client to clay, parafango, paraffin, honey, shea butter, or diluted seaweed instead. Refer the client to a dermatologist.
Eczema and dermatitis	These terms are used to describe many chronic and inflammatory disorders of the skin. Scaling and papule formation as well as red oozing vesicles may accompany burning and itching sensations.	If the condition is mild, the massage therapist can proceed with full-body massage or the application of a product to the body. Essential oils of German chamomile, Roman chamomile, yarrow, frankincense, *Helichrysum*, lavender, and myrrh can be used in shea butter, sweet almond oil, hemp oil, or borage oil. Seaweed may cause irritation, so it should be diluted. Mud and peat should be avoided, but clay or Parafango can be used. Avoid products with synthetic fragrances or dyes. Refer the client to a dermatologist.

rify the skin before a second product, such as a mask (treatment product), is applied. A cleanser applied with warm water provides enough lubrication for Swedish massage strokes to be used. This relaxes muscles, stimulates circulation, and adds a textural experience for the client. The use of water with the massage strokes stimulates and energizes the body.

Toners and Astringents

Toners complete the cleansing process and help to restore the skin's acid mantle. They are usually glycerine-based and do not contain alcohol; therefore, they are suitable for dry skin types. Astringents are a stronger form of toner designed for oily skin. Astringents usually contain alcohol to dissolve excess oil. Toners leave the skin feeling fresh and cool. Alcohol is very drying for the skin, but a gentle toner applied with massage strokes feels invigorating and refreshing. Readers may notice that a skin toner is often used as a treatment step in the procedures section. This is a good skin care practice but also acts as a safety measure. Toners return the skin to a balanced pH, which decreases the chances of the client's developing skin sensitivity to strong treatment products such as seaweed.

Exfoliation Products

Exfoliation products aim to remove trapped debris while sloughing off dead skin cells, smoothing the skin's surface, stimulating circulation and lymph flow, and relaxing the body. The salt glow is a classic exfoliation treatment that first developed as a friction technique in traditional hydrotherapy. At the time, its primary focus was to increase the vital energy of the body and not to smooth the skin. However, overexfoliation on a regular basis can lead to an increase in epidermal thickness, resulting in a "leathery" skin appearance. The skin should not be exfoliated more than once a week except by estheticians for a specific treatment goal.

Treatment Products

Treatment products or "masks" are usually applied with a specific purpose or treatment goal in mind. Parafango masks relax chronic muscular holding patterns, soothe arthritis pain, and promote greater range of motion. They are also useful in cellulite reduction treatments. A full-body seaweed mask is an effective treatment for fibromyalgia or low energy. The mineral elements in some products are absorbed through the skin and support the general health of

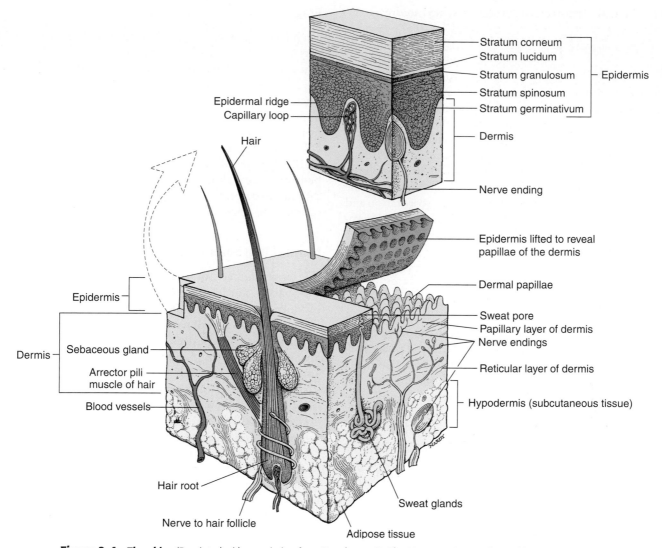

Figure 2-4   The skin. (Reprinted with permission from Premkumar K: *The Massage Connection*. Baltimore: Lippincott Williams & Wilkins, 2004, p. 57.)

the entire body. An esthetician apply masks to the facial or body skin to tighten sagging skin, absorb excess oil, hydrate and moisturize the skin, soothe irritated skin, and beautify the skin. Massage therapists use treatment products to relax or revitalize the body or for a physiological effect on soft tissue structures.

Finishing Products

In this text, finishing products are the last product used in a treatment. A finishing product should contribute toward the goal of the treatment and leave the body feeling refreshed. The therapist might choose a seaweed gel at the end of a seaweed wrap or a detoxifying herbal wrap. Seaweed gel is light, absorbs quickly, and stimulates both circulation and lymphatic flow, so it can contribute to the overall therapeutic goal of the treatment.

A moisturizer is usually used as the finishing product to replace any natural skin oils and moisture lost in the other treatment steps. In general, moisturizers prevent moisture loss from the skin and protect the skin from the environment. They contain oils and emollients with water to soften the skin and prevent premature aging.

IMPORTANT PRODUCT TERMS

Learning to read product labels is an important skill for spa therapists. These labels indicate the type of seaweed or botanical product that has been added, if dyes or fragrances have been added, if the product has ingredients that might be potential allergens for a particular client, or a warning the product has undesirable fillers or chemicals. Milady's *Skin Care and Cosmetic Ingredient Dictionary* by Natalia Michalun is an excellent guide to product ingredients.[12]

The following terms are used widely, so they require a basic explanation.

pH

The pH of a product refers to its level of acidity or alkalinity; pH is measured on a scale of 1 to 14 from acid to alkaline. A pH of 7, which is in the middle of the scale, is considered to be neutral. If the product's pH is lower than 7, it is acidic. If its pH is higher than 7, it is alkaline. The skin is naturally slightly acidic with a pH between 4 and 6, depending on the skin type. In general, the less acidic the skin (the higher the pH number) is naturally, the more prone it is to irritation and sensitivity. The more acidic the skin (the lower the pH number) is naturally, the less prone it is to sensitivity (Fig. 2-5).

Antioxidants

Antioxidants are substances that prevent damage to cells and DNA by free radicals. Free radicals are compounds produced by chemical reactions in the cells that involve oxidation. Normal metabolic reactions and external factors such as ultraviolet radiation, exposure to chemicals like pesticides, air pollution, drugs, and cigarette smoking can produce free radicals. Free radicals interfere with a cell's biochemistry and play a role in some diseases associated with age, including heart disease and cancer. Free radicals attack fats, carbohydrates, proteins, and enzymes, including the collagen in the dermis. This process results in decreased skin elasticity and pliability. Common antioxidants include vitamins E and C, carotenoids (lycopene, lutein, beta-carotene), selenium, green tea, and honey. These ingredients are often found in anti-aging cosmetics and after-sun products.

Botanicals

Botanicals are plant extracts used in spa products to achieve a specific therapeutic goal. The botanical extracts added to a preparation are often chosen because they are anti-inflammatory, soothing, or antiseptic, although they may have a wide range of other actions, depending on the extract. The concentration of the botanical extract and other components in the preparation determine the overall therapeutic value of the preparation. Sometimes an extract is added to a preparation for marketing purposes in very low concentrations, so it adds very little, if anything, to the therapeutic properties of the product. Sometimes the preparation only contains an isolated chemical component of the original botanical extract.

Fragrance

Fragrances enhance the smell of a product, and even products such as seaweed and mud are often fragranced. The fragrance used is either natural or synthetic. Natural fragrances are usually based on natural essential oils or botanical extracts. Synthetic fragrances are usually composed of a small number of artificially synthesized compounds that, on their own, may cause skin irritation or unwanted side effects such as headaches or a slightly sore throat. The popularity of aromatherapy has led to the increased use of essential oils in expensive skin care lines. Although this is a positive trend, it is difficult to determine the quality and purity of the essential oils that are being used.

Natural Ingredients

The term *natural* is not regulated in the cosmetic industry.[13] Companies can legally put just about anything in their products and call them "natural" if they want to. A product line claiming to be "all natural" usually still contains some synthetic ingredients, dyes, or preservatives. In aromatherapy, it is well known that an essential oil may smell differently from batch to batch. The smell of the oil is naturally variable because of the climatic conditions during the year in which it was grown, the time of day at which it was harvested, the skill of the distiller, and the means by which it was stored and shipped. All of these circumstances affect the final chemical composition of the oil and, therefore, its therapeutic properties and its smell. If the oil smells the same from batch to batch, the consumer would be right to wonder if the oil has been adulterated with synthetic additives to achieve a reliable fragrance. Many products claiming to be all natural have a consistent fragrance that is not possible without the addition of other chemicals to standardize the scent.

PRODUCT EXPLORATION

It is important for the therapist to know the products that they are using and to "play" with the products before applying them to clients. Individual seaweeds have different mixing and spreading properties. Some types of mud are difficult to remove from clients' bodies and may require a foaming cleanser to lift them off skin. Some products may dry out quickly and need a plastic cover to keep them moist. It is not a good idea to find these things out during a session. Ordering and trying out new spa products is the best way to discover new treatments and new ways of using prod-

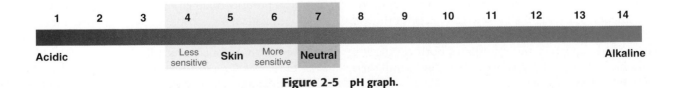

Figure 2-5 pH graph.

ucts. Only by practicing regularly with products will the treatment steps and transitions between the steps become easier. For example, one exfoliation product on the market goes on wet and dries as it is rubbed in. It is brushed away with a dry towel. It requires only one towel for removal on the entire body (eight towels would normally be required). This is faster and easier than a "wet" exfoliation requiring hot towel removal, and it feels more satisfying than dry skin brushing.

Summary

Although luxurious surroundings enhance the mood and character of the spa experience, spa treatments can be delivered satisfactorily in small spas or to private massage clients without great expense. Regardless of the size of the facility, all therapists and employees play a role in preventing the spread of harmful pathogens by using appropriate sanitation procedures. Sanitation protocols should be based on the guidelines and standards of the OSHA, CDC, state board of cosmetology, state board of massage, and department of health in the state where business is conducted.

To ensure the client's safety, a health intake and treatment record should be kept on file and updated for each return visit. Usually, if massage is contraindicated, then spa treatments are also contraindicated, although this is not always the case. A current medical dictionary, drug reference, and pathology reference should be available for therapists to look up unfamiliar conditions and medications. If a client experiences increased pain, discomfort, agitation, nausea, headache, or dizziness from a treatment, the treatment should be discontinued and a physician should be consulted.

A basic understanding of the skin and its care is important for every therapist working in a spa regardless of the scope of practice. Massage and body products affect the skin, even if it is not the massage therapist's aim. Some skin care products penetrate the skin and may produce a physiological effect on the body. Understanding spa products and their ingredients is important to the successful delivery of good spa treatments.

REFERENCES

1. The Centers for Disease Control: *Guideline for Hand Hygiene in Health-Care Settings. Recommendations of the Healthcare Infection Control Practices Advisory Committee and the HICPAC/SHEA/APIC/IDSA Hand Hygiene Task Force.* Available at http://www.cdc.gov.
2. The Centers for Disease Control and Prevention. Available at http://www.cdc.gov
3. The Occupational Safety and Health Administration. Available at http://www.osha.gov
4. Potts RO, Francoeur ML: The influence of stratum corneum morphology on water permeability. *J Invest Dermatol* 1991(Apr);96(4): 495–499.
5. Tanojo H, Bouwstra JA, Junginger HE: In vitro human skin barrier modulation by fatty acids: Skin permeation and thermal analysis studies. *Pharm Res* 1997;14:42–49.
6. Loftsson T, et al. Effect of various marine lipids on transdermal drug delivery: In vitro evaluation. *Bollettino Chimico Farmaceutico* 1997;136: 640–650.
7. Shao Jun J, Young Koo K, Seung Hun L. The ultrastructural changes of stratum corneum lipids after application of oleic acid in propylene glycol. *Ann Dermatol* 1998(July);10(3):153–158.
8. Kaplun-Frischoff Y, Touitou E. Testosterone skin permeation enhancement by menthol through formation of eutectic with drug and interaction with skin lipids. *J Pharm Sci* 1997(December);86(12): 1394–1399.
9. Kunta JR, et al: Effect of menthol and related terpenes on the percutaneous absorption of propranol across excised hairless mouse skin. *J Pharm Sci* 1997(December);86(12):1369–1373.
10. Dreher F, Maibach H: Protective effects of topical antioxidants in humans [abstract]. *Curr Probl Dermatol* 2001;29:157–164.
11. Aiol A, et al: Effects of vitamin E and squalene on skin irritation of a transdermal enhancer, lauroyl sarcosine. *Int J Pharmacol* 1993;93:1–6.
12. Michalun N, Michalun MV: *Skin Care and Cosmetics Ingredients Dictionary*, 2nd ed. Albany, NY: Milady, Thomson Learning, 2001.
13. *Paula Begoun: The cosmetic cop.* Myth Busters Available at http://www.cosmeticcop.com
14. McFadden R: *Cleaning and Maintenance Management Online. Dealing with Blood-Borne Pathogens.* Available at http://www.cmmonline.com
15. U.S. Environmental Protection Agency. Available at http://www.epa.gov

REVIEW QUESTIONS

1. A hot wrap requires which type of materials to achieve its purpose?
   a. A cotton blanket and flannel sheet
   b. A wool blanket and specialized linen sheet to trap body heat
   c. A wool blanket and thermal space blanket to trap the most heat
   d. An electric blanket and flannel sheet

2. As part of good therapist hygiene, the therapist's fingernails should be:
   a. Painted with nail polish to smooth the edges
   b. Clipped short, natural, without polish, and filed to a smooth edge
   c. Long and tapered
   d. Manicured with gel tips to keep them looking attractive

3. Universal Precautions are best described as:
   a. The use of Material Safety Data Sheets to identify potentially harmful chemicals
   b. The proper sanitation of countertops after every treatment
   c. The use of gel hand sanitizers throughout treatments
   d. The CDC's policy regarding blood and body fluids

4. _____ soap that has been used by more than one client is unsanitary and should not be kept in the shower or where hands are washed. _____ soap should be used instead.

5. A _____ application of seaweed would be more dangerous than a spot treatment for a client in a weakened condition.

6. Mild nausea and headache are usually signs of accelerated _____, but if these symptoms persist, a physician should be consulted.

7. Spa clients should always be draped. _____ undergarments can be used by the client during treatments that require more exposure.

8. If a client has moderate to severe hypertension their systolic blood pressure will be above _____ and their diastolic blood pressure will be above _____.

9. When a massage therapist encounters a client with a skin condition that could benefit from regular treatment, the therapist should:
   a. Choose appropriate essential oils and treat the skin.
   b. Refer the client to an esthetician for advanced skin care advice and treatment.
   c. Use seaweed on the condition because seaweed regularly heals problem skin.
   d. Refer to a skin care book before treating the client's skin.

10. Toners are used:
   a. Only by estheticians as a skin care step
   b. By both estheticians and massage therapists in spa treatments as a safety measure to return the skin to a more normal pH and prevent skin irritation
   c. By physicians only directly before a face lift
   d. By clients after they have received a face lift to protect their skin from the sun

Foundation Skills for Spa Treatment Delivery

Chapter Outline

Key Terms

Atomizer: A device that breaks down a watery product into a fine mist for spraying onto the body.

Dry room: A treatment room in which there is no shower or hydrotherapy equipment. Instead, hot towels are used to remove products from the clients' body or clients take showers in a different area.

Herbal infusions: Herbs steeped in water to produce an infusion. Sheets, bath towels, or hand towels are soaked in herbal infusions and applied to the body for therapeutic purposes.

Parafango: A product composed of paraffin and mud. It is mainly used to apply heat to body parts.

Swiss shower: A shower stall that has pipes in all four corners with 8 to 16 water heads coming off each pipe.

Vichy shower: A horizontal rod with holes or water heads that rain water from above a wet table down onto clients.

Wet room: A treatment room that contains specialized hydrotherapy equipment such as showers that remove spa products from clients' bodies, hydrotherapy tubs, and Scotch hoses.

This chapter focuses on the basic skills needed to deliver spa body treatments. It begins with a discussion on the scope of practice restrictions that each therapist must research and consider before providing a spa treatment. Next the chapter discusses draping clients elegantly and efficiently. The goal is to preserve the client's modesty without being overly fussy when applying spa products. Then the chapter explores different ways to apply spa products to the body and how to position clients on the treatment table while products are being applied. Finally, **dry room** and **wet room** removal techniques are discussed. After mastering these foundation skills, readers can choose and match different treatment steps to develop more creative spa services.

Scope of Practice Considerations

The spa industry has grown so rapidly that it has created some confusion about the scope of practice for therapists delivering spa services. Much of this has centered on massage therapists and estheticians. In many states, the board of cosmetology has raised concerns that massage therapists are encroaching on the scope of practice of estheticians when they provide such services as seaweed wraps or body polishes. On the other hand, in some states, massage therapists are concerned that estheticians are using massage techniques that manipulate soft tissue while applying products, therefore encroaching on the scope of practice for massage therapists. The basis of such concerns is that many of the products used in the spa industry affect the physiological health of the muscle tissue and body, as well as the health and appearance of the skin. A seaweed wrap could be used for relaxation or as an active treatment to support a client with fibromyalgia, sore muscles, or low energy (general massage scope of practice). A seaweed wrap can also be used to soften, hydrate, and beautify the skin (general esthetics scope of practice). Body polishes stimulate circulation and lymph flow, tone muscle tissue, or increase the vital energy of the body as in a classic friction rub (general massage scope of practice). They are also an exfoliation treatment that deep cleans, softens, smoothes, and beautifies the skin (general esthetics scope of practice).

This issue is further complicated because laws and regulations vary widely from state to state. A treatment that is within the scope of practice for massage therapists in one state may be banned for massage therapists in another state. For example, massage therapists cannot cleanse, exfoliate, mask, or tone the facial tissue in most states. They can apply creams or lotions (including essential oils) to the face to perform massage. In many states, massage therapists cannot use the word "facial," even when describing a facial massage (they must say "face massage"). In a few states, however, massage therapists can provide facials using certain types of products only. Usu-

ally (but not always), massage therapists can use an exfoliation product such as salt on the body (except the face) to increase circulation, stimulate lymph flow, and relax the body. Products such as seaweed and mud can be used to promote changes in soft tissue or for relaxation or revitalization.

In many states, estheticians cannot apply products with any stroke other than effleurage. They can use various strokes on the face, arms to the elbows, feet to the knees, and on the décolleté (upper chest) for beautification purposes only. They cannot manipulate soft tissue, so they should avoid strokes that lift, knead, or broaden the muscles. Again, in certain states, the above is not true, and estheticians even receive training in full body massage.

This textbook is written on the premise that spa body treatments are a shared practice. It assumes that massage therapists will focus on the benefits of a treatment for the body and estheticians will focus on the benefits of the treatment for the skin. The treatment steps for massage therapists may be the same steps that an esthetician uses, but the goals of the treatment (i.e., the therapist's intention) will be different. This may also be expressed in the promotional descriptions used to sell the treatments to the public: whereas massage therapists market the benefits of the treatment for the body, estheticians market the benefits of the treatment for the skin.

Throughout the treatment chapters, esthetically orientated information is included in "broaden your understanding" boxes. This information has been separated from the main body of the text to avoid confusing new spa therapists who are still unclear about their scope of practice. Estheticians who are using the book as a reference should be aware of the properties of products such as mud and seaweed for the skin. Massage therapists who want the broadest possible understanding of a treatment should understand its implications for the skin, even though they will probably not market these effects to their clients.

Therapists should check to see if any treatments or practices are not allowed by the regulatory body in the state where they are practicing. They should also check to see if their liability insurance policy covers the treatments they are offering. Table 3-1 provides a brief overview of the coverage of spa treatments by some common providers in the massage industry as of July 2005.

Spa Draping

In a massage session, range of motion techniques require a tight drape that is tucked in, wrapped around the limb, and sometimes held taut by the client. Clients receiving spa treatments are draped slightly differently than they would be in a normal massage. Although the client is always draped, the aim is to preserve modesty and warmth without being too fussy. Spa draping should be quick, elegant, and

Table 3-1	Common Liability Insurance Providers and Spa Coverage			
INSURANCE PROVIDER AND CONTACT INFORMATION	**AROMATHERAPY**	**HYDROTHERAPY**	**SPA TREATMENTS**	**EXCEPTIONS**
North American Studio Alliance (NAMASTA), http://www.namasta.com, 877-626-2782	Yes	Yes	Some	Does not cover a spa treatment if it is restricted by state laws
USMTO Insurance, http://www.usmto.lockton-ins.com, 877-240-2670	No	Basic hydrotherapy such as hydroculator packs	No	Does not cover hot stone massages
The International Massage Association, http://www.holisticbenefits.com/ima/international-massage-association.htm, 866-243-1707	Yes	Yes	Herbal wraps only	Spa treatments by massage therapists are not covered
Massage Magazine Hands-On Trades Protection Plan, http://www.massagemag.com/insurance.htm, 800-533-4263	Yes	Yes	Some	Check restrictions before providing treatments
American Massage Council, 800-500-3930	Essential oils when applied with massage only	Some	No	Check restrictions to hydrotherapy before providing treatments
Associated Bodywork and Massage Professionals, http://www.abmp.com/membership/index.html, 800-458-2267	Yes	Yes	Yes	Does not cover spa treatments that are restricted by state laws
American Massage Therapy Association, http://www.amtamassage.org/membership-intro.html, 877-905-2700	Yes	Yes	Yes	Does not cover spa treatments that are restricted by state laws

efficient. Disposable undergarments can be used for treatments in which clients are more exposed. Some spas and clients are more relaxed about draping than others. Good draping sets up good professional boundaries, so it is encouraged. Therapists should discuss the spa's draping policy during the job interview to decide if they are comfortable with it. The following draping methods work well. Draping methods are shown in Figure 3-1.

POSTERIOR LEG

To undrape the posterior leg, gather the drape at the greater trochanter and at the ankle. Fold the bottom end of the drape at an angle across the opposite leg while holding the drape at the greater trochanter as a pivot point. With the lower hand, grab the fold of the drape and tuck it under the opposite thigh. Fold the top section of the drape across the back, leaving the gluteals exposed. With practice, this draping can be accomplished in three moves and provides a clean line for the application of spa products from the toes to the top of the posterior superior iliac spine (PSIS).

ANTERIOR LEG

To undrape the anterior leg, gather the drape at the anterior superior iliac spine (ASIS) and at the ankle. Fold the bottom section of the drape at an angle across the opposite leg using the upper hand to hold the drape at the ASIS as a pivot point. With the lower hand, grab the fold of the drape and tuck it under the opposite thigh. Fold the top section of the drape across the belly, leaving the ASIS exposed.

BREAST DRAPE

Align the top edge of the main drape with the bottom edge of the hand towel or pillow case that will be used for the breast drape. As the main drape is pulled down, the breast drape will take its place.

ANTERIOR PELVIC DRAPE

After the breast drape is in place, continue to pull the main drape down until the stomach is uncovered. Align the fold of the main drape with the bottom edge of the hand towel

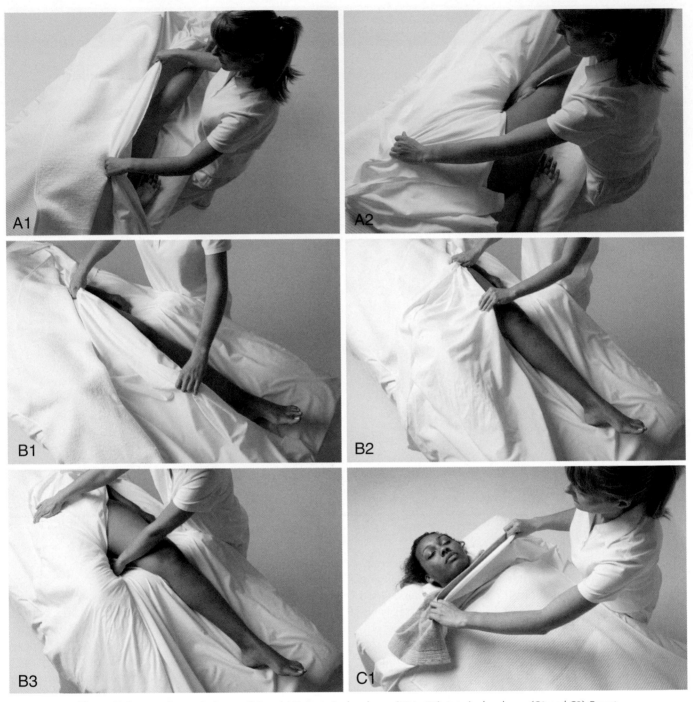

Figure 3-1 Draping techniques. (A1 and A2) Posterior leg drape. (B1 to B3) Anterior leg drape. (C1 and C2) Breast drape. (D1 to D3) Anterior pelvic drape. (E1 and E2) Turban drape. (F1 and F2) Gluteals drape.

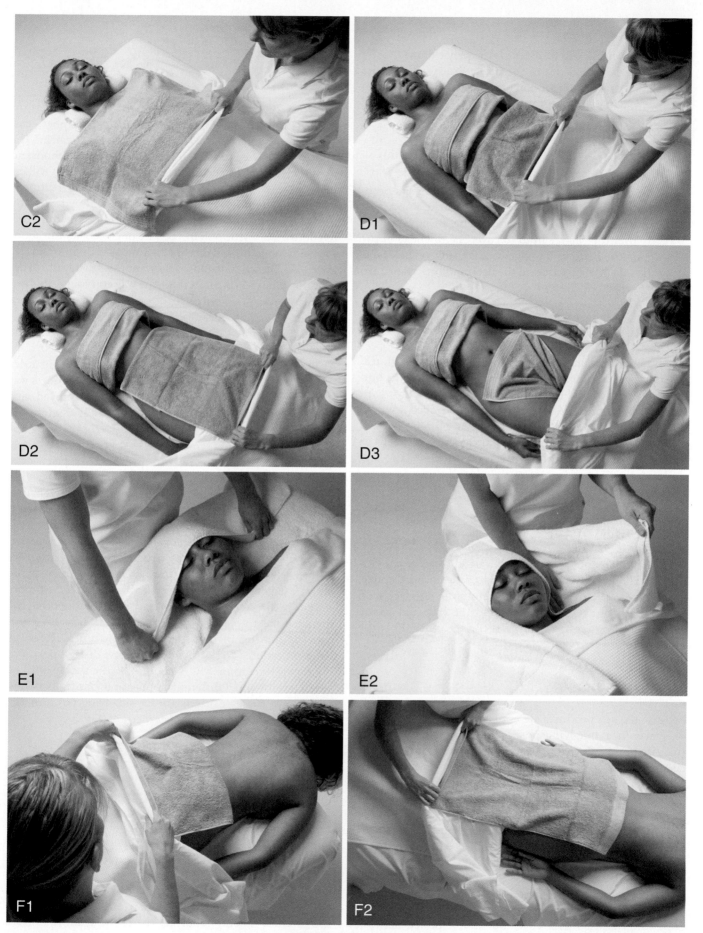

Figure 3-1 *continued*

or pillow case that will be used for the pelvic drape. As the main drape is pulled down, the pelvic drape will take its place. Tuck the bottom section of the pelvic drape between the legs, leaving a safe distance between the tucking hand and the genitals.

TURBAN DRAPE

This type of drape protects the client's hair from spa products and prevents heat loss during a treatment. Put a bath towel on the table before the treatment. Bring the bath towel up over the client's head to cover the forehead or the eyes. Using the hand as a wedge on each side of the drape, bring the side portions around the neck and tuck them into the top of the body drape.

GLUTEAL DRAPE

Uncover the back and fold the drape down to the gluteal cleft. Grasp the folded edge of the main drape and the bottom edge of the hand towel or pillow case that will be used for the gluteal drape. As the main drape is pulled down to expose the gluteals, the hand towel or pillow case will replace it. Tuck the bottom of the gluteal drape between the legs leaving a safe distance between the tucking hand and the genitals. Fold the edges of the gluteal drape to create clean lines for product application.

SIMPLE HAIR DRAPE

Hold diagonally opposite ends of a hand towel at the corner and allow the rest of the towel to drop into a triangle. Place this on the treatment table before the client gets on it, and then bring the edges around the hair and secure with a bobby pin or by tucking the end into the fold of the towel.

SIDE-LYING DRAPE

Because the spa products are applied to the client while he or she is in a side-lying position, this drape is different than it would be for a massage. It is important to ask the client to wear disposable undergarments to preserve modesty. The sheet is kept over the client until he or she is moved into the side-lying position. Undrape the client's upper body (females should either wear a disposable bra or hold a towel over their breasts) and place a bath towel across the client's hip. Grasp the folded edge of the main drape and the bottom edge of the bath towel. As the main drape is pulled down to expose the gluteals, the bath towel will replace it, and the sheet is removed completely. The client needs to be in disposable briefs because the bath towel is used as a cover but is not pulled between the legs.

Positioning the Client for Product Application

Rumi (1207–1273 C.E.), the well-known Sufi poet, said "There are a thousand ways to kneel and kiss the earth." The same could be said for spa treatments. There are a thousand ways to deliver the same treatment. A good therapist will explore a treatment thoroughly and arrange the treatment steps in different ways until they can be delivered perfectly with maximum fluidity. Each therapist brings something different to a treatment, and in a private practice, they can adapt the basic steps and enhance the treatment in unique and creative ways. By contrast, most spas want their therapists to deliver the same treatment in the same way every time. It is important to maintain this sort of consistency for returning clientele. The techniques described below work well, but each can be done in many different ways. Again, exploration is the best way for therapists to find out what works for them.

The choices made when delivering a treatment in a dry room setting may well be different to those made for a wet room setting. In a wet room, spa products are removed with a specialized or handheld shower. Shower removal is quicker and easier for the therapist than removal using hot towels. Still, hot towel removal feels wonderful if the towels are hot (rather than lukewarm) and the therapist works with purpose, flow, and attention to detail.

Many body treatments, regardless of their therapeutic objectives, have the same basic steps: exfoliation, application of the treatment product, time for the treatment product to absorb and work, removal of the treatment product, and application of a finishing product (usually a moisture lotion, gel, or cream). Sometimes it is better to treat the body in segments, which helps the treatment to flow more smoothly through the product transitions. More often the therapist has to plan how to apply several different products without turning the client too many times. The treatment procedures sections in each chapter discuss positioning for each treatment. It is helpful for the therapist to be familiar with three different application positions before continuing; these positions are the side-lying position, the sit-up method, and the flip-over method (Fig. 3-2).

THE SIDE-LYING POSITION

The client begins the treatment in the supine position for the exfoliation step. After exfoliation on the anterior body, turn the client into a side-lying position for the posterior exfoliation. The client remains in the side-lying position while the treatment product is applied. After the product has been applied, roll the client onto his or her back again before wrapping the client. The client needs to stay alert throughout the treatment and roll from side to side. As the spa product is being removed, the client again rolls from side to side to be toweled off (in a dry room).

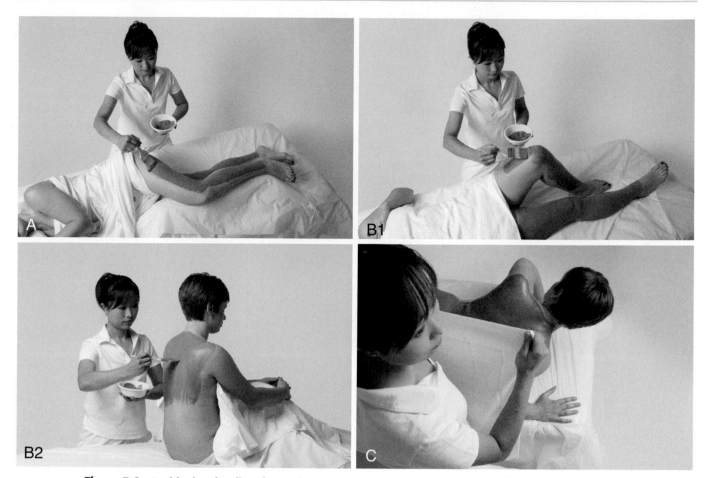

Figure 3-2   Positioning the client for product application. (A) The side-lying position. (B1 and B2) The sit-up method. (C) The flip-over method.

THE SIT-UP METHOD

The client begins the treatment in a prone position so that the posterior body can be exfoliated. Then the client is turned into a supine position so the anterior side of the body can be exfoliated. The knees are bent and the treatment product is applied to both the anterior and posterior sides of the legs. Flatten the client's legs against the plastic body wrap and then wrap the legs in the body wrap. Remove the bolster and then ask the client to sit up. Apply the treatment product to the back and gluteals and then ask the client to lie back down again. Finally the belly, upper chest, and arms are treated, and then the client's upper body is wrapped. The product is removed using the same method, and the client is only turned over once during the entire treatment. For some clients, sitting up is impossible because of lower back problems or weak abdominal muscles. In these cases, choose the safest and easiest application method for the individual client.

THE FLIP-OVER METHOD

In the flip-over method, the client starts the treatment in the prone position for the exfoliation step. Apply the treatment product before turning the client. Ask the client to flip over (the goal is to make sure that the client makes a clean flip and does not get spa product all over the place). The therapist holds up a drape and looks away to protect the client's modesty. Exfoliate the anterior body and apply the treatment product before the client is wrapped. This application method can be messy if the client does not make a clean flip. Sheets or bath towel drapes are difficult to use because they will become covered in product. For this reason, the client should probably use disposable undergarments. The treatment product will be on the client's back and posterior legs for an extra 10 minutes while the anterior body is being treated. This may be problematic with some products (e.g., very strong seaweed).

Basic Application Techniques

When choosing an application technique, the thickness of the product, the speed at which it needs to be applied, and the way the product should feel as it goes onto the body need to be considered. The following methods work well and are shown in Figure 3-3.

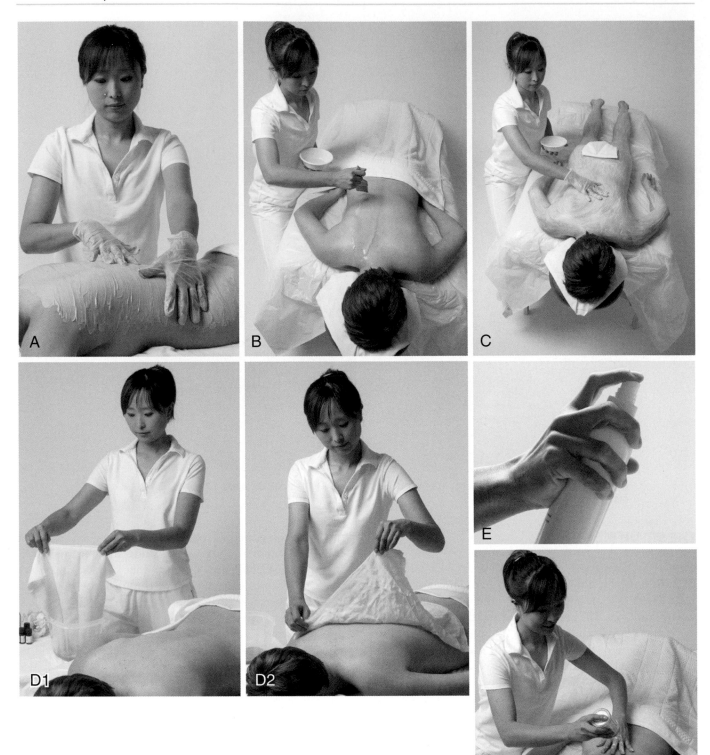

Figure 3-3   Application methods. (A) By hand. (B) Using a brush. (C) With one hand gloved. (D1 and D2) Using gauze or fabric. (E) Using a mist. (F) Using a shaker.

APPLICATION BY HAND

Smooth the product onto the skin using effleurage strokes. Some products provide enough lubrication to massage into the skin with a full range of strokes. The use of massage enhances the treatment and is more enjoyable for the client. If applying the spa product by hand, the therapist has to decide if he or she will use gloves to apply it or wash it off the hands after the application. Gloves are quickest.

APPLICATION WITH ONE HAND GLOVED

Sometimes the product is applied with one hand wearing a glove while the ungloved hand is used to undrape body areas as needed or hold the container of product. This technique works well with the flip-over position already described.

APPLICATION BY BRUSH

If the client is sunburned or has delicate skin, using a brush works well as long as the product is thin enough to be applied with a brush. A large brush is quicker and more efficient than the smaller brushes used for facials. If massage is included as part of a different treatment step, applying the product with a brush will provide a different sort of texture and give the overall treatment greater tactile variety. Using a brush also keeps the therapist's hands clean if needed to drape and undrape body areas during the application process.

APPLICATION WITH GAUZE OR FABRIC

For some spa products, a piece of gauze or light fabric is dipped into the product and then applied to the body area. This method is used with paraffin, **parafango**, **herbal infusions**, and mud, although it can be used with many different products. It allows the therapist to cover body areas rapidly and precisely. Paraffin and parafango drip easily. The use of the gauze prevents the product from getting onto the floor or dripping onto the client. If the product is too warm, it may burn the client or be very uncomfortable because the heat feels intense when a large area is being covered at once. This is the main drawback of this method of application.

APPLICATION BY MIST

Very thin or watery products can be sprayed onto the body with an **atomizer** or mister. Products that are misted onto the body feel cool, even when the product has been heated.

APPLICATION WITH A SHAKER

Dry products such as ground herbs, salt, sugar, medicated powder, and flour can be applied to the body through a sugar shaker. This is a unique sensory experience for the client; it is often described as feeling like raindrops.

Dry Room Removal Techniques

Use hot, moist towels to remove the treatment product from the client's body in a dry room setting. This is a warm and satisfying experience when the towels are steamy hot and the therapist uses long, elegant strokes. To prepare the towels, pull off all the tags, fold the towels in half (the long way), and roll them up like a sausage. It is important that all the tags are removed because they could scratch the client. Place the towels in a hydroculator, hot towel cabinet, or roaster oven for 20 minutes at 165°F. With thermal gloves, remove a towel from the water, ring it out, and place it in the soda cooler. Close the lid of the cooler and remove the next towel. Keep the lid of the cooler shut as much as possible so the towels stay hot throughout the treatment. Towels can be enhanced by soaking them in herbal infusions or adding essential oils just before use. Some therapists color coordinate their towels for the treatment (e.g., green towels for seaweed treatments, brown towels for mud treatments, beige towels for herbal infusions) to camouflage any product stains.

STEAMY ROSEMARY TOWELS

Add 3 to 5 drops of rosemary essential oil to the soda cooler full of towels. As each towel is removed, it will fill the treatment room with a refreshing scent. Most single oils such as eucalyptus, common sage (*Salvia officinalis*), Spanish sage (*Salvia lavandulifolia*), thyme, and lemon oil smell good, but floral scents such as ylang ylang and jasmine are not as pleasant in steam. The essential oil on the towel is not likely to cause any skin irritation because essential oils are volatile substances and begin to evaporate rapidly the minute they are placed on the hot towels in the cooler, and most of the oil is burned off before the first towel is used, leaving only some of the scent behind. Therefore, potential skin irritation is minimized.

HERBAL-INFUSED TOWELS

Muslin bags filled with fragrant herbs can also be used to scent towels. A muslin bag of herbs is added to the water in which the towels are heated. A nice combination is eucalyptus leaf, rosemary, clove buds, and juniper berry. A half a cup of herbs to around 16 quarts of water provides a nice concentration, although more or less herbs can be used according to preference. Towels heated in herbal solutions will be lightly stained.

HOT TOWEL REMOVAL

Legs

Remove a towel from the soda cooler and hold it by the edges because it is hot. Let it cool slightly and place it on the proximal portion of the leg (anterior or posterior). Allow it to sit on the leg and do not touch it again until it cools down (about 30 seconds). Place both hands on the towel and pull it toward the distal portion of the leg and off the foot. Turn the towel over and use the clean side to make another sweep (Fig. 3-4A).

Feet

Place a hot towel around each foot to steam the feet and provide a nice sensation. Then remove the product from one foot at a time (Fig. 3-4B).

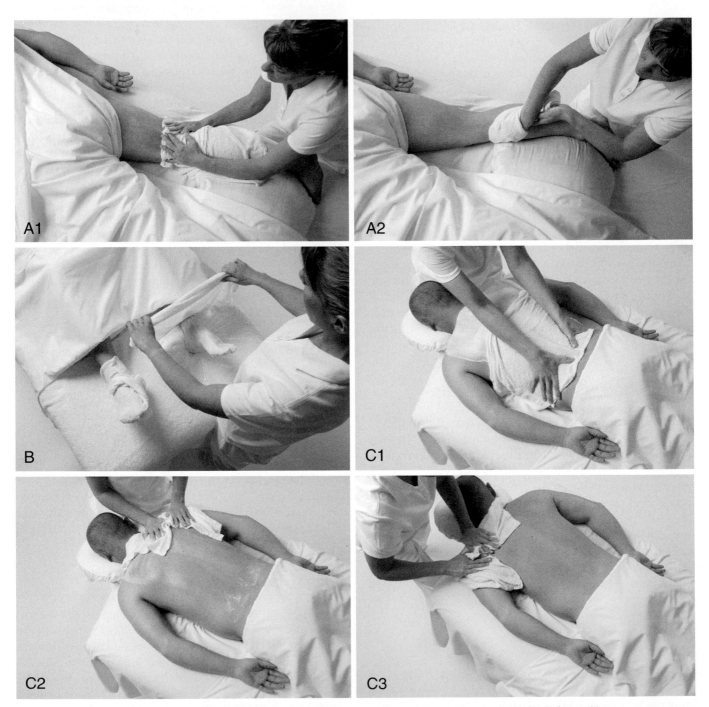

Figure 3-4 **Hot towel removal.** (A1 and A2) Legs. (B) Feet. (C1 to C3) Back. (D) Arm. (E) Abdominal area. (F) Upper chest. (G) Product removal with sponges and hot water.

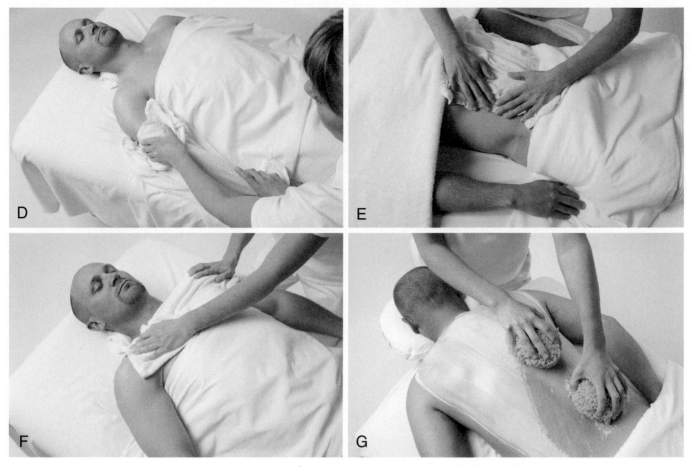

Figure 3-4 *continued*

Back

Place the hot towel horizontally on the lower back and allow it to cool slightly without touching it. Place both hands on the towel and pull it toward the client's head. As the towel gets to the neck, pull it off to one side, removing the product from the shoulder without getting it into the client's hair. Turn the towel over and use the clean side to make a second sweep, removing the product from the second shoulder (Fig. 3-4C).

Arms

Place the hot towel vertically on the proximal portion of the arm and pull the towel toward the hand in one sweep. Lift the arm by holding onto the client's hand, and use the clean side of the towel to wipe down the other side of the arm (Fig. 3-4D).

Abdominal Area and Upper Chest

Place the hot towel horizontally on the belly and pull it from the left side to the right side. Turn the towel over and use the clean side to remove the product from right to left. Place a hot towel across the upper chest and remove the

product by pulling the towel from one side to the other (Figs. 3-4E and F).

OTHER DRY ROOM REMOVAL TECHNIQUES

Sponges and warm water can be used to remove the product in a dry room setting (Fig. 3-4G). In this case, place a bucket of warm water close to the treatment table on a rolling cart. Dip a sea sponge, large cosmetic sponge, or a washcloth into the water and use it to wipe off the product. Dry the client with a hand towel after the product has been removed. The only problem with sponge removal is that it is difficult to keep the linens under the client dry. Some therapists put a thick bath towel on top of the linens before the treatment and get the client to lift his or her body so that the towel can be removed after the sponge bath.

MOVING A CLIENT FROM PLASTIC TO A PRESET MASSAGE SHEET

In many different types of body wrap, the client is covered in a spa treatment product and then wrapped in plastic. After the treatment product has been removed, a finishing product is applied to the client, often in a full-body massage. In

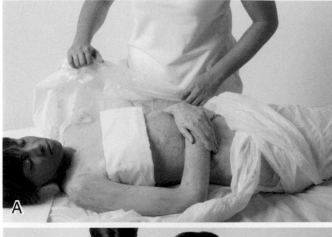

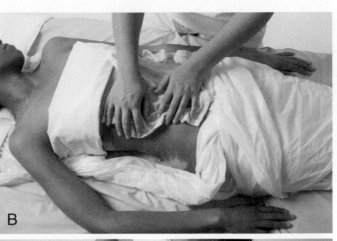

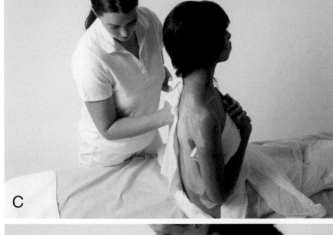

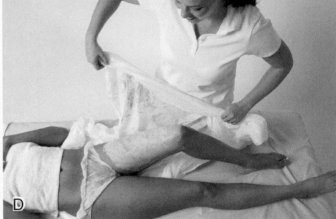

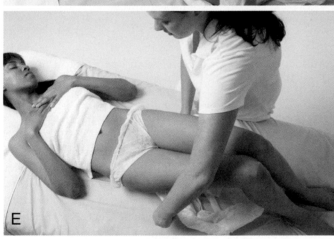

Figure 3-5   Moving a client from plastic to a preset massage sheet. (A) Unwrap the client. (B) Remove the product from the arms, upper chest, and abdominal area. (C) Remove the product from the back and roll up the plastic. (D) Remove the product from the legs and roll up the plastic. (E) Remove the plastic from under the client.

a dry room setting, the therapist has to get the dirty plastic out from underneath the client without asking the client to get off the treatment table (a clean massage sheet has been preset under the plastic). To do this, unwrap the plastic, leaving the client covered by the breast drape and anterior pelvic drape (or disposable undergarments) that were put on before the client was wrapped up (Fig. 3-5). Remove the product from the client's arms, upper chest, and abdominal area and ask him or her to hold onto the breast drape and sit up. Remove the product from the back and the posterior arms. Roll up the plastic sheet so that the dirty side is rolled in until it sits as close to the gluteals as possible. Then ask

the client to lie back down (onto the clean massage sheet). Move down to the lower legs and wipe the feet with a hot towel. Ask the client to bend the knees and hold up the feet. Roll up the dirty side of the plastic that is underneath the client's feet. Place the client's clean feet on the massage sheet, which is underneath the plastic (the knees are still bent). Remove the spa product from both legs with hot towels and roll the plastic up as high as possible under the gluteals. Place the clean legs flat on the massage sheet and cover the client with a sheet or towel for warmth. The client then lies back down on the massage sheet and slightly lifts the hips so that the plastic can be removed.

Wet Room Removal Techniques

In a wet room, a specialized shower is used to remove spa products from the client's body. Specialized showers include a handheld shower, a standard shower, the **Swiss shower**, and the **Vichy shower**. Always read the manufacturer's instructions for the particular piece of equipment beforehand. It is important to practice a treatment at least two to three times when using a specialized shower so that the temperature and pressure of the shower are safe and comfortable for the client. Wet room removal techniques are shown in Figure 3-6. Wet room equipment is also described in Chapter 4.

THE HANDHELD SHOWER

A handheld shower is used in combination with a wet table for the easy removal of spa products. Some handheld showers can deliver a pulsating water massage and may also have

an attachable body brush for exfoliation. A wet table has a special surface to channel water into a receptacle under the table, or it has a drain in the wet room floor. The table is often constructed of heavy plastic or acrylic for easy cleanup and sanitation. A soft, waterproof insert makes the table comfortable for the client. Sometimes a bucket of warm water is poured over the client to remove the spa product. This type of removal provides an invigorating experience for the client, but the client should be dried quickly so he or she does not get too cold.

THE STANDARD SHOWER

A standard home shower is less expensive than a Swiss or a Vichy shower, but it does not allow the same range of control. The pressure of the water, the degree of pulsation, and the temperature of the water cannot be controlled by the therapist. The client is moved between the massage table and the shower as needed during the treatment. For example, if

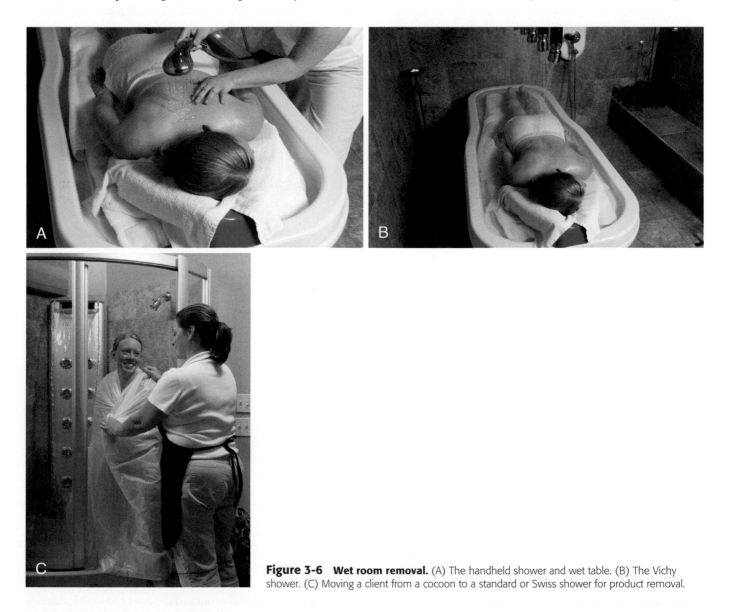

Figure 3-6   Wet room removal. (A) The handheld shower and wet table. (B) The Vichy shower. (C) Moving a client from a cocoon to a standard or Swiss shower for product removal.

seaweed is applied after exfoliating the client with a dry brush, the client will be moved off the massage table after the seaweed has been allowed to process and taken to the shower so the seaweed can be washed off. While being moved, the client stays loosely covered in the plastic wrap until he or she gets into the shower. The client then passes the plastic wrap to the therapist to throw away. The therapist then places clean linen sheets on the massage table while the client finishes showering. The client returns to the massage table for a massage or to have a finishing lotion or cream applied.

THE SWISS SHOWER

A Swiss shower surrounds the client with jets of water directed at specific areas of the body. Usually the shower stall has pipes in all four corners with 8 to 16 water heads coming off each pipe. Adjust the position of the water heads for the client's height. A control panel outside the shower stall allows the therapist to control contrasting warm and cool jets of water. A shower can be used for product removal, as an active treatment in itself, or to provide the heating phase of the treatment for products such as cellulite cream.

THE VICHY SHOWER

A Vichy shower is a horizontal rod with holes or water heads that rain water down onto the client from above the wet table. Vichy showers are used to rinse off spa products, but these showers can also be used as a treatment in themselves. A control panel allows the therapist to alternate between hot and cool water, which increases the therapeutic benefits of some products and uses the mechanical effects of water on soft tissue. Vichy showers have an adjustable face guard that is meant to keep water off the client's face, although some water invariably gets through. A soft, lightweight washcloth can be used to cover the client's face and protect it from water droplets. Care must be used when moving the client off the wet table because the area around the table may be slippery with water. Although a finishing lotion or cream can be applied while the client is on the wet table, it is nicer to move the client to a dry room massage table for this final step. Wet rooms may feel a little cold and can echo because of the tiled floor.

 Sanitation

The shower stall or wet table, the floor outside the shower, the shower curtain (if there is one), and any other surface that touches the client or water must be cleaned, disinfected, and dried between clients. Towels and floor mats also need to be changed between clients.

The Spa Massage and Treatment Enhancers

Massage in a spa setting is just like massage in any other setting: it is usually customized to fit the needs of the individual client and can take many forms. All types of massage, including Swedish, Lomi Lomi, Thai, manual lymphatic drainage, craniosacral, Shiatsu, deep tissue, myofascial release, ayurvedic marma point therapy, stone massage, sports massage, neuromuscular therapy, and many others are offered in spas across the country. Sometimes the whole massage routine is based on one style (e.g., Lomi Lomi), and sometimes a combination of techniques from other styles (e.g., Thai, marma point massage) are included in, for example, a Swedish-style massage. The spa may train everyone to deliver the same massage or may allow each therapist to do his or her own massage routine. Therapists who would like to work in an established spa should make sure that their Swedish massage is flowing and elegant. They should work to engage the tissue so that the strokes have depth and intent. Practice draping efficiently and incorporating a variety of strokes so that the massage feels complete. When developing a "spa massage," try to make the service as luxurious as possible by adding several small but exceptional enhancers. These enhancers may include the use of steamy aromatic towels, aroma mists, a simple hand and foot treatment, paraffin dips, the use of warm packs, an eye pillow, or a firming face massage. The spa massage outlines presented in Table 3-2 are meant to provide some structure for those developing relaxation spa massages. The outlines help therapists see how massages are enhanced with little extras to make them special. Step-by-step directions for some useful enhancers are described below and shown in Figure 3-7.

WARM PACKS

Chapter 4 describes the use of hot and cold packs to facilitate changes in muscle tissue and to achieve a physiological effect on the body. In a relaxation massage, the goal is to get clients to relax completely, to breathe deeply, to reflect on their inner thoughts, and to feel revitalized and rested at the end of the session. Warm packs of rice, corn, or flax seed keep clients warm but do not generate enough heat to produce perspiration. These warm packs are used to make clients feel pampered and cozy and are placed on the back and on the feet in the prone position. In the supine position, a warm pack can be placed on the belly, around the feet, and if the shape is appropriate, under the neck. Eye pillows filled with fragrant herbs can be warmed or cooled and placed over the eyes to block out excess light. A Fomentek water bottle can be placed under the bottom massage sheet to provide warmth, or the table can be heated with an electric table warmer. However, many therapists do not use electric table warmers because they feel that they disrupt clients' electromagnetic (energy) fields. Hot placement stones can also be used during a relaxation massage

Table 3-2	Spa Massage and Enhancers: Sample Outlines

SIMPLE AND SUMPTUOUS	EFFORTLESS INDULGENCE
1. The client is supine, semi-reclined, and bolstered.	1. The client is prone and bolstered.
2. Place a warm pack on the belly.	2. Place a warm pack on the back and on the bottom of the feet.
3. Place 1 drop of lemon oil in the hands and pass the hands in an arc over the client's nose for one or two breaths.	3. Place 1 drop of lavender oil on a tissue and tuck it into the bottom of the face cradle so that the client can smell a light fragrance.
4. Place an aromatic hot towel over each foot and steam the feet. Remove the towel and proceed with the foot massage.	4. Massage the posterior legs and gluteals. Undrape the back and place a steamy rosemary towel on the back.
5. Massage the anterior legs.	5. Massage the back. At the end of the back massage, apply a body wash gel with warm water and work it into a lather. Remove the lather with a hot towel. Redrape the back.
6. Massage the arms and hands. Apply an exfoliation product to the hands and then remove it with a hot towel. Paraffin dip the hands and wrap them in cellophane and a warm towel.	6. Remove the warm pack that is sitting on the feet. Turn the client into a supine position. Place a warm pack under the neck and an eye pillow over the eyes. Rebolster the client.
7. Remove the pillows from under the client's head and proceed with a neck and face massage. Place a steamy aromatic towel on the face at the end of the massage.	7. Massage the feet. At the end of the foot massage, apply exfoliation cream to the feet and scrub the feet. Remove the exfoliation product with hot towels.
8. Remove the paraffin from the hands, remove the warm packs, and turn the client into the prone position.	8. Massage the anterior legs and abdominal muscles.
9. Rebolster the client and massage the posterior legs and gluteals.	9. Massage the arms and hands.
10. Massage the back. Apply a foaming exfoliation product to the back and work it into lather. Remove with steamy aromatic towels.	10. Massage the neck and face. Place a steamy aromatic towel over the face to end the massage. Remove the towel and use an aroma mist spritzed high over the client.
11. Spritz an aroma mist over the client and throughout the treatment room to complete the massage. When the client gets off the table, he or she will smell the fresh scent.	11. Allow the client to relax on the treatment table for an extra 10 minutes before getting up.

to bring a sense of weight and heat to clients. For instruction in the use of placement stones, refer to Chapter 12.

STEAMY AROMATIC TOWELS

Earlier in the chapter, the use of steamy rosemary towels and towels infused with herbs was described for product removal. These steamy aromatic towels also make a pleasing enhancer for a full-body relaxation massage. For example, a steamy aromatic towel can be applied to the back right before the back massage is done. This warms the body tissue and feels especially satisfying. Another way of using a hot towel on the back is to apply a bit of body wash gel or foaming exfoliation cream with warm water at the end of the back massage. Lather it with the hands and then remove the lather with a hot towel. This takes only 1 minute out of the massage but becomes a

memorable moment for the client and prevents the client from feeling oily at the end of the treatment. A steamy aromatic towel can be used in the same way on the feet before the foot massage, on the face before the face massage, or on the face at the end of the service as a closing gesture.

A SIMPLE HAND OR FOOT TREATMENT

During a relaxation massage, a simple hand or foot treatment can be added to make the massage special. These enhancers take up very little massage time and are a memorable part of the experience for the client. For a simple foot treatment, prepare by placing a bath towel at the end of the treatment table where the client's feet will sit and put two hot moist hand towels in a soda cooler. Just before the foot massage, simply undrape the client's feet and apply a little

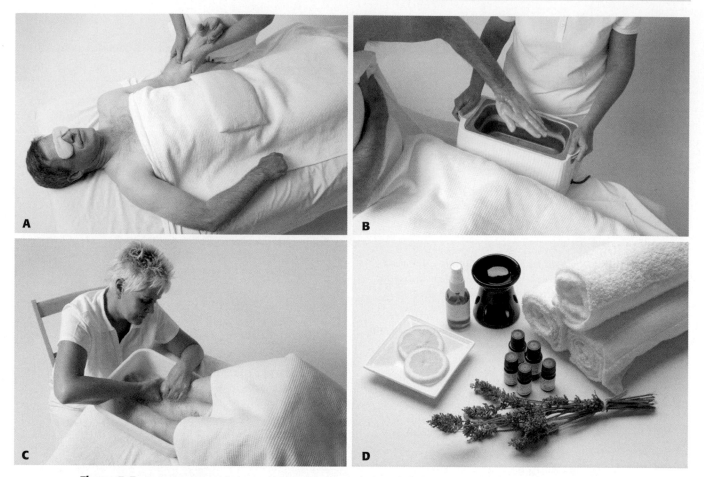

Figure 3-7   Spa massage enhancers. (A) Warm packs, including a belly pack and eye pillow. A warm neck ring or foot warmers might also be used. On the posterior body, the therapist might use a warm pack on the back and on the bottoms of the feet. (B) A simple foot and hand treatment. A complementary foot or hand treatment such as a paraffin dip make a client's experience special. (C) Foot soak. A foot soak can be used at the beginning of the session before the client gets on the table or during the session, as shown here. (D) Aromatic enhancers. Steamy aromatic towels, aroma mists, and aroma inhalations enhance the session with delightful scents.

exfoliation cream to each foot. Scrub the feet with the exfoliation cream and then place a hot towel over each foot. After the feet have steamed in the towels, use them to remove the exfoliation product and proceed with the foot massage. The hand treatment is conducted in the same way. An exfoliation cream is massaged into the hand and up to the elbow. A hand towel is placed over each hand and the product is removed directly before the hand massage.

PARAFFIN DIP

Paraffin is a waxy substance obtained from the distillates of wood, coal, petroleum, or shale oil. It is used to coat the skin and trap heat and moisture at the skin's surface. This increases circulation, which improves joint mobility and increases absorption of spa products whenever they have been applied before using the paraffin. It is an effective treatment for chronic arthritis, tight muscles, and painful joints. It also leaves the skin soft, and it feels warm and sumptuous.

To apply paraffin to the hands or feet, wash the area to be dipped or mist the area with alcohol so that it is properly sanitized. Dip the hand or foot into the paraffin and allow the paraffin to harden slightly before dipping the area again. Dipping the area up to five times should be sufficient. Wrap the paraffin-covered hand or foot in cellophane wrap or a plastic bag before placing it into a heated mitt or a warm towel. To remove the paraffin, simply peel off the cellophane wrap together with the wax in one piece. The hands can be dipped while the client is on the table in the prone or semi-reclined position. The feet can be dipped while the client is on the table in the supine position. Paraffin can also be applied with a brush or on gauze strips that are wrapped around the body area.

EASY AROMATHERAPY ENHANCEMENTS

Small aromatherapy enhancements stand out as moments of particular radiance in a good relaxation massage. Essential oil massage blends create an olfactory reaction that may facilitate deeper relaxation in the client. It is a good idea to provide a selection of three to five blends so that the client can choose which ones he or she likes best. Aroma mists are another way to bring the pleasure of good smells into the massage. An aroma mist is usually made from distilled water with some added essential oils, but a hydrosol (flower water) can also be used. The mist is spritzed high over the client while he or she is in a supine position to fill the treatment room with a refreshing scent. The scents used in the treatment can be varied to keep the client's olfactory "palate" stimulated.

Aroma inhalations are used either at the beginning or end of the massage. One drop of an oil or one drop of a blend of different oils is quickly rubbed together in the hands before being passed over the client's nose in an arc so that the oil can be enjoyed on a deep inward breath. The therapist then proceeds with the massage. Table 3-3 provides some nice aromatherapy blends that are generally popular with clients. These blends can be mixed

Table 3-3	Easy Aromatherapy		
MASSAGE BLENDS		**AROMA MISTS**	**INHALATIONS**
The following blends can be added to 1 fluid oz of an expeller-pressed oil (i.e., hazelnut, sweet almond, sunflower) or plain massage cream. The numbers refer to drops.		The following blends can be added to 1 oz of distilled water.	The following blends can be mixed up and used undiluted (1 drop) in the hands for an aroma inhalation.
Relax Factor		**Radiance**	**Inspiration**
Frankincense 4		Atlas cedarwood 5	Rose 1
Mandarin 8		Neroli 2	Mandarin 10
Ylang ylang 2		Lavender 4	Clove 1
Cypress 2		Grapefruit 6	
Refreshing		**Revitalize**	**Verve**
Rosemary 3		Grapefruit 8	Rosemary 2
Clary sage 2		Eucalyptus 1	Geranium 1
Lemon 7		Cypress 2	
Geranium 1		Sweet orange 6	
Citrus Star		**Summer**	**Sparkle**
Grapefruit 11		Mandarin 6	Peppermint 1
Jasmine 1		Lemon 7	Grapefruit 8
		Geranium 1	
Muscle Ease		**Rain**	**Siesta**
Sweet Birch 3		Juniper berry 4	Lime 7
Juniper berry 2		Thyme 2	Jasmine 1
Lavender 6		Lavender 6	
Lemon 6		Cypress 3	
Detox		**Mental Boost**	**Quietude**
Sweet fennel 5		Rosemary	Neroli 2
Juniper berry 4		Basil	Clary sage 5
Grapefruit 10		Lemon	Sandalwood 10
Body Boost		**Sweet Dreams**	**Wake Up**
Peppermint 1		Neroli 2	Peppermint 2
Tea tree 2		Lavender 7	Rosemary 2
Lavender 6		Mandarin 10	Basil 1
Lemon 6			

into a plain massage cream or in expeller pressed vegetable oil for the massage, or they can be mixed with water for an aroma mist. The table also includes a list of blends that work well for aroma inhalations. Aromatherapy and blending techniques are discussed in Chapter 5.

FIRMING FACE MASSAGE TECHNIQUES

In massage school, students are often taught to work into the muscle tissue during a face massage. This is especially appropriate if the client suffers from conditions that cause tension in the jaw or forehead. In a spa, where skin care is frequently a priority, the therapist may be directed to use lighter massage techniques. Firming face massage is a series of lifting, toning, and stimulating massage strokes that are deeply relaxing for the client. They leave the face feeling firm, tingly, and renewed. The following routine is meant to be delivered with light and gentle fingertips and is shown in Figure 3-8.

If the client comes to the massage session wearing makeup, ask if a face massage is going to be included in the session. If the answer is yes, send the client to the bathroom with a makeup remover to clean the face (unless the therapist works in a state where they can legally cleanse the client's face). Rich emollient face cream or whipped shea butter is recommended for this treatment. Massage oil, massage cream, or massage gel are not recommended because these products may leave the facial skin feeling clogged and bogged down.

Before touching the client's face, the therapist's hands should be sanitized with an alcohol-based sanitizer. This prevents any microbes that were picked up on the body or in the treatment room from being transferred to the delicate facial skin and ensures that the therapist's hands smell clean to the client. The therapist may want to drape the client's hair to protect it from face cream using the simple hair-draping method described earlier in the chapter.

Step 1: Apply an Aromatic Towel to the Face

Remove a steamy rosemary- or herbal-infused towel from a cooler and drape it on the face by spreading it from under the chin to the forehead. Allow the towel to sit on the face for up to 1 minute and than gently press it into the client's face to increase the sensation of heat. Remove the towel from the face and repeat with a second towel if desired.

Step 2: Massage the Face

Apply a rich emollient facial cream starting under the chin, coming up around the mouth, around the nose, up the nose to the forehead, and down the sides of the face to the chin. Repeat this technique six to eight times to spread the cream evenly over the surface of the skin.

- Perform gentle cross strokes between the eyebrows. Transition into s-bows, covering the whole forehead with s-bow strokes (Fig. 3-8B&C).
- Transition to glides down either side of the nose and activate the pressure points at the top of the nose and bottom of the nose as the fingers circle. Repeat this technique three to six times (Fig. 3-8D).
- Transition into small figure eights using light finger pressure. Glide over the entire face, chin, and forehead with this technique (Fig. 3-8E).
- Slide a relaxed hand over one eye in a circular motion and finish the stroke with pats at the side of the eye. Repeat this four times and transition to the other eye (Fig. 3-8F).
- Make small circles around both eyes at the same time and then transition to the chin using small finger circles.
- Lightly petrissage the jaw line and s-bow the chin. Then use a crossed thumb technique at the chin.
- Use the index finger and the thumb on both hands to apply a lifting technique around the upper and lower lips (Fig. 3-8G&H).
- Bring the thumb and index finger of one hand around the mouth in five to seven strokes to smooth the tissue at the sides of the mouth (Fig. 3-8I).
- Using soft hands and relaxed wrists, apply a gentle slapping tapotement to the underside of the jaw. Bring the gentle slapping tapotement up the jaw line and cheek area and then transition back to underneath the jaw (Fig. 3-8J1–J2).
- Transition from the slapping tapotement into a "snapping" tapotement and apply the stroke to the jaw line and cheek area on both sides of the face. To learn this stroke, make a pinching movement with the thumb and index finger but instead of meeting the fingers, lift them up off the face (Fig. 3-8K1–K2).
- Soothe the sides of the face with gentle upward strokes toward the top of the forehead (Fig. 3-8L).
- Gently massage the outer edge of the ear and push the ear forward to stretch it. Massage the area directly behind the ear and finish the area by laterally flexing the neck to one side during a long stoke down the neck, over the shoulder, and down the arm. Repeat this stroke on the opposite side (Fig. 3-8M1–M2).
- The facial sequence can be repeated up to three times for a longer face massage. To end the face massage, place 1 drop of peppermint or lemon oil in the hands and rub them together, and cover the nose lightly for 30 seconds. A second steamy aromatic towel can be placed over the face or a cool towel can be placed over the face to finish the service.

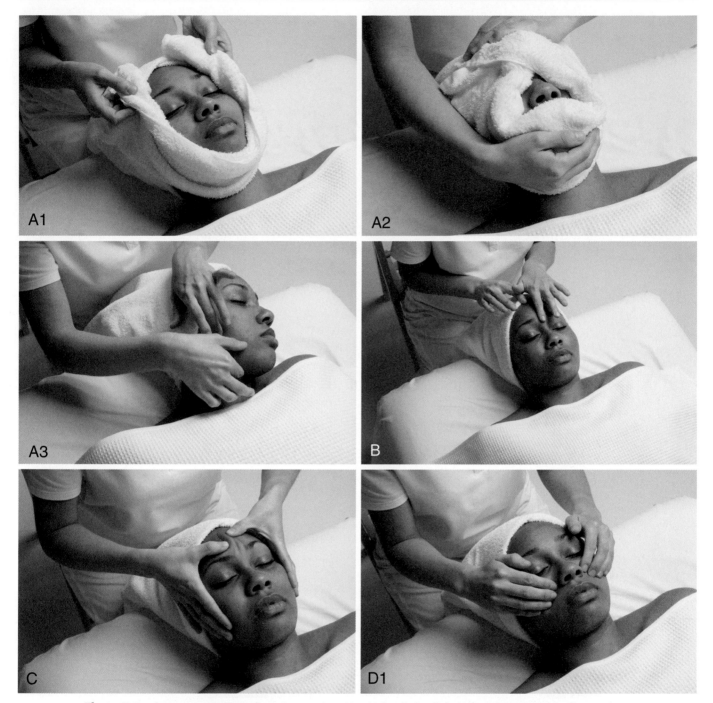

Figure 3-8 Face massage procedure. (A1 to A3) Sanitize the hands directly before touching the face and steam the face with an aromatic towel. Apply a rich face cream from below the jaw line, up over the cheeks, and to the forehead. (B) Cross strokes between the eyebrows. (C) S-bows on the forehead. (D1 and D2) Glides down the side of the nose and along the cheek bones activate pressure points. (E) Figure eights across the surface of the face. (F1 and F2) Circular hand around the eye. Transition to circular hands around both eyes. (G) Petrissage the jaw line. (H) S-bow the chin. (I) Crossed-thumb technique at the chin. (J1 and J2) "Slapping" tapotement. (K1 and K2) "Snapping" tapotement. (L) Soothing upward strokes from the jaw line to the forehead. (M1 and M2) Flex the neck. Flex the neck to one side and stroke down the arm while you stretch the neck. Repeat on the other side, and finish the session with an aroma mist or inhalation.

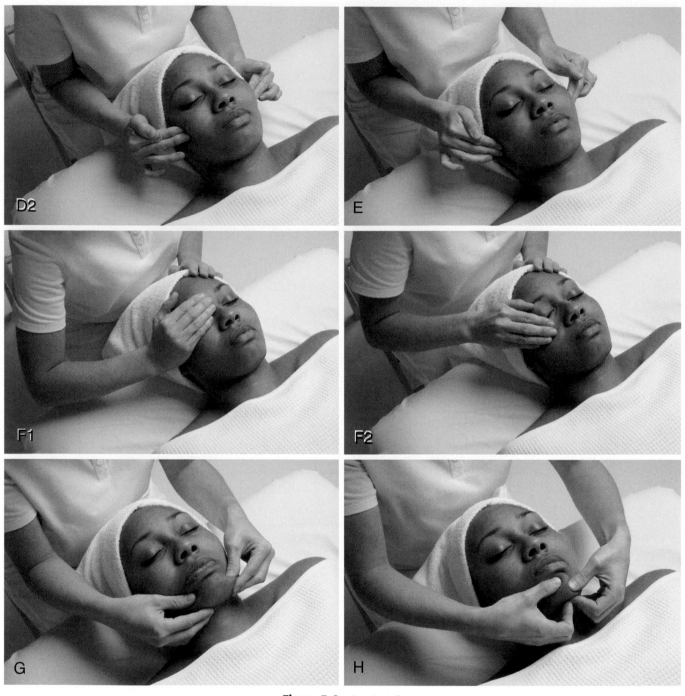

Figure 3-8 (continued)

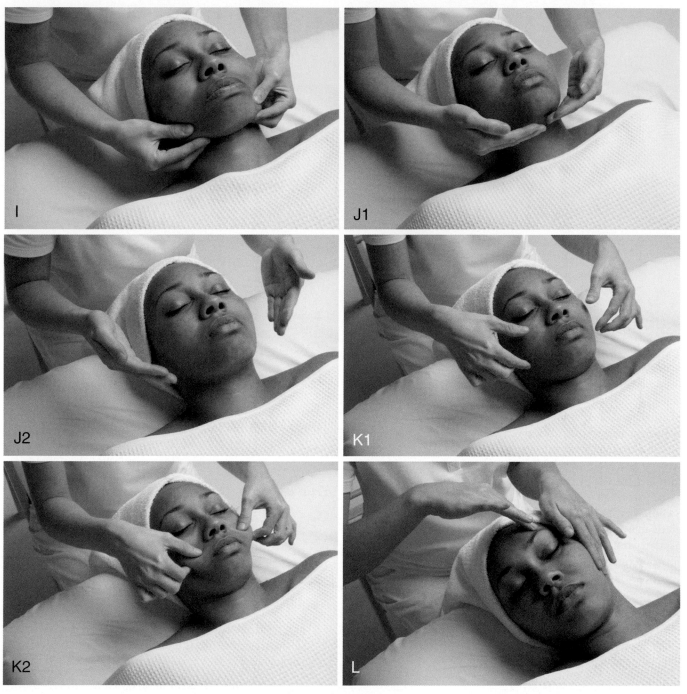

Figure 3-8   (continued)

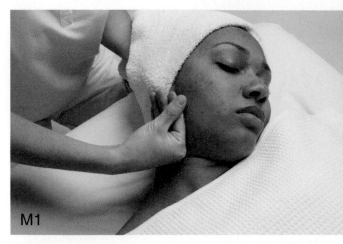
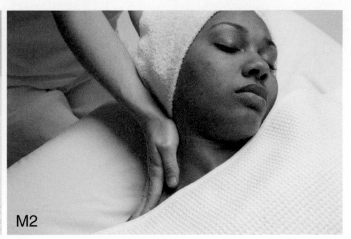

Figure 3-8 *(continued)*

Summary

Student spa therapists should practice basic spa skills in preparation for the delivery of core spa treatments. These skills include elegant spa draping, appropriate positioning of the client for product application, the use of a variety of application methods, and the smooth and efficient removal of spa products with hot moist towels. Enhancers such as steamy aromatic towels, firming face massage, and simple foot treatments provide moments of particular radiance in a spa massage. New spa therapists should perfect their Swedish relaxation massage and offer several enhancers while maintaining the flow of the massage. If a wet room is used to remove products, practice with the specialized equipment to ensure that the water temperature and pressure are safe and comfortable for the client. As soon as these skills have been mastered, new spa therapists will be able to work more creatively with treatment steps to develop unique services. Every therapist is responsible for checking the laws and regulations in their particular state to ensure that they are delivering services that are within their scope of practice.

REVIEW QUESTIONS

Matching

1. Vichy shower   _____ A. A shower with pipes (each pipe has 8 to16 water heads) in each corner of the stall

2. Swiss shower   _____ B. A handheld shower that is used with a wet table

3. Hand shower   _____ C. A regular shower that might be found in someone's home

4. Standard shower   _____ D. A shower that rains water down from above a wet table

True or False

5. _____ In a spa treatment, the body is draped just as it is for a regular massage.

6. _____ The therapist must decide how to best position the client for the treatment. Some clients are not able to sit up easily, so either the side-lying or flip-over method should be used.

7. _____ If the client is sunburned, the product is thin, or the therapist needs to keep his or her hands clean, the product is best applied using a large brush.

8. _____ The use of essential oils with hot towels is not recommended. Essential oils added to hot towels always cause skin irritation.

9. _____ The sit-up method works well in a dry room setting because the client only has to turn over once during the treatment.

10. _____ A spa product should never be massaged into the skin because its purpose is to sit on top of the skin and not to act as a lubricant for massage.

Water Therapies

Chapter Outline

Key Terms

Cryotherapy: The therapeutic application of cold temperatures.

Father Sebastian Kneipp: A Bavarian priest who streamlined Priessnitz's treatments and combined herbal treatments with water cures.

Homeostasis: The body's ability to maintain a relatively constant internal environment despite changing external conditions.

Hunting reaction: Alternating cycles of vasoconstriction and vasodilatation in response to cold.

Mechanical effect: The effect on the body of water that is pressurized in sprays, whirlpools, or through jets.

Thermotherapy: The therapeutic application of heat

Vasoconstriction: When the lumen of a blood vessel is contracted, reducing the diameter of the vessel and decreasing blood flow to a region of the body.

Vasodilatation: When the lumen of a blood vessel is relaxed, increasing the diameter of the vessel and increasing the blood flow to a region of the body.

Vincent Priessnitz: An Austrian farmer who became famous for the cold-water cure, which consisted of drinking large amounts of cold water, and applications of cold water by packing, immersions, and douches.

The use of water for health and wellness (hydrotherapy) is a historical cornerstone of the spa experience. As discussed in Chapter 1, the revitalizing effects of water were well known in ancient cultures around the world. **Vincent Priessnitz** and **Father Sebastian Kneipp** developed methods and procedures that advanced the understanding of hydrotherapy. Although spa treatments can be offered without wet room equipment such as Vichy showers and hydrotherapy tubs, it is helpful to be well versed in hydrotherapy principles. For therapists working in spas that offer hydrotherapy treatments, this understanding is essential to providing safe and effective client care.

Basic Principles of Hydrotherapy

Hydrotherapy is the use of water for healing. Traditionally, water is used in one of its three forms: solid (ice), liquid (water), and vapor (steam). It may be applied either externally (e.g., baths) or internally (e.g., drinking mineral water, douches). Except for the common practice of advising clients to increase their overall water intake after a massage, the use of water internally (e.g., enemas, douches) is out of the scope of practice for massage therapists.

The principles of hydrotherapy are not difficult to understand because they are experienced on a daily basis by anyone who takes a hot shower, rinses their face in cold water, or drinks a cup of hot herbal tea. Every winter, many people take part in a polar bear plunge. They race into freezing cold water and race out again. The excitement that is generated at such an event is partially because of the invigorating effects of cold water. A cold plunge is a classic example of a hydrotherapy treatment. The core principles of hydrotherapy are discussed below.

PRINCIPLE 1: THE GREATER THE TEMPERATURE DIFFERENCE BETWEEN THE BODY AND THE WATER, THE GREATER THE PHYSIOLOGICAL EFFECT ON THE BODY

In hydrotherapy, the environment of the body is changed by the application of water at a temperature above, close to, or below that of the body. If a person is placed in a bath at 97°F (close to natural body temperature), neither the therapist nor the client will notice much of a physiological difference (although a mild tonic effect occurs with neutral applications). If the same person is placed in a bath at 110°F, however, the physiological changes in the body will be readily apparent to both. The pulse rate increases, the skin flushes, the body temperature increases, the metabolism picks up, the blood becomes more alkaline, and the white blood cells increase in number.[1] The client may feel nervous or even agitated by the application and will probably want to get out of the hot water.

PRINCIPLE 2: THE LENGTH OF THE APPLICATION INFLUENCES THE PHYSIOLOGICAL EFFECT ON THE BODY

If a client is placed in very cold water (32° to 55°F), he or she will have two very different reactions based on the length of the treatment. If the application is brief (< 1 minute), the body will experience **vasoconstriction** to prevent heat loss, followed by **vasodilatation** shortly afterwards as the body tries to warm itself. Muscle tone is increased, and the client may describe a feeling of well being.

If the application is longer, the body experiences vasoconstriction of the capillaries and arteries as blood is held in the body's core. After about 20 to 30 minutes of continuous cold, vasodilatation occurs, which increases circulation (the **hunting reaction**). It should be noted that this increase in circulation does not increase above the baseline when the cold was first applied. The physiological processes of the body are depressed, and if the client is not removed from the cold water, death could result.

PRINCIPLE 3: THE LARGER THE BODY AREA TREATED, THE GREATER THE PHYSIOLOGICAL EFFECT ON THE BODY

Hydrotherapy applications may be used over the entire body or locally. If the body is immersed in a bath, as in the examples above, the effect will be more profound than if a cold pack is applied to one local area, such as the hamstring. If the cold application is a full-body immersion, the hunting reaction is potentially deadly because it uses heat from the body's core to delay tissue loss at the periphery.[2] If the cold is applied just to the hamstring, the hunting reaction acts as a pump to flush out metabolic wastes in the tissue and bring fresh oxygen and nutrient-rich blood to the area.

The hunting reaction involves alternating cycles of vasoconstriction and vasodilatation. When an ice pack is applied to an area, the body undergoes a series of distinct physiological responses. In the first phase, the blood vessels constrict, and blood flow to the area is reduced. This decreases local edema and causes the skin to appear pale. In the second phase, the body attempts to warm the area through vasodilatation that increases circulation. If the cold persists, vasoconstriction resumes, and the cycle repeats itself.

PRINCIPLE 4: HYDROTHERAPY APPLICATIONS HAVE REFLEXIVE AS WELL AS PHYSIOLOGICAL EFFECTS ON THE BODY

Humans are able to maintain internal physiological stability because intricate regulatory mechanisms continually monitor and adjust the body's internal environment (i.e., homeostasis).[3] The body's core temperature is relatively constant, even in the face of widely varying environmental temperatures. The body produces heat when the core is cooled and increases heat loss when the core is heated.

Table 4-1	Degrees of Hot and Cold		
NEUTRAL TO VERY COLD		**WARM TO VERY HOT**	
Neutral	90° to 98°F	Warm	98° to 100°F
Cool	70° to 90°F	Hot	100° to 104°F
Cold	56° to 70°F	Very hot	104° to 110°F
Very Cold	32° to 56°F	Too hot (do not use)	*110°F and above

*Some products such as paraffin (122°F), parafango (120° to 122°F), and therapeutic mud and peat (115°F) are applied at temperatures above 110°F. These products transfer the heat slowly to the body area, so they do not burn the client.

Physiological effects occur as a result of the body's attempt to return to a constant state. A common physiological effect of the application of heat is vasodilatation (which cools the core) and increased blood flow to the area. A common physiological effect of cold is decreased local edema and decreased pain. The edema is reduced through vasoconstriction (which warms the core), and pain is reduced by a decrease in nerve conduction velocity.[4]

Hydrotherapy applications also produce reflexive effects (sometimes referred to as a consensual response) that occur because of a nervous system reaction to the treatment. Reflexive effects happen in an area removed from the point of local application, usually between the skin and the viscera, although heat applied to one limb increases circulation in the contralateral limb. The reflex relationship between the skin and the internal organs is caused by a segmental connection. Both receive sensory innervation from the same segment of the spinal cord. For example, heat applied to the abdomen causes the activity of the intestines to decrease. A hot or cold application to the sternum affects the function of the esophagus.[1]

Different reflex and physiological effects are based on the temperature of the water applied to the body. Table 4-1 provides an overview of common water temperatures used in hydrotherapy.

Effects of Heat

The physiological responses of the body to heat are an attempt to prevent an increase in body temperature (Table 4-2). Whereas brief applications stimulate the body, applications of longer duration sedate the body. The use of external applications of heat for therapeutic purposes is sometimes referred to as **thermotherapy**.

When heat is applied to the body with a full-immersion bath, steam bath, hot pack, or partial bath (e.g., foot bath), the peripheral blood vessels dilate, and the body begins to perspire. The blood flow to the area increases significantly

Table 4-2	Effects of Hot and Cold	
HOT	**COLD**
Perspiration	Decreased local blood flow
Increased local blood flow	Decreased tissue metabolism
Tissue will flush	Decreased edema
Increased heart rate	Increased numbing
Increased pulse rate	Decreased pain
Increased metabolism	Initial increase in respiratory rate
Increased oxygen consumption in the body tissues	Initial increase in heart rate
	Initial increase in BP
Increased white blood cell count	Respiratory rate, heart rate, and BP gradually decrease
Stimulates the immune system	Increased muscle tone
Relaxes muscles	Short applications stimulate
Decreased muscle spasm	Long applications sedate
Increased range of motion	
Decreased pain	
Short applications stimulate	
Long applications sedate	

and flushes the tissue. The heart rate, pulse rate, respiratory rate, and overall rate of metabolism increase, which increases the consumption of oxygen in the tissues. The increase in core body temperature creates an artificial fever, which, in turn, stimulates the immune system and causes the body's white blood cell count to increase, inhibiting the growth of some bacteria and viruses. The higher blood flow to the area relaxes muscles, reduces muscular spasm, increases the extensibility of collagen, "melts" the superficial fascia, increases the range of motion in joints, reduces pain, and is generally relaxing.

Effects of Neutral Applications

Neutral applications are administered at or close to normal body temperature and produce a tonic and balancing effect in most individuals. They soothe the nervous system and are an effective treatment for insomnia, nervous irritability, anxiety, or depression.[5] They are sometimes used at the beginning or end of a hot or cold application to help the body ease into or out of the more intense temperatures. The use of external applications for therapeutic purposes at temperatures close to the body's normal temperature is sometimes called neutrotherapy.

Effects of Cold

The physiological responses of the body in reaction to cold are an attempt to prevent a decrease in body temperature. Similar to heat, brief applications of cold stimulate the body, and applications of longer duration sedate the body. The use of external applications of cold for therapeutic purposes is sometimes referred to as **cryotherapy**.

Cold penetrates more deeply into the tissues than heat because vasoconstriction causes a decrease in local circulation and tissue metabolism. There is also a decrease in leukocytic migration through the capillary walls, which aids in the reduction of edema and pain. Initially, there is an increase in respiratory rate, heart rate, blood pressure, and muscle tone. These gradually decrease if the application of cold is prolonged. The reduction of nerve conduction velocity leads to a numbing that significantly reduces pain. If the cold persists, vasodilatation and circulation are briefly stimulated.

Effects of Contrasting Temperatures

Contrasting applications involve applying a hot pack and then a cold pack to the same body area. This creates a *vascular flush* in which the tissues are "pumped" free of "toxic"

buildup because of the alternating vasoconstriction and vasodilatation of the peripheral blood vessels.[4] Often the treatment follows a pattern of 3 minutes of hot to 1 minute of cold for three rounds. The treatment always ends with a cold application to prevent congestion in the local tissue. Sometimes a longer rotation is used in which the ratio is 10 to 15 minutes for the hot pack followed by 10 to 15 minutes with a cold pack. Again, the treatment ends with a cold application. An alternative method is to place a cold pack on the area of injury and a hot pack proximal to the injury site close to the cold pack. This helps to relax clients and help them deal with their reaction to cold.

Mechanical Effects of Water

When water is pressurized in sprays, showers, hydrotherapy jets, or whirlpools, the force of the water on the skin's surface and on the muscle tissue below reduces muscular tension, stimulates general function, and gives vital energy to the body. This is referred to as the **mechanical effect** of water.

Hydrostatic Effects of Water

The hydrostatic effect of hydrotherapy is movement of fluid from one body area to another, reducing congestion in the tissues. A classic example is the use of a hot foot bath to decrease congestion in the sinuses caused by a cold. In folk medicine, migraines are treated with a warm foot bath and an ice pack on the back of the neck. The dilation of the blood vessels in one body area reduces the fluid congestion in another area.

Contraindications to Hydrotherapy

Some specific contraindications for hot and cold applications are listed in Table 4-3. In general, hydrotherapy is contraindicated for individuals who have serious heart, circulatory, nervous system, or systemic conditions. Open wounds and skin rashes are also contraindications when using extremes of hot or cold. Moderate temperature applications may be used in combination with specific products for the treatment of such conditions by estheticians or dermatologists.[6]

The length of time that the client is exposed to the treatment depends on the client's overall state of health and vitality. Those who are in a weakened condition or elderly should not spend more than 15 minutes in hydrotherapy tub treatments, steam rooms, and saunas. Healthy individuals can remain in such treatments for 20 to 30 minutes. Very cold applications for longer than 20 minutes are not

Table 4-3	Contraindications to Hydrotherapy

CONTRAINDICATIONS TO HOT APPLICATIONS	CONTRAINDICATIONS TO COLD APPLICATIONS
High or low BP	High or low BP
Acute injury or inflammation	Heart conditions
Heart conditions	Circulatory conditions
Circulatory conditions	Pregnancy
Pregnancy	History of CVA (stroke)
Burns, including sunburns	Diabetes
History of CVA (stroke)	Raynaud's disease
Systemic conditions (i.e., lupus)	Hypothyroidism
History of seizure	Poor kidney function
Diabetes	Hypersensitivity to cold
Varicose veins	Open wounds or skin conditions
Open wounds or skin conditions	Osteoarthritis
Phlebitis	Rheumatoid arthritis
Edema	Obesity, debility, or weakened condition
Rheumatoid arthritis	Certain cancers or cancer treatments
Obesity, debility, or weakened condition	Decreased sensory awareness
Certain cancers or cancer treatments	Mental conditions
Decreased sensory awareness	Asthma
Mental conditions	
Autoimmune conditions	

BP = blood pressure

recommended because they can cause tissue damage, frostbite, or even hypothermia. A client who is already cold will not benefit from a cold treatment.[7]

If a client feels lightheaded, nauseous, headachy, or dizzy at the end of the treatment, monitor the client while he or she relaxes in a quiet environment at a normal temperature. Offer the client cool water and chart the reaction in the file. If the symptoms increase or persist, consult a physician.

Common Methods of Application

Common methods of application include hot or cold packs, therapeutic showers and baths, friction treatments, and wet sheet wraps. In a general spa setting, hydrotherapy is most often used to relax the client, revitalize the body, and remove a product. In medical spas, certain types of wellness

centers, and many European spas, hydrotherapy applications are used for specific conditions or pathologies under the guidance of a physician.

HOT OR COLD PACKS

Pack is a general term for any local hydrotherapy treatment that uses a compress, gel pack, hydrocollator pack, fomentation pack, or commercially made chemical hot or cold pack. Some packs are electric, some are heated in the microwave, and some require specialized equipment. Probably the most effective hot pack is the hydrocollator pack (Fig. 4-1). This pack has a canvas casing that is filled with either silicon granules or clay particles that can hold heat for up to 30 minutes. The packs are submerged in water kept at 165°F in a specialized heating unit called a hydrocollator. The pack is removed from the hydrocollator (with tongs or thermal gloves) and wrapped in a minimum of four to six

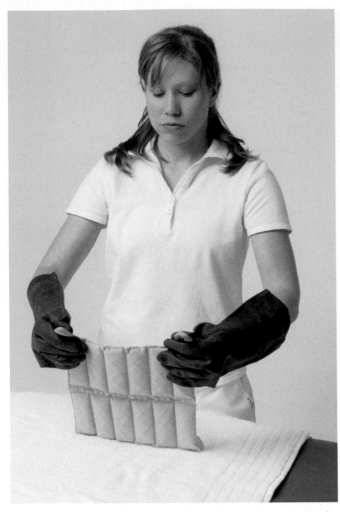

Figure 4-1   Hydrocollator packs. Hydrocollator packs are removed from the hydrocollator with tongs or gloves. They are wrapped in four to six layers of thick towels before they are placed on the area to be treated.

layers of thick towels. The bundle is placed on the area to be treated for up to 20 minutes. Hydrocollator packs are often used to relax chronic muscular conditions before the area is massaged. The pack should be monitored constantly so that it does not burn the client. Clients should never lie on top of hydrocollator packs.

Gel-filled commercial packs or homemade ice packs can be used effectively as cold packs. Cold packs are applied on top of a thin layer of insulation (as opposed to the thick layer used with a hot pack) for up to 20 minutes. In an ice massage, a Styrofoam cup is filled with water and frozen. The edges of the cup are peeled away, but the base of the cup is left intact. The base of the cup can then be used to hold onto the ice while it is applied to the affected area in a circular motion. Ice massage of an area can last for up to 20 minutes. Cold packs and ice massage are an effective treatment for acute inflammation or after a massage treatment using friction techniques. These types of treatments are most likely to be used at massage clinics specializing in injury rehabilitation massage or sports massage or by physical

therapists. Unless the spa specializes in the treatment of soft tissue injury, it is unlikely that the therapist will give an ice massage.

THERAPEUTIC BATHS

Therapeutic baths (sometimes called balneotherapy) may make use of a range of different hydrotherapy methods, including whirlpool baths, steam baths, saunas, full-immersion baths, partial baths, and sitz baths (Fig. 4-2). A sitz bath is a bath that comes up to the navel but no higher and is often used to treat reproductive or urinary disorders by naturopathic doctors. The main type of tub used in a spa setting is a hydrotherapy tub. These tubs are designed for professional use with multiple air and water jets. Essential oils (aromatherapy bath), herbs (herbal bath), seaweed, seawater or algae (thalassotherapy or algotherapy), and mud or clay (fangotherapy) are common additives that increase the therapeutic benefit of the water treatment. In a warm to hot bath, the superficial capillaries dilate, which improves product absorption through the skin. With some products, this dilation of the capillaries can also lead to an increased risk of skin irritation. When using a bath additive like those mentioned above, follow the manufacturer's suggested guidelines for products and amounts. Only products especially formulated for the tub should be used or they may damage the tub's jets and plumbing.

Sanitation

Modern hydrotherapy tubs usually come with a self-cleaning function that makes sanitizing the tub's jets easier. The therapist puts a concentrated disinfectant (formulated by the manufacturer of the tub) in a special holder and then pushes a button. At the end of the cleaning cycle, the tub is dried and fresh bath mats and towels are put out for the next client. The area outside the tub, such as the floor and hand rails, should be wiped down with a disinfectant.

Professional hydrotherapy tubs have an underwater massage hose that uses air pressure aimed at specific body areas to improve circulation and lymph flow. The therapist begins the underwater massage on the plantar surface of the foot and works in small circles up and over the top of the foot. The therapist continues up the medial leg and then returns to the foot and repeats the process, this time working up the lateral leg. The air flow is then directed from the distal area of the body toward the proximal area (heart) of the body. As the therapist works up the lateral leg, he or she asks the client to shift slightly to the side so that the gluteals and back are treated. Both sides of the lower body are treated

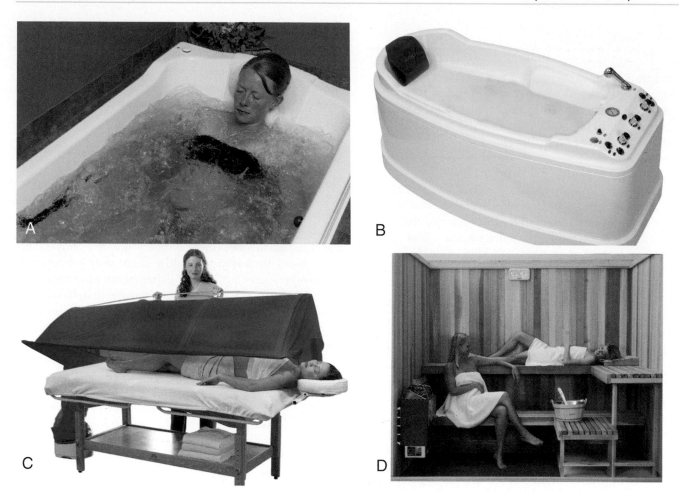

Figure 4-2   Therapeutic baths. (A) A full-body immersion could be offered in a whirlpool, professional hydrotherapy tub, or soaking tub. It may contain additives such as seaweed, fango, or herbs. **(B)** Professional hydrotherapy tub with underwater massage. **(C)** Steam baths can take place in a single-person steam cabinet, steam room, or under a steam canopy, as shown here. **(D)** A sauna.

before moving to the upper body. The client is asked to lie low enough in the water for the shoulders and neck to be treated because the hose will splash if it is not kept under the surface of the water.

Steam baths, steam showers, and steam cabinets are considered baths because the client is "bathing" in water vapor. The heat and moist air of steam facilitate perspiration and help the body to detoxify. Steam baths can be used before another treatment to warm and relax the body or before the application of a spa product. They are also used to clear the sinuses and respiratory congestion. They also help to open blocked pores, which is useful for treating chronic skin conditions.

A steam canopy fits over the top of a wet table or massage table and can be used in place of a blanket or thermal space blanket for wraps. The heat and moisture under a steam canopy helps with product absorption and keeps the client warm. Essential oils that support the respiratory system (e.g., eucalyptus, rosemary, pine, juniper, thyme, lemon, and Spanish sage) work well in a steamy environment. Floral scents such as jasmine, neroli, rose, and geranium tend to be overpowering in the confines of a steam bath. After

steaming it is important to rehydrate the skin with a moisturizer. Elderly or weakened clients should stay in a steam bath no longer than 5 to 15 minutes.

Saunas combine hot air (170° to 210°F) with low humidity to stimulate metabolism, increase core body temperature, and facilitate detoxification. It is important that the humidity in a sauna is not allowed to decrease below 10% or else the hot air will start to dry out the mucous membranes. Weakened individuals and those who have not experienced a sauna before should leave after 15 minutes. Healthy individuals can remain for up to 30 minutes. Water should be consumed throughout the sauna treatment. Similar to a steam bath, a sauna can be used to preheat the body in preparation for another treatment. Essential oil recommendations for the sauna are the same as for the steam bath. They are added to the water that is ladled onto the heat source (approximately 3 drops of essential oil to 1 gallon of water). The water is ladled on the heat source from a bucket, and only small amounts of water are used at one time. Essential oils should never be placed directly on the heat source without first being diluted in water because they are flammable and might catch on fire or "pop" if used incorrectly.

Sanitation

Small, one-person steam cabinets should be completely wiped out with a disinfectant between clients. For larger steam rooms or steam showers, the floor and seat should be disinfected between clients, but the walls can be left until the end of the day.

In traditional hydrotherapy, hot foot baths (100° to 104°F) are used to pull congestion from internal organs and the head, relieving congestive headaches and chest congestion. They are warming, promote sweating, and can be used at home to offset an oncoming cold or flu. In a traditional hot foot bath, the feet are submerged for up to 25 minutes and hot water is continuously added to maintain the temperature. To end the foot bath, cool water is poured over the feet, and the feet are dried briskly. Individuals with migraines, cluster headaches, and tension headaches respond well to hot foot baths if a cool compress is placed on the back of the neck at the same time. Hot foot baths should not be used in clients with diabetes, arteriosclerosis, frostbite, hypertension, renal disease, gastric ulcers, cancer, sciatica, neuralgia, prostate disease, rheumatoid arthritis, gouty arthritis, recent pelvic inflammatory disease, or cystitis. In most spa settings, a warm foot bath is used to preheat the body before a second treatment such as a herbal body wrap is performed. It might also be used as a pampering step while the client fills out a health history form or to provide a transition from one treatment to another in a spa package.

Cold foot baths (59° to 78°F) are traditionally used to treat inflammation of the feet and ankles, but the feet should only be immersed for very short periods of time. If the client has any vascular insufficiency, cold foot baths, even for short periods of time, are contraindicated. Relaxing foot baths are discussed in detail in Chapter 8.

Sanitation

Soaking containers without jets are simply washed with hot, soapy water; dried; sprayed with alcohol and left to air dry. If the soaking tub has jets, they must be flushed with an approved disinfectant.

THERAPEUTIC SHOWERS

Therapeutic showers are used to remove a spa product from the client, facilitate a desired physiological and reflex effect, warm the body in preparation for another treatment, or cool the body at the end of a treatment. In a spa wet room, four main types of showers are used. These are the handheld shower used in combination with a wet table, the standard shower, the Swiss shower, and the Vichy shower (Fig. 4-3). A Swiss or Vichy shower have control panels so that the temperature can be directed by the therapist. In a standard shower, clients can control the water temperature themselves, so the temperature is not exact. These specialized showers are described in Chapter 3.

Shower Temperatures

Hot showers (100° to 104°F) are stimulating and pain relieving. They may also be used to increase the core body temperature of the client in preparation for another service (e.g., herbal wrap). A hot shower begins at 100°F. As the client acclimates to the temperature, the temperature is gradually increased. A healthy client may tolerate very hot temperatures up to 110°F (temperatures should not exceed 110°F). The hottest temperature that is safe and tolerable to the individual client is held for 2 minutes and then decreased rapidly to a neutral temperature to end the shower.

A graduated shower is used to cool the body after a prolonged heating treatment such as a steam bath or sauna. The water temperature begins at 102°F and is increased quickly to the tolerance of the client. The elevated temperature is held for 2 minutes and then lowered at intervals. Each interval is held for 1 to 3 minutes. The final ending temperature is in the range of 80° to 85°F. This temperature is held for 4 minutes to finish the shower.

Cold showers (56° to 70°F) are stimulating and toning for the muscles and skin. They are often used to refresh the body after the application of a treatment that heats the body (i.e., hot sheet wrap, cellulite treatment). They are brief in duration and only used on healthy individuals who have no contraindications.

Hot and cold contrast showers stimulate metabolism, increase circulation, and revitalize the body. They are effective for fatigue, mental burnout, and low energy. Hot and cold temperatures are reversed for three sets of one interval each (timing per interval can range from 1 to 3 minutes). The treatment ends on the cold water setting.

SCOTCH HOSE

A Scotch hose directs a strong stream of water at the client to increase circulation, stimulate function, tone muscles, decrease pain, and decrease congestion in a particular body area. It is an effective treatment to use on areas that are prone to stagnation (e.g., cellulite). Clients stand at the end of the wet room holding onto handles that are attached to the wall while a therapist directs the pressurized stream in a specific sequence over the client's body (Fig. 4-4). The water begins at a warm temperature and graduates to a hot and cold contrast. The pressure of the hose can also be controlled. Avoid the breast and face and use long, smooth movements from the feet to the shoulders.

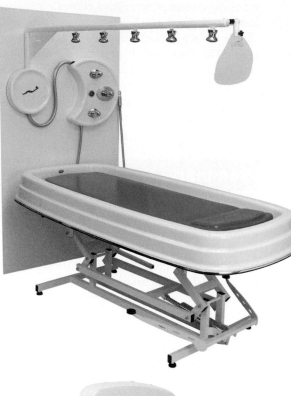

A

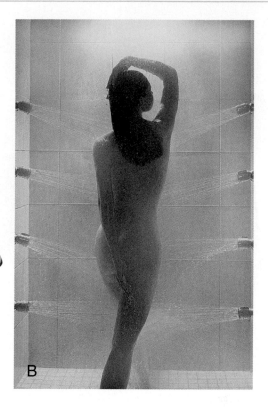

B

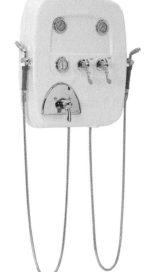

C

Figure 4-3   Therapeutic showers. (A) The Vichy shower. **(B)** The Swiss shower. **(C)** The Scotch hose. (Part B photo by Rick Raphael; Courtesy of the Avanyu Spa at the Equinox Resort and Spa, Mancheser, VT.)

FRICTION TREATMENTS

In classical hydrotherapy, the type of friction treatment that a client received was carefully considered. Friction treatments were either soft and dry (delivered with powder) or brisk and invigorating (perhaps delivered with wet salt, vinegar, or rubbing alcohol). The temperature of the treatment and the client were constantly monitored to achieve the desired therapeutic effect. Often the client was in a severely weakened condition, so the friction treatment had to be exact in its delivery to ensure the client's safety.[5] Cold mitt friction is a treatment that is still widely used to prevent colds,

boost immunity, increase circulation, increase endurance, and invigorate the body. The client is placed on a treatment table and draped with a sheet and a blanket. Terry mitts are worn on the therapist's hands and dipped into icy water. The mitts are rubbed vigorously over a body area in a back-and-forth motion, and then the area is dried with towels. The therapist redrapes the area and moves onto the next area. Depending on the client's health and the goal of the treatment, one body area or many areas can be treated in a session. If the client is shivering and cold, the treatment should end. A rule of hydrotherapy passed down from Kneipp is that a cold client should never receive a cold treatment.

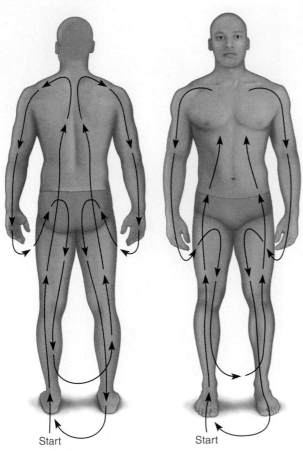

Figure 4-4 Direction of Scotch hose treatment.

Today, friction treatments can take many different forms and either target the skin or act on circulation, lymph flow, and muscle tone. As with the classical form of friction treatment, modern friction treatments can be used to invigorate and revitalize or to soothe and relax. Soft, natural bristle brushes; loofahs; rough-textured cloths; or grainy products may be used on either dry or wet skin. Whereas friction services for beautifying the skin are usually delivered by an esthetician, friction treatments meant to tone muscle, increase circulation, and increase lymph flow while promoting detoxification are provided by massage therapists. Common friction treatments such as body polishes, loofah scrubs, dry skin brushing, and salt and sugar glows are the topic of Chapter 6.

WET SHEETS

Kneipp used the cold, wet sheet treatment as a means of strengthening the patient's body in a number of different conditions. In this early form of a body wrap, the client either lies on a cold, wet sheet or is covered with a cold, wet sheet and then wrapped in blankets for up to 1 hour.[4] The patient experiences a vascular flush effect that increases the core body temperature and stimulates the body to cool itself through perspiration. Kneipp used cold, wet sheets for

menstrual cramps, digestive complaints, fever, weakness, lower back pain, and for general complaints. Modern spas offer a variety of body wraps to treat a wide range of conditions. The cold, wet sheet wrap is probably not the most popular offering at these spas. The herbal hot sheet wrap, also used by Kneipp, is widely offered, as are wraps that target skin health, detoxification, and body slimming. Chapter 7 discusses many different body wrap treatments in depth.

Summary

Hydrotherapy is the use of water for healing. Its use was formalized in modern times by Vincent Priessnitz and Father Sebastian Kneipp. Hydrotherapy is traditionally applied externally (i.e., baths, packs) or internally (i.e., enemas, douches), although internal application is outside the scope of practice of massage therapists. Water is used in one of its three forms for external applications: liquid (water), solid (ice), or vapor (steam).

The effect of a hydrotherapy application is based on the temperature of the application, the length of the application, the amount of body area that is treated, and the overall condition of the client. Hydrotherapy affects the body physiologically and reflexively. Physiological effects are produced as the body tries to maintain a stable internal state (**homeostasis**) when a hot or cold application is applied. Reflexive effects are produced because of a nervous system response to the application. Areas that share sensory innervation from the same segment of the spinal cord are connected reflexively. For example, heat applied to the abdomen causes the activity of the intestines to decrease.

Thermotherapy (heat), neutrotherapy (temperatures close to that of the body), and cryotherapy (cold) applications come in the form of packs, baths, showers, frictions, and sheet wraps. These treatments may be contraindicated in clients with serious heart, circulatory, nervous system, or systemic conditions; those with open wounds or skin rashes; and those who are in a weakened condition. Symptoms of nausea, headache, and dizziness are signs that the treatment should stop and its appropriateness for the client should be reevaluated. Even in healthy clients, rest time after a treatment should equal the amount of time used during the treatment.

REFERENCES

1. Moor FB: *Manual of Hydrotherapy and Massage.* Boise, ID: Pacific Press Publishing Association, 1964.
2. Bjerke HS, Tevar A: *Frostbite.* Available at http://www.emedicine.com/med/topic2815.htm
3. Premkumar K: *The Massage Connection, Anatomy and Physiology,* 2nd Ed. Baltimore, MD: Lippincott Williams & Wilkins, 2004.
4. Fahey T, Romero J: *Thermal modalities.* Available at http://www.sportscience.org/encyc/drafts/thermal-modalities.doc

5. Kellogg JH: *Rational Hydrotherapy*, Vol. 2, 2nd Ed. Philadelphia, F.A. Davis Company, 1903.
6. Miller ET: *Salon Ovations: Day Spa Techniques*. Albany, New York: Milady Publishing, 1996.
7. Kneipp S: *My Water-Cure*, 3rd Ed. (English). Kempten, Bavaria: Jos. Koesel Publishers, 1894.

REVIEW QUESTIONS

Multiple Choice

1. Hydrotherapy is best defined as:
   a. The use of wet sheet wraps for healing
   b. The use of hot temperatures for healing
   c. The use of hydrocollator packs for healing
   d. The use of water for healing

2. Hydrotherapy is traditionally used in three forms. These are:
   a. Solid, liquid, vapor
   b. Vapor, syrup, herbal concoction
   c. Ice, herbal rub, liquid
   d. Steam bath, friction rub, ice

3. The polar bear plunge is a form of hydrotherapy. It is best described by the word:
   a. Thermotherapy
   b. Cryotherapy
   c. Neutrotherapy
   d. Aromatherapy

4. The hunting reaction could best be described as:
   a. Never-ending vasoconstriction
   b. Never-ending vasodilatation
   c. Vasoconstriction of the heart with prolonged applications of cold
   d. Alternating cycles of vasoconstriction and vasodilatation with prolonged applications of cold

5. There are two types of effects that occur with hydrotherapy applications. These are:
   a. Cold and hot effects
   b. Tonic and nontonic effects
   c. Physiological and reflexive effects
   d. Reflexive and psychosomatic effects

Fill in the Blank

6. The greater the _____ differences between the body and the water, the greater the physiological effect on the body.

7. The _____ of the application influences the physiological effect on the body.

8. The _____ the body area treated the greater the physiological effect on the body.

9. A _____ effect occurs because of a nervous system response to the treatment.

10. Physiological effects occur with hydrotherapy applications because the body is trying to maintain _____.

Introduction to Aromatherapy for Spa

Chapter Outline

Key Terms

Aromatherapy: The use of essential oils for healing.

Essential oils: Volatile plant oils extracted from certain aromatic plants that have both physiological and psychological effects on the human body.

Fixed oils: Vegetable oils that are nonvolatile such as sweet almond or sunflower. Essential oils readily dissolve into fixed oils, so fixed oils are often used as carriers for essential oils.

Functional group: A reactive oxygen or nitrogen-containing unit of a chemical compound (in an essential oil).

Learned-odor response: A response that occurs when an odor is paired with a person, place, or thing and a memory link is formed.

Limbic system: The oldest part of the brain where olfactory signals activate smell-related responses.

Olfactory response: Olfaction is the sense of smell. An olfactory response includes the mental, emotional, or spiritual changes that may be elicited by an aroma.

Oxidation: A reaction that occurs when the chemicals in essential oils interact with the oxygen that is present in the air. This results in degradation of the oil.

Quenching: Process that occurs when the action of one compound in an essential oil is suppressed by another compound, thereby making the oil safer for use.

Synergy: When the whole is greater than the sum of its parts and those parts are mutually enhancing.

Volatility: The rate at which a compound turns from a liquid to a gas at room temperature (i.e., when it evaporates).

Aromatherapy is both a complex area of study and a simple enhancing technique that can be added to any spa service. The goal of this chapter is to provide an overview of the topic and some guidance on safe and effective ways to use **essential oils** in a spa for those without extensive training. The National Association of Holistic Aromatherapy (NAHA) suggests a formal course of study of no less than 230 hours for professional therapists.[1] A number of comprehensive programs are described in the resources section at the back of the book. Also at the back of the book is a chart listing common names of essential oils with their botanical names to help therapists order the correct oil indicated in the text. In certain instances, the Latin names are given in the text to provide clarity. This is to prevent confusion because sometimes the common name refers to more than one botanical species or very similar common names are used for different species. For example, the common name *sage* can cause problems. Common sage (*Salvia officinalis*) is used differently than clary sage (*Salvia sclarea*) and Spanish sage (*Salvia lavendulifolia*). Common sage contains up to 42% thujone, a potentially dangerous ketone that is contraindicated for elderly individuals, pregnant women, people who are in a weakened condition, and children. Although common sage is not dangerous when applied topically in low concentrations to healthy individuals, it does contain methyl chavicol, which can cause skin irritation. Clary sage contains 75% esters, which support relaxation and stress reduction and is safe for liberal use. Spanish sage contains camphor and cineol, making it the best of the three oils for respiratory support.

It is important to note that essential oils are not meant to take the place of professional medical treatments and should be used by massage therapists to provide general support for their clients. Although blends can be created that directly address the symptoms of many conditions, therapists must always be careful not to make false claims or go beyond their scope of practice.

Aromatherapy: An Art and Science

Looking at the many definitions of aromatherapy offered by different authors, one that comes very close to describing the reality of practice is that of Jade Shutes, president of NAHA (2000-2004). She defines aromatherapy as follows: "Aromatherapy is the *art* and *science* of healing *body*, *mind*, and *spirit* through essential oils."

Each client is unique, so an aromatherapist must reflect on and synthesize numerous pieces of information when determining the best form of essential oil support for a client. This requires intuition, creativity, and the ability to process information abstractly and then "mold" it into a support plan. In other words, the practice of aromatherapy is an *art*.

Aromatherapy is also a *science*. Essential oils are composed of complex mixtures of chemical compounds, and

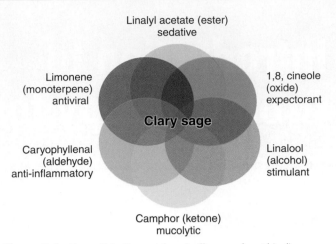

Figure 5-1 Essential oils are chemically complex. This diagram represents some of the chemical components that are found in clary sage and their general properties.

skilled aromatherapists select oils for a treatment based on their known biological effects (Fig. 5-1). Understanding the effects of different oils on the human body requires rigorous study and careful observation over time. Experienced practitioners know that some compounds can have negative effects on the human body under particular conditions. Understanding how to select and blend different oils is both an art and a science.

Lastly, aromatherapy not only affects the body but also the *mind* and the *spirit*. The psychological effect of essential oils on the mind and spirit are based on the often powerful emotions and memories elicited by aromas.

Essential oils are regularly used for their relaxing effects and to ensure that the treatment area is clean and healthy. It is important to point out that different types of health care providers may use essential oils in quite different ways. Medical doctors in France can legally prescribe essential oils to be taken internally for a specific pharmacological effect.[2] This type of use is not often seen in a spa setting. More often, the oils are used by massage therapists, counselors, life coaches, and estheticians. Massage therapists focus on topical applications of essential oils for stress reduction, injury rehabilitation, detoxification, and to help reduce chronic symptoms associated with an underlying soft tissue pathology. Psychologists, counselors, and life coaches focus on inhalations of essential oils to reduce anxiety, facilitate emotional clearing, dissipate defensive relating, improve moods, or associate a scent with a positive experience for use as a resource in later sessions. Finally, estheticians often use professional skin care lines (e.g., Aveda, Decelor) that incorporate essential oils as active ingredients to increase the therapeutic benefits of skin care applications.

Aromatherapy can be viewed as the primary treatment (e.g., aromatherapy massage, aromatherapy wrap) or as accent notes in treatments with a different focus (e.g., aroma mists, cellulite cream, aromatic foot soak). All of these uses enhance the spa experience. Figure 5-2 lists six easy ways that aromatherapy can be added to any treatment, and Figure 5-3

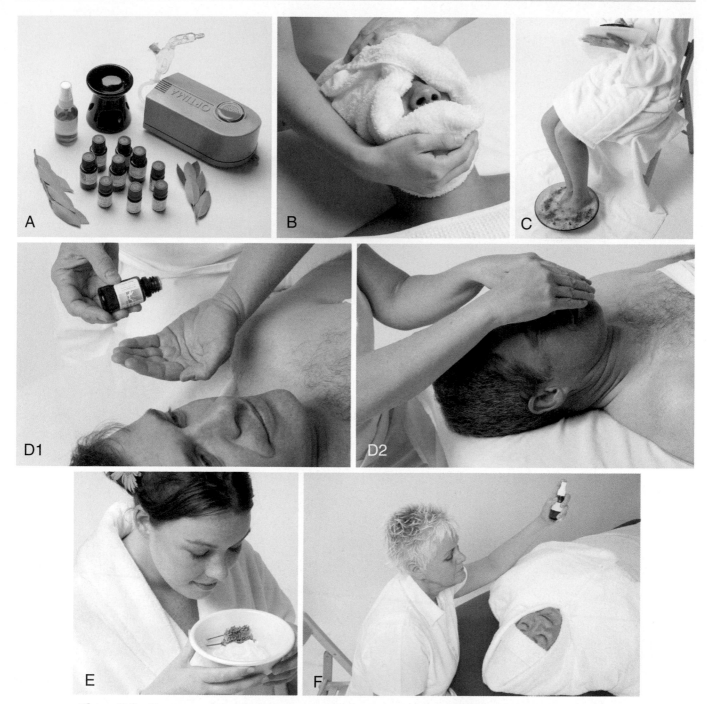

Figure 5-2   Six easy ways to add aromatherapy to any treatment. (A) Diffuse oils in the treatment room. When a client enters a clean and fragrant treatment room, his or her perception of the business and the treatment is enhanced. Use light scents such as lemon, mandarin, or lavender and avoid heavy fragrances such as ylang ylang or jasmine that some clients might dislike. **(B)** Steamy aromatic towels. Scent hot moist towels with essential oils. These towels can be used for product removal or as an accent before a step in the treatment (e.g., steamy rosemary towel before the face massage). **(C)** Fragrant foot soaks. While the client fills in the health history form, it is nice to offer an aromatherapy foot bath. Foot soaks are warming and relaxing. **(D1** and **D2)** Aromatherapy inhalations. At the beginning of the treatment, place 1 drop of essential oils between your hands. Rub the hands together and then hold them in an arc over the client's nose while the client takes a deep breath. **(E)** Smell-scapes. Smell-scapes are aroma landscapes that are created to fit the theme of the treatment. Essential oils are carefully chosen and added to base product to treat the client to a unique olfactory experience. **(F)** Aroma mists. At any time during a treatment, an aroma mist can be spritzed over the client to refresh the body and fill the treatment room with a revitalizing fragrance.

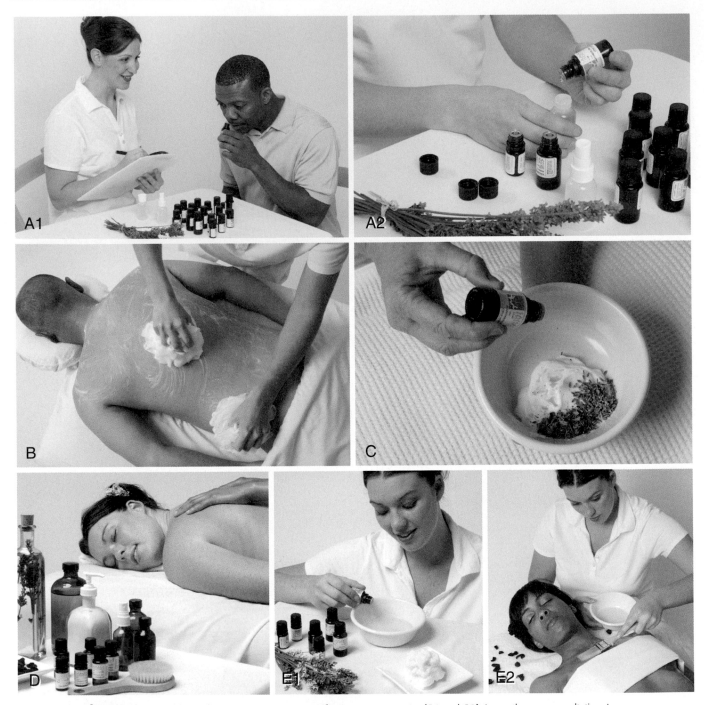

Figure 5-3   Overview of some common aromatherapy treatments. (A1 and **A2)** Aromatherapy consultation. In a consultation, a blend of oils is created especially for a client. The blend can then be applied in numerous ways such as in a bath or through massage. **(B)** Aromatherapy body shampoo. Essential oils are added to a foaming cleanser for a revitalizing body shampoo. **(C)** Aromatherapy body polish. Essential oils may be added to a variety of granulated exfoliation products for a fragrant body polish. **(D)** Aromatherapy massage. Essential oils are well known to balance the central nervous system and relax the body. A popular way to use essential oils is in a massage. **(E1** and **E2)** Aromatherapy body wrap. Essential oils can be used in numerous types of body wraps. For example, essential oils might be added to melted shea butter and brushed on the body before it is wrapped.

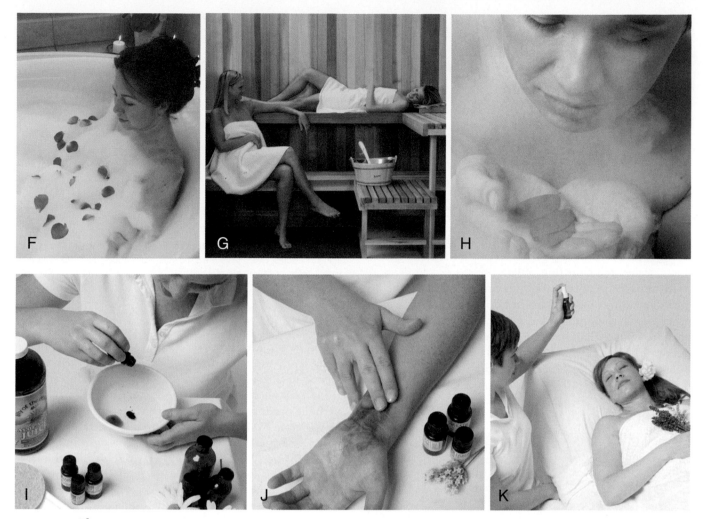

Figure 5-3 *(continued)* **(F)** Aromatherapy baths. Essential oils can be added to hydrotherapy tubs or standard soaking tubs for therapeutic baths. The oils are usually mixed first into an emulsifier or carrier product to prevent skin irritation or "pooling" of the oils. **(G)** Aromatic saunas. Essential oils are added to the water that is used on the sauna's heat source. Respiratory support oils such as pine and eucalyptus are usually preferred. **(H)** Aromatic steams. Essential oils can be used in steam rooms, steam cabinets, or under a steam canopy. **(I)** Sunburn relief. Anti-inflammatory and skin-soothing essential oils are added to aloe and brushed on the skin to heal the tissue after it has been burned by the sun. **(J)** Spot application. Certain essential oils such as German chamomile can be used at full strength for specific conditions such as carpal tunnel syndrome. Oils from grapefruit, juniper berry, or thyme might be used as an application for cellulite. **(K)** Guided meditation with aromas. Essential oils can be used during a guided meditation session or hypnotherapy session for the psychological effects.

provides an overview of aromatherapy treatments that are common in spas. As Susan Irvine writes in The Mystery of Perfume, "Scent passes under doors, seeps through walls, crosses boundaries. It is the un-containable, the symbol of being between one State and another."[3]

Essential Oils

Essential oils are complex mixtures of chemical compounds that are found in aromatic plants. The compounds contained in essential oils are mostly terpenes, a class of chemical compound that is quite toxic to living plant tissues and so must be stored in specialized structures such as glands, ducts, scales, and hairs (Fig. 5-4).

Most essential oil compounds are volatile to some degree, depending on how many carbon atoms they have or, in other words, their molecular size. Small molecules tend to be more volatile than larger molecules. The term **volatility** refers to the rate at which compounds turn from a liquid to a gas at room temperature and evaporate.

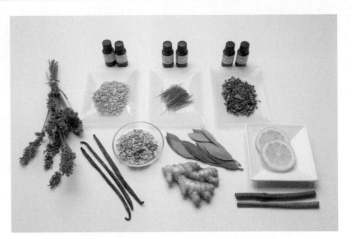

Figure 5-5   Essential oil storage sites. Essential oils are stored in leaves, needles, twigs, resin tears, flowers, fruits, roots, bark, wood, heartwood, zests, or the whole plant.

The specialized structures storing essential oils can be found in the leaves or needles, twig, bark, flowers, flower buds, fruits, stems, roots, or sometimes, as in the conifers, all organs of the plant (Fig. 5-5). They are usually extracted from fresh plant material using steam distillation, CO_2 hyperbolic production, solvent extraction, or physical expression (Table 5-1). On average, most essential oil species contain about 1% to 2% of their fresh weight in essential oils. In some species of *Eucalyptus*, up to 10% of the fresh weight of the leaves consists of essential oil (100 pounds of *Eucalyptus* leaves may yield up to 1 lb of oil). In rose and jasmine, the essential oil is nearly all found in the petals, so the yields are very low. For example, 60,000 whole rose flowers produce about 1 fluid oz (or 30 ml) of oil, a yield of about 0.05% of the fresh weight on average. It is no surprise, then, that whereas rose and jasmine are quite expensive, *Eucalyptus* is inexpensive and readily available.

Many factors affect the chemical composition and, therefore, the therapeutic value of an essential oil. The chemical composition can vary greatly depending on climate, soil conditions, air quality, and the variety or cultivar of the plant being grown; the cultivation, harvesting, and extraction methods being used; the storage and transportation conditions; and the age of the oil. No chemical compound is likely to be present in any essential oil in exactly the same proportion from one year to the next. The acceptable range in the percentage of the main chemical constituents present in most commercial essential oils has been defined by the International Standards Organization (ISO). The purpose of the ISO standards is to describe the normal range of variability in the oil so that users can compare samples with an agreed standard. Essential oils are costly to produce, so they are often adulterated to increase the profit margin of the grower or supplier.

Professional aromatherapists notice that the human body responds differently to natural oils than to synthetic oils. This is probably because of the relative chemical

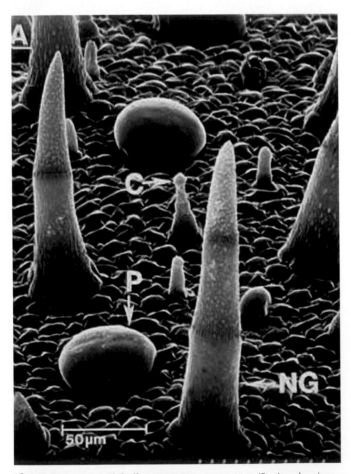

Figure 5-4   Essential oil storage structures. Magnification showing essential oils storage in a trichome (hair) of basil (*Ocimum bascilicum*).

Table 5-1	Methods of Extraction of Aromatic Materials	
METHOD	**DESCRIPTION**	**COMMENTS**
Expression ("essence" or essential oils)	Citrus fruit peels are subjected to lateral compression (squeezing) or machine abrasion (puncturing or grating) to extract the "essence" or essential oil from the rind.	This method of extraction is used to obtain essential oils from citrus fruits. Because no heat is used in the process, the composition of the expressed oil is very similar to that of the oil in the plant, and the smell is not affected by high temperatures.
Steam distillation (essential oils and hydrosols)	Steam is used to rupture the storage sites of volatile essential oils. The oils vaporize in the steam and are passed through a condenser, which cools the vapor so that it becomes a liquid. The water (from the steam) and the essential oils that have been condensed are separated. Some oils, such as rose oil, are slightly soluble in water, so the infused water, known as a flower water or hydrosol, is also sold as a valuable product.	Different plant species may require slightly different distillation conditions. Sometimes the plant is placed in the still directly after harvesting, sometimes it is left to dry, sometimes it is placed on a grate above the water, or sometimes it is mixed with the water. A variety of methods are used.
Solvent extraction (concrete, resinoid, and absolute)	Aromatic plant material is extracted by means of a hydrocarbon solvent. Solvent extraction yields either a concrete or a resinoid, which is further processed with pure alcohol to produce an absolute.	Solvent extraction is used with aromatic plants whose delicate fragrances would be damaged by the heat used in steam distillation. This includes jasmine, narcissus, and violet. Some plants are offered as either an absolute or an essential oil. Absolutes smell closer to the original plant than essential oils.
CO_2 hyperbolic production (CO_2 oils)	Under high pressure, hypercritical (in a state between a liquid, vapor, and gas) carbon dioxide is used as a solvent to extract essential oils.	This is considered by many as an ideal form of extraction because it happens at low temperature with no chemical reactions between the solvent and aromatic substances.[7]

simplicity of synthetic oils compared with natural oils. A pure, natural oil is so chemically complex that it is not economically viable to synthesize in a laboratory all of the compounds present. Instead, only the most important aroma compounds are synthesized. Even the best synthetic oils used in perfumery seldom have more than about 30 chemical compounds compared with 100 to 400 or more present in a natural oil. Although little is known about how the chemical constituents interact with each other and thereby affect the body, it is likely that both the trace compounds as well as major constituents play a role in the overall therapeutic action of the oil. Also, any quenching effects of particular compounds may be compromised if the oil has been synthesized or adulterated with synthetic compounds. Quenching effects occur when the action of one compound (usually negative) in an essential oil is suppressed by the presence of another compound, making the

oil safer to use. For example, citral in a pure and isolated form is a strong skin irritant, but when it is combined with the other compounds in lemon oil, it is rarely irritating. (Lemon oil contains approximately 5% citral and 95% other terpenes.) The other terpenes present (particularly *d*-limonene and α-pinene) have a *quenching* effect on citral, and so any side effects caused by the presence of citral are minimized. Synthetic oils often cause nausea, headaches, skin sensitivities, and emotional irritation. These symptoms are rarely, if ever, seen when pure oils are used.

Lastly, some companies specialize in supplying therapeutic-grade essential oils for the aromatherapy market, and some small suppliers import oils based on close relationships developed with producers. The oils sold through such companies are more expensive but are much more attractive to professional aromatherapists. Even with the best of intentions, it should be noted that adulterated oils can sometimes be sold unknowingly by the most knowledgeable and reputable suppliers. A number of reputable suppliers who carry high-quality, therapeutic-grade essential oils can be found in the resources section at the back of the book.

When oils are exposed to light, heat, and oxygen, their chemical compositions are altered (oxidation), and their therapeutic properties may change. To slow the rate of **oxidation**, oils should be kept in dark bottles with as little air at the top of the bottle as possible. They should be stored in a refrigerator and replaced if they have not been used within 1 year. Citrus oils oxidize more rapidly than other oils, so they should be replaced every 6 months.

SAFETY CONSIDERATIONS

When therapeutic-grade essential oils are used at low concentration (1% to 3% or 6 to 18 drops to every fluid ounce [1 oz = 30 mL] of carrier) and applied externally, negative reactions are minimal. It is important for therapists to understand the potential undesirable effects that may occur if the oils are used inappropriately or without understanding. It should be emphasized that before using any oil, the aromatherapist should identify any possible contraindications for use of the oil by checking safety data sheets or reliable textbooks.

It is out of a massage therapist's scope of practice to recommend the internal use of essential oils unless he or she is also a doctor because all essential oils are potentially toxic when taken internally, especially when taken in doses that are larger than those used therapeutically by doctors. For this reason, oils must be kept out of the reach of children and not used internally. Some oils contain chemical components that may cause liver or kidney irritation when used for prolonged periods of time (even when they are applied topically). The general rule of thumb is that an oil should not be used continuously for longer than 2 weeks to prevent sensitization of the kidneys, liver, or skin.

It is believed that most essential oil compounds are able to pass through the placenta to the developing fetus. It is also possible that certain essential oils may disrupt the delicate hormonal balance of the body and cause unwanted effects during pregnancy. With the exception of mandarin and lavender (used at 1% concentrations = 6 drops per fl oz of carrier), those without formal training in aromatherapy should avoid the use of essential oils with pregnant clients.

The most likely undesirable effect that a spa therapist will see when using essential oils is skin irritation or phototoxicity. Skin irritation is rare if the therapist is using standard concentrations of 1% to 3% of therapeutic-grade oils (irritation is more likely with synthetic oils). When large amounts of certain oils are used topically or when oils are used with heat (e.g., stone massage, hot packs, hot sheet wraps), irritation is more likely to occur.

The term *phototoxicity* refers to an increased sensitivity to the sun. Oils containing compounds called coumarins and furocoumarins increase the skin's tendency to burn. Clients should avoid suntanning and tanning booths for 24 hours after the application of these oils. Figure 5-6 lists some general best practices for the safe use of essential oils. Table 5-2 lists oils that should be avoided or used with caution.

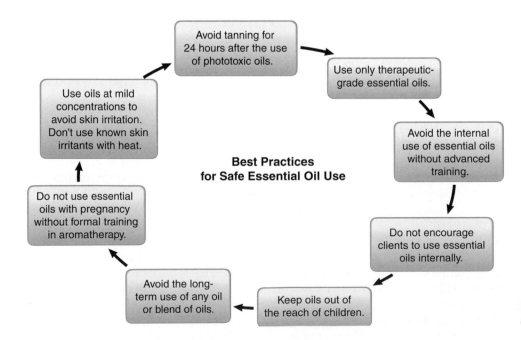

Figure 5-6 **Best practices for safe essential oil use.**

Table 5-2	Essential Oils to Avoid or Use with Caution

ESSENTIAL OILS TO COMPLETELY AVOID
Bitter almond, boldo leaf, buchu, yellow camphor, brown camphor, sassafras, calamus, horseradish, mugwort, mustard, pennyroyal, rue, savin, savory, tansy, thuja, wormseed, wormwood

ESSENTIAL OILS TO AVOID WITH PREGNANCY
Aniseed, basil, birch, wintergreen, cedarwood, clary sage, cypress, geranium, sweet fennel, jasmine, juniper berry, sweet marjoram, myrrh, peppermint, rosemary, common sage, thyme, hyssop

ESSENTIAL OILS THAT ARE SKIN IRRITANTS
Ajowan, cinnamon bark, cinnamon leaf, sweet fennel, cassia, clove leaf, clove bud, costus, oregano, basil, fir needle, lemongrass, lemon verbena, Melissa, peppermint, thyme

ESSENTIAL OILS TO AVOID WITH CLIENTS WHO HAVE HIGH BLOOD PRESSURE
Pine, hyssop, rosemary, common sage, thyme

ESSENTIAL OILS TO AVOID WITH CLIENTS WHO ARE TAKING HOMEOPATHIC REMEDIES
Rosemary, eucalyptus, peppermint

ESSENTIAL OILS TO AVOID WITH CLIENTS WHO HAVE EPILEPSY OR A HISTORY OF SEIZURES
Sweet fennel, bitter fennel, common sage, hyssop, basil

ESSENTIAL OILS TO AVOID WITH A HISTORY OF ESTROGEN-DEPENDENT CANCER
Aniseed, basil, birch, wintergreen, cedarwood, clary sage, cypress, geranium, sweet fennel, jasmine, juniper berry, sweet marjoram, myrrh, peppermint, rosemary, common sage, thyme, hyssop

ESSENTIAL OILS THAT ARE PHOTOTOXIC
Bergamot, lime, bitter orange, lemon, grapefruit, sweet orange, mandarin, ginger, angelica root

PATHWAYS INTO AND OUT OF THE BODY

Essential oils enter the body by absorption through the skin, inhalation, and ingestion. They are eliminated through the kidneys, through perspiration, and through exhalation.

Absorption Through the Skin

Compounds in essential oils that are absorbed through the skin enter the capillary network of the bloodstream. Although many aromatherapists take skin absorption for granted, the research supporting this is not clear. A number of studies indicate that essential oils promote penetration of other substances through the skin.[4] Some show that although certain compounds in essential oils pass through the skin, others do not.[5]

Absorption of essential oil compounds is affected by both the viscosity of the carrier product (thicker products slow the rate of absorption) and by the thickness of the adipose layer in the skin, which varies from individual to individual (the thicker the adipose layer, the slower the rate of absorption is likely to be). The most permeable areas of the body are the armpits, forehead, scalp, hands, feet, and inguinal areas.

Inhalation

When an essential oil is inhaled, the scent triggers an **olfactory response**, which is discussed in the section on the psychology of oils.

Inhaled essential oil molecules travel down the respiratory tract to the lungs, where they are either absorbed by the mucous membrane lining of the respiratory tract or are transferred to the blood circulating in the lungs at the point of gaseous exchange between air and blood in the alveoli and respiratory bronchioles. In the nose, where the endothelium is thin, it is assumed that essential oil molecules reach local circulation in the brain fairly quickly and easily.[6]

Ingestion

Ingestion of essential oils is a form of treatment that is mainly used by medical doctors in Europe. When an oil is ingested, it is taken internally by placing 1 to 3 drops in water, on a sugar cube, or in honey. Ingestion is not commonly used by anyone other than doctors because all of the essential oil is rapidly absorbed by the body, making this a potentially toxic and dangerous practice.

Physiological and Psychological Effects of Essential Oils

Aromatherapy has significant therapeutic potential because each essential oil has a unique combination of chemical compounds that interact with the body's chemistry and thereby affect specific organs, systems, or the body as a whole (physiological effects). The inhalation of essential oils also triggers an olfactory response that can lead to powerful mental and emotional behavioral changes (i.e., psychological effects).[7] Holistic aromatherapy is concerned with both the symptoms of a condition and its underlying causes. Its aim is to address the body, mind, and spirit for mental, emotional, and physical wellness.

PHYSIOLOGICAL EFFECTS

Each essential oil has a set of potential therapeutic properties based on its chemical composition (Fig. 5-7). Sometimes the properties of the individual compounds present may seem to oppose each other. This is the case with lavender, which contains esters (generally sedative), and alcohols (generally stimulating). In fact this "checks and balances" system of chemicals with opposing physiological effects allows essential oils to act in a balanced manner without side effects.[6]

Therapists use oils with specific properties (actions) to improve the functioning of a particular body system and, therefore, support health. For example, if the treatment aims to decrease muscular tension and increase relaxation, oils that are antispasmodic, pain relieving, warming, and sedative will probably be chosen. Essential oils are often used in a spa setting to treat the symptoms of mild lymphatic stasis. These treatments can be focused on a cosmetic goal such as the reduction of cellulite, or they can aim to boost immunity, facilitate detoxification, and support general wellness. Lymph flow is hindered by a sedentary lifestyle or whenever a person sits or stands in one place for a long period. When lymph flow is slow, excess fluid may accumulate in the tissues and gradually overwhelm the lymph nodes and liver. This metabolic buildup may lead to infection and disease.

Citrus oils (e.g., lemon, grapefruit, sweet orange) and warming oils (e.g., clove, black pepper, ginger) are good choices for lymph stimulation. Diuretics applied topically (e.g., sweet fennel, grapefruit, juniper berry) support elimination through the kidneys and increase the flow of urine. This accelerated elimination helps to detoxify the body and reduce water retention. All of the oils mentioned here could be used in various ways to support detoxification treatments such as slimming wraps or herbal wraps. The oils might be applied to the body before a warming soak, or they might be applied in a massage at the end of the wrap. A blend of three to four of these oils might be massaged into target areas to further stimulate circulation and lymph flow.

A key benefit of using essential oils regularly is that they kill many strains of pathogenic microorganisms. They either destroy the pathogen or disrupt its life cycle so that it cannot reproduce. Oils that kill pathogenic organisms are known as antiseptic, antibacterial, antifungal, and antiviral agents. Certain essential oils also stimulate the production and activity of white blood cells, which boosts immunity. This cytophylactic activity was noted by Gattefossé and Valnet and has been observed by many other researchers.[8,9] Phagocytosis, the ability of white blood cells to ingest foreign bodies and wastes, is increased by essential oils known as depuratives or by the popular name of blood cleansers. Although a massage clinic or therapist would not sell or

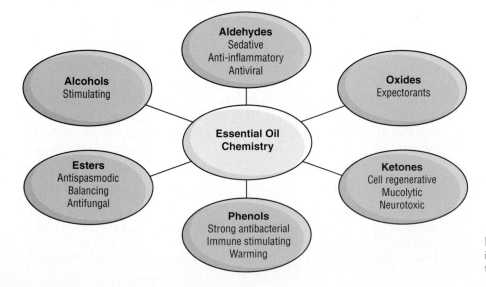

Figure 5-7   Essential oil chemistry. Chemical components in essential oils have therapeutic effects on the body.

market essential oils to boost immunity because this would be out of their scope of practice, they will probably notice that clients feel energized, rested, and revitalized by treatments that include essential oils.

Aromatherapy massage is a popular treatment at many spas, and a wide variety of essential oils can be used in massage to achieve a broad spectrum of treatment goals. Essential oils are often used for their pleasant aromas and to decrease stress. Oils high in a **functional group** known as the esters are usually effective antispasmodic agents. These oils, including Roman chamomile, clary sage, and petit-grain, are especially helpful in balancing the nervous system.[10] Phenylpropane ethers—especially estragole, which is found in basil—are thought to stabilize an overactive sympathetic nervous system, and cypress, basil, and sweet marjoram are noted for skeletal muscle spasm.[6] Caution should be used with basil because of its methyl chavicol content, which may cause skin irritation.

White birch (*Betula alba*), German and Roman chamomile, frankincense, wintergreen, clove, lavender, and mint oils are all effective analgesics.[11] White birch, yellow birch (*Betula alleghaniensis*), sweet birch (*Betula lenta*), and wintergreen (*Gaultheria procumbens*) all contain a high percentage (≤ 98%) of methyl-salicylate (an ester). Methyl-salicylate is the active ingredient used in pain rubs such as Bengay. These oils are effective in blends used in sports treatments or to decrease general muscular soreness. They may also be used in medical spas to decrease pain from a musculoskeletal condition such as osteoarthritis or Osgood-Schlatter disease.

Mint oils contain menthol, which has been used traditionally for headache pain. It should be noted that peppermint oil should not be applied undiluted to the temples to decrease headache pain. Used in this manner, it may cause a burning sensation and skin irritation. However, it is very effective for headaches when massaged, diluted in lotion or oil, into the posterior neck and shoulders. Mint oils are often used in treatments that aim to refresh the body because menthol increases the peripheral circulation and affects cold receptors in the skin, resulting in a cooling sensation.

Essential oils that support the respiratory system are effective when used in steam rooms and saunas. In a study by Eremenko et al.,[12] 96 patients suffering from chronic bronchitis showed significant clearing of the airways as well as reduced infection levels when inhaling vapors of camphor and menthol and particularly oils of *Eucalyptus* and peppermint. The oils improved the function of the lungs and bronchi by reducing mucous congestion and dealing with chest infections, colds, and influenza.[12] When inhaling essential oils in steam, smaller doses are more effective than large amounts of oils.[13] Pine, rosemary, *Eucalyptus*, and thyme oil work well in both saunas and steam rooms. Although spa massage therapists do not focus on respiratory pathologies, a basic understanding of core respiratory oils allows therapists to support their clients' overall health and wellness. For example, floral oils would not be used in a sauna or steam room because they may cause a headache in a close, hot environment.

Oils with a high sesquiterpene content are likely to have good anti-inflammatory properties. The most important anti-inflammatory compounds in essential oils are chamazulene and α-bisabolol (a sesquiterpene alcohol), both of which are found in German chamomile and in *Helichrysum*. The more effective compound of the two is α-bisabolol, which works mainly by inhibiting some of the enzymes involved in the inflammation response.[2] Anti-inflammatory oils are most often used in spas for skin irritations such as sunburn. They can be used in medical spas for soft tissue pathologies such as carpal tunnel syndrome, plantar fasciitis, and tendonitis. Table 5-3 gives an overview of some of the properties of essential oils and some of the treatments they support.

PSYCHOLOGICAL EFFECTS

In a therapeutic setting, good smells can be used together with massage, hydrotherapy soaks, meditation, hypnotherapy, or any other treatments to promote relaxation. This is important because stress is at the core of many modern diseases, and studies suggest that by simply decreasing stress, health and immunity can be improved. Smells can evoke intense emotional reactions and can even be used to change behavioral patterns. This psychological use of aromas has ancient roots. Incense has been burned for thousands of years to connect the human spirit with the gods and to shift consciousness from the everyday to the divine. There is credible evidence that agreeable fragrances can improve our mood and sense of well being.[14] This is not surprising because the olfactory receptors are directly connected to the **limbic system**, the oldest and most emotional part of the human brain (Fig. 5-8).

One way that smells can be used for healing is through a **learned-odor response**. In learned-odor responses a smell is used to form memory links to a person, place, or thing (e.g., a positive experience or relaxed state). Hiramoto et al. paired camphor with fever induction and found that a fever response could be elicited by camphor afterwards.[15] Whole memories, complete with all their associated emotions, can be prompted by smell.[16] This is entirely unconscious and cannot necessarily be prompted voluntarily, although countless studies have shown that recall can be enhanced if the learning was done in the presence of an odor and that same odor is presented at the time of recall. This information can be used by therapists to help clients recall "resource" states from a body treatment or meditation session. For example, if a therapist uses an exfoliation or body wash product scented with an uplifting mint fragrance in the treatment room, the client will remember the session every time he or she uses a home care product with the same fragrance. Not only will the client remember the session mentally, but his or her body will "remember" and through that memory, feel more relaxed.

Table 5-3	Therapeutic Actions and Properties of Selected Essential Oils

ACTION	DEFINITION	SELECTED INDICATION	SELECTED ESSENTIAL OILS	SELECTED METHOD OF APPLICATION
Alterative	An agent that corrects disordered body function and supports balance in the body	Stress, for recent trauma such as a car accident, as part of a detoxification regimen, burnout, anxiety	Lavender, Melissa, geranium, fir, juniper berry, petitgrain, lemongrass, valerian	Bath, body lotion, massage, as part of any relaxation treatment, mist inhalation, room scent, foot bath, aromatherapy wrap, etc.
Analgesic	An agent that reduces the sensation of pain	Soft tissue pain (use analgesics that are also anti-inflammatory during acute injury)	Bay laurel, bay rum, bergamot, birch, cajeput, German chamomile, Roman chamomile, clove, coriander, *Eucalyptus*, fir, ginger, jasmine (mild), lavender, lemongrass, sweet marjoram, peppermint, nutmeg, black pepper, rosemary, rosewood (mild), turmeric, wintergreen	Local application for an area of pain, massage, compress, muscle blends, sports massage blends
Anti-depressant	An agent that helps to alleviate depression	Depression, stress, anxiety	Basil, bergamot, geranium, jasmine, lavender, lemongrass, neroli, sweet orange, patchouli, rose, rosewood, clary sage, Spanish sage, sandalwood, vanilla, ylang ylang	Massage, bath, mist, inhalation, room scent, foot bath, with hypnosis or guided meditation
Anti-inflammatory	An agent that decreases inflammation	Recent soft tissue injury, skin irritation or sensitivity, neuritis	Benzoin, birch, camphor (white), German chamomile, frankincense, geranium, *Helichrysum*, jasmine, peppermint, myrrh, bitter orange, sweet orange, patchouli, common sage, Spanish sage, spikenard, tea tree, turmeric, wintergreen, yarrow	Local application for area of inflammation, skin lotion, cool bath, sunburn wrap
Antimicrobial	An agent that destroys or inhibits the life cycle of pathogenic micro-organisms	Onset of a cold or the flu, for skin infections, in natural cleaning products	Most essential oils to some degree	Massage, body lotion, lymph rub, bath, foot bath, body wrap
Antineuralgic	An agent that relieves or decreases pain from irritated nerves	Neuralgia	Bay rum, cajeput, Roman chamomile, clove, *Eucalyptus*, *Helichrysum*, Scotch pine	Application to the nerve path, massage to associated areas
Antipruritic	An agent that relieves or prevents itching	Itchy skin, insect bites, skin irritation, itchy scalp, sunburn	Birch, peppermint, wintergreen	Cool bath, skin lotion, hair rinse, body wrap
Antirheumatic	An agent that decreases or relieves rheumatism	Rheumatic conditions, stiff, sore muscular conditions	Bay laurel, bay rum, birch, clove, coriander, cypress, *Eucalyptus*, juniper berry, lavender, lemon, lime, nutmeg, Scotch pine, rosemary, thyme, turmeric, yarrow	Massage, body wrap, dry skin brush, body lotion, bath

Table 5-3 *(continued)*

ACTION	DEFINITION	SELECTED INDICATION	SELECTED ESSENTIAL OILS	SELECTED METHOD OF APPLICATION
Antisclerotic	An agent that helps to prevent the hardening of tissue	Scar tissue, mature skin, wrinkles	Lemon, carrot seed	Spot treatment, application to scars, massage with cross-fiber friction
Antiseborrheic	An agent that controls the production of sebum	Oily skin, dandruff	Atlas cedarwood, clary sage (sebum regulator), Spanish sage (sebum regulator), valerian (anti-dandruff), ylang ylang	Skin lotion, bath, hair rinse, in skin care products for oily skin
Antiviral	An agent that destroys or disrupts the life cycle of a viral pathogen	Onset of a cold or the flu or to generally boost immunity	Camphor (white), clove, *Eucalyptus*, hyssop, lime, sweet marjoram, peppermint, oregano (caution), patchouli, Scotch pine, tea tree, thyme	Inhalation, massage, lymph rub, body lotion, body wrap, bath
Astringent	An agent that firms or tightens tissue	Saggy skin, skin lacking in tone, oily skin, as a support for inflammatory conditions	Balsam fir, bay rum, benzoin, birch, atlas cedarwood, cypress, frankincense, geranium, grapefruit, *Helichrysum*, hyssop, juniper berry, lemon, lemongrass, linden, peppermint, myrrh, bitter orange, patchouli, rose, rosemary, clary sage, common sage, Spanish sage, sandalwood, spruce (*tsuga*), tea tree, thyme, wintergreen, yarrow	Skin care products, massage, cellulite and firming treatments, body wraps, body lotion
Cicatrisant	An agent that promotes healing through the formation of scar tissue	Wounds, skin conditions, skin revitalization treatments	Balsam fir, German chamomile, Roman chamomile, elemi, *Eucalyptus*, geranium, *Helichrysum*, hyssop, jasmine, juniper berry, lavender, lemon, myrrh, neroli, palmarosa, patchouli, rose, rosemary, clary sage, sandalwood, thyme, yarrow	Skin care products, skin care treatments, massage, baths
Cytophylactic	An agent that increases the activity of leukocytes in the body, therefore boosting immunity	To boost general immunity	German chamomile, frankincense, lavender, oregano (caution), rosemary, tea tree	Massage, reflexology, baths, foot baths, lymph rubs, dry skin brushing, detoxification treatment
Depurative	An agent that combats impurities in the blood and organs and aids detoxification	Detoxification treatments, revitalization treatments, to support a diet	Angelica, birch, carrot seed, coriander, *Eucalyptus*, grapefruit, juniper berry, lemon, rose, Spanish sage, vetiver	Massage, reflexology, baths, foot baths, lymph rubs, dry skin brushing, detoxification treatment

Table 5-3   (continued)

ACTION	DEFINITION	SELECTED INDICATION	SELECTED ESSENTIAL OILS	SELECTED METHOD OF APPLICATION
Diuretic	An agent that promotes the production of urine and aids water retention	Detoxification treatments, water retention, revitalization treatments	Angelica, balsam fir, bay laurel, benzoin, bergamot, birch, camphor (white), cardamom, atlas cedarwood, cypress, *Eucalyptus*, frankincense, geranium, grapefruit, *Helichrysum*, hyssop, juniper berry, lavender, lemon, linden, mandarin, sweet marjoram, patchouli, black pepper, scotch pine, rosemary, common sage, sandalwood, spruce (*tsuga*), thyme, turmeric, valerian	Massage, bath, body lotion, dry skin brush, body wrap, detoxification treatment
Emollient	An agent that softens the skin	Dry skin, mature skin, dehydrated skin, rough skin	Linden (other oils are not specific emollients but support dry skin: frankincense, myrrh, elemi, rose, lavender)	Skin lotion, massage, bath, skin care products, body wraps
Expectorant	An agent that promotes the removal of mucus from the respiratory system	These oils can be used for general respiratory support to prevent congestion and aid breathing	Angelica, balsam fir, bay rum, benzoin, cajeput, camphor (white), atlas cedarwood, *Eucalyptus*, fir, frankincense, ginger, *Hyssop*, sweet marjoram, peppermint, myrrh, scotch pine, Spanish sage, spruce (*tsuga*), tea tree, thyme, yarrow	Inhalation, chest rub, steam bath, shower, sauna
Fungicidal	An agent that combats fungal infection	Fungal foot infections	Angelica, bay laurel, atlas cedarwood, coriander, geranium, *Helichrysum*, lemongrass, sweet marjoram, myrrh, bitter orange, rosemary, sandalwood, spikenard, tea tree, thyme	Direct application to the local area of fungus, in cleaning products used at the spa
Hepatic	An agent that tones and stimulates the function of the liver	As a support for liver cleansing or detoxification treatments	Carrot seed, German chamomile, Roman chamomile, cypress, *Helichrysum*, peppermint, rose, rosemary	Body wrap, dry skin brush, body lotion, bath, massage
Hypotensive	An agent that lowers blood pressure	Stress, anxiety	Bay laurel, lavender, lemon, sweet marjoram, neroli, sweet orange, clary sage, Spanish sage, turmeric, valerian, yarrow, ylang ylang	Massage, body lotion, room scent, with guided meditation, hypnosis, inhalation, mist
Nervine	An agent that strengthens and tones the nerves and nervous system	Stress, nervous tension, burnout, neuritis, neuralgia	Angelica, basil, *Helichrysum*, hyssop, juniper berry, lavender, lemon, lemongrass, linden, sweet marjoram, peppermint, patchouli, petitgrain, rosemary, clary sage, Spanish sage, spruce (*tsuga*), thyme, ylang ylang	Body wrap, massage, body lotion, bath, direct application to an area of nerve pain
Relaxant	An agent that soothes and relieves tension	Stress, anxiety, insomnia	German chamomile, Roman chamomile, lavender, neroli, nutmeg, sandalwood, vanilla, ylang ylang	Body wrap, massage, bath reflexology, body lotion, room scent, mist, inhalation

Table 5-3 *(continued)*

ACTION	DEFINITION	SELECTED INDICATION	SELECTED ESSENTIAL OILS	SELECTED METHOD OF APPLICATION
Restorative	An agent that revitalizes and strengthens the body	Low immunity, burnout, mental exhaustion, stress	Basil, coriander, lavender, lemon, lime, myrrh, Scotch pine, rosemary, tea tree	Body wrap, massage, bath reflexology, body lotion, room scent, mist, inhalation
Rubefacient	An agent that increases local circulation to the skin and is warming; may lead to skin irritation	Tight muscles, detoxification, cellulite treatments, muscle pain and soreness	Birch, camphor (white), *Eucalyptus*, fir, ginger, juniper berry, oregano (caution), black pepper, Scotch pine, rosemary, spruce (*tsuga*), thyme, turmeric, vetiver, wintergreen	Cellulite application, massage, spot treatment, muscle blends, sports massage blends
Sedative	An agent that sedates or calms the central nervous system, a body system, or the body in general	Relaxation treatments, stress, anxiety, insomnia	Balsam fir, bay laurel, benzoin, atlas cedarwood, German chamomile, Roman chamomile, frankincense, *Hyssop*, jasmine, juniper berry, lavender (balancing), lemongrass, linden, mandarin, sweet marjoram, myrrh, bitter orange, sweet orange, rose, clary sage, sandalwood, spikenard, tuberose, valerian (depresses central nervous system), vanilla, vetiver, yarrow, ylang ylang	Body wrap, massage, bath reflexology, body lotion, room scent, mist, inhalation, with hypnosis or meditation
Stimulant	An agent that increases the function of a body system or the body in general	Mental and physical burnout, stress, to revitalize and energize	Angelica, bay rum, bergamot, camphor (white), clove, cardamom, carrot seed, atlas cedarwood (circulatory), coriander, elemi, *Eucalyptus*, fir, geranium, ginger, grapefruit (lymphatic), lavender (balancing), lemon (lymphatic), mandarin (lymphatic), peppermint, nutmeg, neroli (nerve), sweet orange (lymphatic), palmarosa (circulatory), patchouli, black pepper, petitgrain, Scotch pine, rosemary, rosewood (immune), common sage, Spanish sage, spruce (*tsuga*), thyme, turmeric, vetiver (circulation)	Body wrap, massage, bath, reflexology, body lotion, room scent, mist, inhalation, dry skin brushing
Sudorific or Diaphoretic	An agent that promotes or increases perspiration	To warm an area, detoxification treatments, cellulite treatments, sore muscles	Bay laurel, cajeput, German chamomile, Roman chamomile, cypress, ginger, *Hyssop*, juniper berry, sweet marjoram, rosemary, tea tree, thyme, yarrow	Body wrap, massage, body lotion, spot treatment

Table 5-3	*(continued)*			
ACTION	**DEFINITION**	**SELECTED INDICATION**	**SELECTED ESSENTIAL OILS**	**SELECTED METHOD OF APPLICATION**
Vasoconstrictor	An agent that causes narrowing of the blood vessels	Varicose veins, broken capillaries	Cypress, lemon, peppermint (rose, lavender, German chamomile can be used as support oils)	Direct application to the local area
Vulnerary	An agent that is healing for the skin	Skin conditions, wounds	Balsam fir, benzoin, bergamot, German chamomile, Roman chamomile, *Eucalyptus*, geranium, hyssop, juniper berry, sweet marjoram, rosemary, rosewood (tissue regenerator)	Massage, body lotion, skin care products

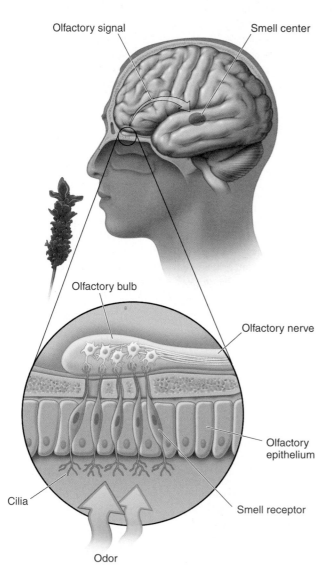

Figure 5-8 The limbic system. Olfactory receptors are directly connected to the limbic system, the oldest and most emotional part of the brain.

Olfactory signal

Smell center

Olfactory bulb

Olfactory nerve

Olfactory epithelium

Cilia

Smell receptor

Odor

Therapists interested in designing treatments that would encourage their clients to relax completely should turn to oils known as sedatives, calmatives, and relaxants. These oils help the body to let go of mental, emotional, and physical tension. For example, in one study, when the sedative essential oils of lavender, rose, and valerian were dispersed in the air, rats took longer to perform tasks.[17] This shows that these oils have the ability to sedate the central nervous system. Oils such as lavender, Roman or German chamomile, and sweet marjoram sedate the body and decrease stress because they stimulate the raphe nucleus, which releases serotonin. Ambient lavender was also shown to increase sleep and lead to better waking moods in psychogeriatric patients under long-term treatment for insomnia.[18] During stressful magnetic resonance imaging medical testing, a vanilla-like scent was used successfully to help patients relax and to reduce anxiety at Memorial Sloan-Kettering Cancer Center in New York.[19]

Stimulating scents are being used by many companies to promote alertness and increase the efficiency and precision of their workers.[20] In one study, there was an increase of cerebral blood flow in humans after inhalation of 1,8, cineol (rosemary, *Eucalyptus* oil).[21] Rosemary, lemon, basil, and peppermint offer a quick energy pickup because they stimulate the locus ceruleus, which releases noradrenalin. People do much better in tasks that require sustained attention if they receive regular puffs of an uplifting aroma.[22]

In one study, peppermint, which is often the oil chosen to promote alert states, enhanced the sensory pathway for visual detection, which allowed subjects more control over their allocation of attention. Ambient peppermint aroma increased word learning and recall.[22] A spa therapist could use stimulating oils in treatments aimed at energizing the body or at the end of a relaxation treatment to help wake up the client.

Spas spend large amounts of money to influence their clients' perceptions of their business. Perception can only be created or altered through one of the five senses because these are the means by which we interpret our environment. The positive emotional effects of agreeable fragrances can be used to affect our perception of other people, of a business, or of a product. In a study done to show that scent impacts social relationships, people in photographs were given a higher "attractiveness rating" when the test subjects were exposed to a pleasant fragrance. In a test on shampoos, the product originally ranked last in performance was ranked first in a second test after its fragrance was adjusted.[23]

Smell-Scapes

Olfaction provides spa therapists with another form of communication. It creates connections to the spiritual aspect of self; to the cultural background of a treatment; and to the natural world of field and forest, sea and desert. It adds dimension and texture to the treatment and provides an emotionally satisfying experience for the client.

When a designer plans a service, one of the aspects that should be considered is the smell-scape. A smell-scape is the aroma landscape that is planned for the treatment. The therapist should keep all the scents in a particular category but vary them in such a way that they maintain the client's interest. For example, a citrus salt glow would obviously include citrus oils. If the therapist used the same scent for all of the products (e.g., massage oil, body mist, finishing lotion), the client will register the scent for the first 10 minutes of the treatment but then forget it. A therapist that wants aroma to be an integral part of the treatment will vary the smell-scape. He or she might use grapefruit in the massage oil, mandarin with a floral accent in the body mist, and lemon in the finishing lotion. Each time the product is changed, the room is filled with a new scent, and the client's olfactory enjoyment is enhanced.

For culturally inspired treatments, the smell-scape creates a powerful emotional link to the region where the service originated. In Ayurveda, the traditional medical system of India, medicated oils called *taila* are used.[24] Traditional *taila* smell very strange to the Western nose, and some clients take time to adjust to the new aromas. As this adjustment takes place, it often brings a deeper curiosity about ayurveda, which, in turn, enriches the client's experience of the treatment. Culturally influenced treatments must be designed carefully. It makes sense that a treatment named the Nile body wrap would use plant products that were known and used in ancient Egypt. North American pine oil would be out of place in such a treatment, but frankincense, myrrh, and rose are appropriate. In Chapter 13, a table of different themes, smell-scapes, accents, and associations provides more ideas on scents that might be used in a particular smell-scape.

One easy way to create interest is to contrast distinct smell categories against their opposites. If the massage oil is scented with essential oils that have deep, pungent, heavy, and spicy aromas, the body polish product might be scented with oils that smell light, green, and of citrus. Table 5-4 breaks essential oils into smell categories for easy scent contrasts.

When therapists use smell-scapes in treatments, they are using oils psychologically. Blending oils for a physiological effect requires a different set of considerations. Eventually, therapists find that they can achieve both a physiological and psychological balance in their blends. This type of blending is called *holistic blending* because the formulations aim to address the needs of the body, mind, and spirit.

Blending Essential Oils

The techniques outlined in this chapter are keys to blending only. They are meant to provide structure for those who are learning how to blend by providing a way to think about the blend and the many considerations to be kept in mind when blending. Like smell itself, the blending process is personal, biased, and inspired by private memories and relationships with past events. There is no such thing as a bad blend, and there are many different ways, beyond those outlined here, for therapists to approach blending. Before the blending begins, the therapist needs to choose the type of carrier product that is to be used.

CARRIER PRODUCTS

A carrier product (some therapists refer to them as a vehicle) is a general term for the product that is used to "carry" the essential oil to the client. Essential oils are rarely applied at full strength. More often, they are diluted into a carrier product before they are used in a treatment. Massage therapists most often use an expeller-pressed **fixed oil** as a carrier for essential oils delivered in massage. Expeller-pressed fixed oils are different from essential oils in that they do not evaporate (they are composed of nonvolatile compounds) and are classified as lipids. Fixed oils are sometimes used to adulterate essential oils because essential oils dissolve completely and easily in fixed oils. Fixed oils are lubricating for the skin and often therapeutically useful in their own right. Commonly used fixed oils include expeller-pressed sunflower, sweet almond, apricot kernel, hemp (anti-inflammatory and pain relieving), avocado, borage, jojoba (sebum balancing) and/or hazelnut, although many different types of fixed oils can be used. Some fixed oils such as evening primrose, hemp, jojoba, wheat germ, and pure vitamin E may be added in small amounts to other fixed oils to enhance the therapeutic properties of these oils or act as a natural preservative (1 tbsp of preservative oils to 1 oz of the main fixed oil).

Plain, unscented lotion or massage cream, bath gel, exfoliation product, aloe vera, clay, and body gels can be purchased as carrier products for essential oils. This is especially helpful if the therapist is designing an original service and wants to create a smell-scape for the client, although it is important to avoid products that contain components that block the absorption of essential oils through the skin.

Table 5-4	Basic Scents of Essential Oils and Other Aromatic Materials

SPICY	REFRESHING	HERBACEOUS	SWEET	EXOTIC
Ajowan	Basil	Ajowan	Copaiba balsam	Bay rum
Allspice	Bay laurel	Angelica root	Peru balsam	Copaiba balsam
Angelica seed	Melissa	French basil	Tolu balsam	Peru balsam
Aniseed seed	Fir needle	Calamintha	Benzoin	Tolu balsam
Peru balsam	Bergamot	German chamomile	Sweet birch	CO_2 ginger
Tolu balsam	Cajeput	Roman chamomile	Jasmine	Jasmine
Bay rum	Cypress	*Helichrysum*	Lavender	Myrrh
Caraway	Elemi	*Hyssop*	Lime	Narcissus
Cardamom	*Eucalyptus*	Marigold	Mandarin	Nutmeg
Cascarilla bark	Geranium	Marjoram	Mimosa	Oakmoss
Cassia	Juniper berry	Myrtle	Neroli	Neroli
Cinnamon	Lemongrass	Oregano	Carnation	Patchouli
Clove	Tilia absolute	Patchouli	Rose	Sandalwood
Coriander	Myrtle	Rosemary	Rosewood	Spikenard
Litsea cubeba	Palmarosa	Common sage	Liquidamber	Liquidamber
Cumin	Pine	Santolina	Tonka	Tonka
CO_2 ginger	Rosemary	Tarragon	Tuberose	Tuberose
Nutmeg	Spanish sage	Thyme	Vanilla	Turmeric
Black pepper	Clary sage	Valerian	Wintergreen	Valerian
Turmeric	Common sage	Yarrow	Ylang ylang	Vetiver

LIGHT AND FRESH	POWDERY	EARTHY	FLORAL	WARM AND HOMEY
Rosewood	Copaiba balsam	Angelica root	Gardenia	Almond
Sweet orange	Peru balsam	Carrot seed	Geranium	Honey
Bay laurel	Tolu balsam	German chamomile	Hyacinth	Beeswax
Bergamot	Benzoin	Fennel seed	Jasmine	German chamomile
Grapefruit	Cedarwood	Ginger	Lavender	Cinnamon
Lavender	Frankincense	Myrrh	Tilia absolute	Clove
Lemon	Orris	Oakmoss	Mimosa	Inula
Lemongrass	Sandalwood	Patchouli	Narcissus	Lavender
Lime	Liquidamber	Spikenard	Neroli	Nutmeg
Litsea	Tonka	Vetiver	Rose	Vanilla
Mandarin	Vanilla	Yarrow	Carnation	Mandarin
Clary sage	Violet flower		Tuberose	Rose
Lemon verbena			Violet flower	
			Ylang ylang	

Table 5-4 *(continued)*

LEMONY	CAMPHORACEOUS	MEDICINAL	LEATHERY	ALPINE
Melissa	Exotic basil	Bay laurel	Cade	Fir needle
Elemi	Borneol	Sweet birch	Cypress	Bay laurel
	Cajeput	Cajeput	Guaiacwood	Sweet birch
Lemon	White camphor	White camphor	Labdanum	Cedarwood
Lemongrass	*Eucalyptus*	*Eucalyptus*	Oakmoss	Cypress
Litsea	Niaouli	Niaouli	Opopanax	Juniper berry
Lemon verbena	Oregano	Spanish sage	Patchouli	Pine
		Tea tree	Valerian	Spruce
		Thyme	Vetiver	
			Yarrow	

WOODY	GREEN	MINTY	CITRUS	MUSKY
Amyris	Galbanum	Cornmint	Bergamot	Ambrette seed
Cade	Tilia absolute	Peppermint	Grapefruit	Costus
Cascarilla bark	Myrtle	Spearmint	Lime	Cumin
Cedarwood	Narcissus		Lemon	Labdanum
Cubeb	Tagetes		Mandarin	
Inula	Tarragon		Bitter orange	
Rosewood	Valerian		Sweet orange	
Sandalwood	Violet leaf			

Such products include mineral oil, petroleum, lanolin, coconut oil, and cocoa butter. Sometimes a spa product will be fragranced when it arrives at the spa. If the scent is light, it can easily be modified by adding essential oils. This is not ideal, however, because the fragrance may be synthetic and not appropriate for use in aromatherapy.

ESSENTIAL OIL CONCENTRATIONS

The term *concentration* refers to the amount of essential oil in the final volume of massage oil or carrier product. Table 5-5 outlines how many drops of essential oil are added to a base or carrier for a particular concentration. Figure 5-9

Table 5-5   Carrier Volume to Essential Oil Concentration

CARRIER (OZ)	EO 1% (DROPS)	EO 2% (DROPS)	EO 2.5% (DROPS)	EO 3% (DROPS)	EO 4% (DROPS)
1/2	3	6	7.5	9	12
1	6	12	15	18	24
2	12	24	30	36	48
4	24	48	60	72	96
8	48	96	120	144	192

EO = essential oil.

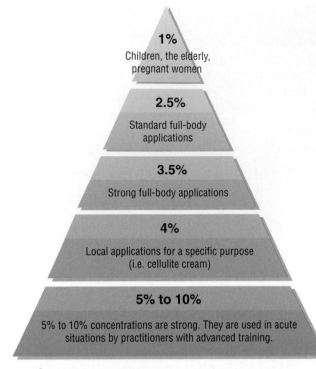

1%
Children, the elderly,
pregnant women

2.5%
Standard full-body
applications

3.5%
Strong full-body applications

4%
Local applications for a specific purpose
(i.e. cellulite cream)

5% to 10%
5% to 10% concentrations are strong. They are used in acute
situations by practitioners with advanced training.

Figure 5-9   Standard concentrations in aromatherapy.

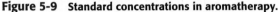

illustrates which concentration to use on a particular type of client or condition. Concentrations of between 1% and 4% are standard in the field of aromatherapy and are low enough to ensure safety and minimize negative reactions. Concentrations of above 4% are used in acute situations or by experienced therapists; 100% (neat) applications are used for spot treatments with specific oils such as tea tree for toe fungus, *Helichrysum* for trigger point therapy, lavender for small burns, German chamomile for inflammation of soft tissue, and lemon, or tea tree or lavender, to dot on a skin blemish.

SYNERGY

A **synergy** is when the whole is greater then the sum of its parts and those parts are mutually enhancing. It is derived from *synergios*, which is a Greek word that means "associate or partner" or literally in this context, working together. Synergistic interactions between chemical compounds create a greater spectrum of action than would be possible using a single oil alone.

When creating synergistic blends, it is important to remember that essential oils are chemically complex, so blending too many oils at once tends to muddy the result. Often only three to four oils are needed to make a good synergistic blend. When you put two, three, or four oils together with similar or complementary therapeutic actions, you create a blend that is much more effective than a single oil working alone.

To create a synergy for relaxation, fir could be chosen for its alterative action, which helps the body to regain balanced function. Sweet marjoram could be added for its nervine qualities, which help to strengthen and support the overall nervous system. Finally, lavender might be added as a restorative that helps with burnout and exhaustion. These three oils will have a broader action on stress than fir on its own.

Therapists can also use the *action/property* words in aromatherapy literature to create a synergy. For example, if a therapist wanted a blend that was antiviral, he or she would simply pick two or three oils that listed *antiviral* in the *action/property* area associated with the essential oil. The chemistry of oils can also be used. For example, if a therapist wants a blend that is a powerful muscular antispasmodic, he or she would turn to essential oils high in esters, such as Roman chamomile (75%), clary sage (70%), and petitgrain (55%).

TOP, MIDDLE, AND BASE NOTE BLENDING

Many perfumers and aromatherapists use the top, middle, and base note classifications of essential oils and perfume materials to achieve a "symphony" of balance in the fragrance. Top, middle, and base notes are determined by their different rates of evaporation. Top notes are generally composed of small molecules (i.e., they are lightweight and evaporate quickly). They are the first aromas to hit your nose and give you the initial impression of the fragrance. Middle notes are slower to evaporate and create the substance or main theme of the fragrance. Base notes appear last because of their larger molecular size and slower rate of evaporation. They also bind all the other ingredients in a scent, holding the scent together. When using notes to create blends, the idea is to include an oil that resonates on each note so that the fragrance smells integrated and whole. If the blend does not harmonize, try to use "bridging oils" such as jasmine and ylang ylang that resonate on more than one note. If the blend smells "rough," you can soften it by adding a blend smoother such as rosemary, marjoram, or a citrus oil. Blend enhancers such as sandalwood, bergamot, clary sage, and lavender bring out the scent of the other oils, bridge gaps, and generally enhance the aroma. Rose and chamomile species often "jump out" of a blend and can be modified with black pepper, geranium, lemon, or clove. Table 5-6 provides an overview of the note classification of some essential oils.

Application Methods

A well-trained, professional aromatherapist is an asset to any spa. He or she can provide custom blending specifically tailored to the needs of the individual client and can develop signature blends for the business and provide smellscape recommendations for specific treatments. But even the simplest aromatherapy treatment can benefit a client immensely by decreasing stress and increasing the pleasure

Table 5-6	Top, Middle, and Base Notes of Essential Oils		
TOP NOTES			
Anise	Fennel	Mandarin	Petitgrain
Bay	Fir	Marjoram	Pine
Bergamot	Galbanum	Mimosa	Rosemary
Birch	Ginger	Nutmeg	Spearmint
Carrot seed	Grapefruit	Orange	Tangerine
Cedarwood	Juniper berry	Oregano	Tarragon
Coriander	Lavender	Palmarosa	Thyme
Cypress	Lemon	Pepper	Wintergreen
Davana	Lime	Peppermint	Wormwood
MIDDLE NOTES			
Allspice	Clary sage	Melissa	Ylang ylang
Basil	Clove	Neroli	
Beeswax	Geranium	Orris	
Benzoin	Jasmine	Osmanthus	
Boronia	Lavender	Pepper	
Carnation	Lemon verbena	Rose	
R. Chamomile	Lemongrass	Tagetes	
Champa	Linden	Tuberose	
Cinnamon	*Litsea cubeba*	Violet leaf	
BASE NOTES			
Ambrette	Fir	Opoponax	Vanilla
Angelica	Frankincense	Patchouli	Vetiver
Benzoin	Galbanum	Peru balsam	
Cassia	Hay	Sandalwood	
G. Chamomile	*Helichrysum*	Seaweed	
Clary sage	Myrrh	Tarragon	
Copaiba balsam	Nutmeg absolute	Tolu balsam	
Costus	Oakmoss	Tonka	

derived from the service. The methods of application described below focus on some of the common ways that essential oils can be used in a spa. Figure 5-3 provides an overview of common aromatherapy treatments.

INHALATIONS

Unless the spa has a medical focus, the therapist will probably use inhalations to facilitate clear breathing in saunas, steams, and showers or to provide mental stimulation or mood enhancement. Some steam baths have a special holder in which essential oils are placed. If this is not available, the oils can be placed directly onto the floor at the edges of the cabinet or room. Four to 6 drops provides a light but detectable scent as the essential oils evaporate into the steam. In the sauna, add the oils to the water that will be ladled on the heat source. Two to 6 drops of essential oil are used, depending on the size of the water container. Oils added to the heat source in a sauna must always be mixed in water because essential oils are potentially combustible and

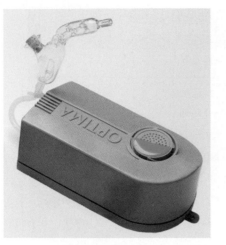

Figure 5-10 Aromatherapy diffuser. A nebulizing diffuser is the best choice if the goal is to decrease airborne pathogens and create a clean and healthy environment.

could "pop" or flame up if added plain. A drop of oil can be placed on a tissue tucked in the face cradle to prevent congestion from lying in the prone position during any treatment.

Diffusing essential oils throughout an area can purify the air, repel insects, enhance mood, or simply make the place smell good. A commercial nebulizing diffuser is the best choice if the aim is to eliminate microbes and promote a clean, healthy living or working space (Fig. 5-10). Earthenware burners, electronic fan diffusers, and items such as lamp rings can be used to scent a room. Spa suppliers have a variety of different types of scenting diffusers. Aromatherapy candles are often scented with synthetics and so should be generally avoided. If the candle is in a base of beeswax, it is more likely to contain a pure oil because essential oils dissolve into beeswax but not into regular candle wax.

Sanitation

Nebulizing diffusers have a glass chamber that should be cleaned out with alcohol once a day to keep the apparatus functioning well. Follow the manufacturer's directions.

AROMATIC EXFOLIATIONS AND BODY SHAMPOOS

Essential oils can be added to a granulated exfoliation product or applied in a foaming bath gel for a fragrant and satisfying body polish or body shampoo. Add 24 drops of an essential oil blend to 2 oz of either exfoliation product or foaming body wash. Aromatic exfoliation can be the first step in a larger treatment (see Chapter 6 for details on exfoliation).

AROMATHERAPY MASSAGE

An aromatherapy massage provides both physiological and psychological benefits for the client. Use a 2% (12 drops/oz of carrier) to 3% (18 drops/oz of carrier) concentration of essential oils in carrier oil or cream for a full body massage. Use a 1% (6 drops/oz of carrier) concentration when massaging elderly individuals, children, or pregnant women. Four percent blends (24 drops/oz) can be used for spot treatments (e.g., trigger-point therapy, cross-fiber friction) or for specific conditions (e.g., carpal tunnel syndrome, lateral epicondylitis). Certain oils such as German chamomile can be used at 100% to decrease pain and inflammation in a specific area.

In a classic aromatherapy treatment, the therapist meets with the client during a "formal" aromatherapy consultation in which the client fills out a health history form and the client and therapist discuss the client's expectations of aromatherapy and health care goals. A custom blend is created and then applied in a full-body massage. Some therapists use methods such as applied kinesiology or "body talking" to choose oils for the client. In such a method, the client holds a bottle of oil, and the therapist uses muscle testing to determine which oil "increases strength." Some therapists let clients pick all of the oils for the blend, believing that they will only be drawn to oils that will support them in their particular healing process. Other therapists take the opposite approach and choose oils that the client mildly dislikes. The assumption in this case is that clients are "out of balance" with what they need for healing and that healing will happen slowly as the client develops an affinity to the oil or blend. Most often, choosing oils for the blend is a joint process between the client and therapist. The therapist suggests oils that have physiological or psychological effects that would support the client's healing needs, and the client shares likes and dislikes until both are satisfied with the oils chosen. The therapist will then check for contraindications before creating the final blend of oils.

Some spas choose not to offer custom blending but create a series of premade blends from which the client chooses a scent. This allows the client to have more massage time for the same amount of money. It also enhances retail opportunities because clients often become attached to a scent and then purchase the body wash, body lotion, and room mist that matches their massage oil. A selection of starter oils and ready-to-blend recipes is offered in Table 5-7 for easy adoption by massage clinics and spas.

AROMATHERAPY BATHS

A hydrotherapy tub is a specialized soaking unit that has multiple air and water jets. Essential oils can be added to the hydrotherapy tub or to a standard soaking tub for therapeutic baths. Sometimes the oils are added simply for the pleasure of their fragrance, or they can be used to treat sore muscles, stress, insomnia, low immunity, skin problems, depression, irritability, or a variety of other conditions. The drawback to

Table 5-7	Starter Oils and Easy-Blend Recipes
21 VERSATILE OILS	**THESE BLENDS ARE FORMULATED AT A 2% CONCENTRATION FOR USE IN 1 OZ OF CARRIER PRODUCT (12 TOTAL DROPS TO 1 OZ OF CARRIER). THEY ARE COMPOSED OF THE 21 STARTER OILS AT THE LEFT**
Bay laurel	Muscle Ease: Bay laurel (3), rosemary (1), lemon (6), juniper berry (2)
Bergamot	Breath Easy: Eucalyptus (3), lemon (7), thyme (2)
Clary sage	Mother-to-Be: Lavender (5), mandarin (7)
Cypress	Clarity: Thyme (1), grapefruit (9), cypress (2)
Eucalyptus	Rain: Cypress (5), thyme (5), geranium (2)
Frankincense	Equilibrium: Clary sage (3), neroli (2), bergamot (7)
Geranium	Girl Power: Clary sage (2), lavender (6), geranium (1), frankincense (3)
German chamomile	Body Boost: Lemon (4), thyme (1), bergamot (4), lavender (3)
Ginger CO_2	Purity: Juniper berry (3), grapefruit (8), thyme (1)
Grapefruit	Revitalize: Bergamot (6), rosemary (2), lavender (4)
Jasmine	Ocean: Rosemary (3), frankincense (7), ylang ylang (2)
Juniper berry	Zen: Ylang ylang (2), ginger CO_2 (2), mandarin (8)
Lavender	Renew: German chamomile (1), rosemary (2), clary sage (4), lavender (5)
Lemon	Shimmer: Bay laurel (3), ylang ylang (1), bergamot (5), frankincense (3)
Mandarin	Meditation: Frankincense (4), jasmine (1), ginger CO_2 (2)
Neroli	Energy: Peppermint (1), thyme (4), bay laurel (4)
Peppermint	Summer: Neroli (2), lavender (4), bergamot (6)
Rose	Refresh: Peppermint (1), eucalyptus (2), lemon (8), geranium (1)
Rosemary	Moon Mist: Jasmine (2), grapefruit (10)
Thyme	Tranquiling: Rose (1), clary sage (2), mandarin (6), frankincense (3)
Ylang ylang	Circulate: Ginger CO_2 (2), grapefruit (9), juniper berry (1)

using essential oils in a bath is that the oils will "pool" on the top of the water. When the client gets into the bath, the oils will stick to the area that hits the water first, or the oils will pool around exposed areas and may cause skin irritation. For this reason, it is best to dilute the oils in carrier oil and massage the blend into the client's skin. After the massage, the client soaks in a warm tub where he or she can enjoy the fragrance of the oils and allow for greater skin absorption. Sometimes essential oils are added to an emulsifier, which disperses them in the body of the water to prevent pooling. In this case, 6 to 9 drops of essential oil are used for a bath.

Aromatic foot and hand baths can be used to treat disorders of the feet and hands such as arthritis and athlete's foot, or they can be used for relaxation, low immunity, or stress-related disorders. The oils are diluted into a carrier product and massaged into the skin before the area is soaked, or the oils are blended into an emulsifier and added directly to the bath. In the case of a foot or hand bath, 2 to 4 drops of oil might be used.

AROMATHERAPY WRAPS

Aromatherapy wraps can take many forms. In the simplest wrap, the client is cocooned in blankets at the end of an aromatherapy massage to relax while the essential oils continue to absorb into the bloodstream. Sometimes essential oils are blended into a very heavy carrier product such as wheat germ oil or shea butter, massaged into the skin, left to absorb during a wrap, and then removed with hot towels, a Vichy shower, or a body shampoo. If a body shampoo is used to remove the excess carrier, a light moisture lotion may be applied at the end of the treatment to rehydrate the skin. These treatments are sometimes called emollient wraps because the heavy carrier product is nourishing for the skin and softens very dry or dehydrated skin. Other carrier products might also be used. For example, aloe vera and anti-inflammatory oils can be brushed on the skin for an effective sunburn relief wrap. Essential oils can be added to body milk (very light and watery lotion) and misted on the body with an atomizer before the body is wrapped. Some therapists soak cotton sheets in hot water and essential oils and apply them in a hot sheet wrap. This is the least effective method of using essential oils in a wrap because the oils tend to evaporate very quickly, so they do not really penetrate the skin. However, this type of sheet wrap does smell nice. Alternatively, hand towels scented with essential oils can be layered on the body after it has been massaged with aromatic oils, and the body can be wrapped. Oils might also be mixed up with clay (e.g., kaolin, French green, Sedona) and applied to the body with a brush before the client is wrapped. There is no end to the ways that different steps can be mixed and matched to form satisfying treatments. Body wrap procedures are covered in Chapter 7.

AROMA MISTS AND AURA MISTS

Aroma mists have a number of different uses in a spa setting. They can be used as air purifiers and fresheners, linen fresheners, mood enhancers, skin toners, or body coolers. In many of the services described in upcoming chapters, aroma mists are used as a treatment step. Aroma mists make nice take-home gifts for clients because they can use them to refresh the car or to mist at any time as an olfactory link to the relaxation they experienced in their spa treatment.

An aura mist is an aromatherapy body mist that is used only at the very end of the treatment. It is misted in a high arch over the client from the head to the toes. It should be scented with an aroma that contrasts with the treatment products and fills the treatment room with a refreshing scent. This helps to wake up the client and stimulate him or her at the end of the session.

A number of different base fluids can be used when creating aroma or aura mists, including purified water, herbal teas, floral waters (hydrosols), lemon juice, witch hazel, and vinegar. Add 30 drops of an essential oil blend to 2 oz of base liquid in a bottle with a spray top. It is best to refrigerate mists between uses to prevent the product from expiring. If tea is used as a base, the product will have a short shelf life (2 to 3 days) and should be made up in small batches only.

SUPPORT LOTIONS

A support lotion is a blend of essential oils mixed into a lotion base that is given to a client to use as a form of self-care. The oils might be chosen to give the client an energy boost, to calm the client if he or she feels anxious, as a link to a positive affirmation or new life choice (quit smoking, take a break, eat healthy), or as a pleasant reminder of the spa stay. The lotion can be used at any time by clients in a variety of ways and gives them a simple way to bring aromatherapy into their lives. They can rub it on their hands and then hold their hands over their nose for a simple inhalation. They can spread the lotion over the anterior neck, down the sternum, under the breast tissue, and behind the neck, where lymph nodes come up close to the surface of the body for a gentle immunity boost. Finally, they can rub the lotion all over their body and take a bath.

Summary

Aromatherapy is the use of essential oils for healing the mind, body, and spirit. Different health care providers use essential oils in diverse ways based on their scope of practice. These modern-day uses mirror those of ancient times, when aromatic substances were used for both medical and spiritual practices.

Essential oils are volatile plant oils extracted from certain aromatic plants that have both physiological and psychological effects on the human body. These oils are chemically complex and may contain as many as 400 different components. The oils are stored in the leaves, needles, twig, bark, flowers, flower buds, fruits, stems, and roots; they are extracted through steam distillation, expression, solvent extraction, or CO_2 hyperbolic production. Essential oils are often adulterated on the international market to increase the profit margin of the grower or supplier. Aromatherapists believe that the human body responds differently to natural oils than to those that are synthetic or adulterated. For this reason, it is important to purchase high-quality, therapeutic-grade essential oils from a reputable supplier.

The oils enter the body via the skin, inhalation through the lungs, and ingestion (which is not used without advanced training). After they have entered the body, the chemical compounds in essential oils interact with the body's chemistry to affect specific organs, systems, or the body as a whole (physiological effects). The inhalation of essential oils also triggers an olfactory response that can lead to powerful mental and emotional behavioral changes (i.e., psychological effects).

Basic blending methods such as synergistic blending and note blending allow the therapist to create interesting smell-scapes to enhance the client's spa experience. Aromatherapy massage, exfoliation, wraps, and hydrotherapy introduce clients to the benefits of essential oils. The pleasing fragrances of the oils also support their use as accent notes in other services.

REFERENCES

1. The National Association of Holistic Aromatherapy. Available at http://www.naha.org
2. Schnaubelt K: *Advanced Aromatherapy: The Science of Essential Oil Therapy.* Rochester, VT: Healing Arts Press, 1995.
3. Irvine SA: *Perfume: The Creation and Allure and Classic Fragrances.* New York: Crescent Books, 1995.
4. Okabe H, et al: Effect of limonene and related compounds on the percutaneous absorption of indomethacin. *Drug Des Deliv* 1989;4:313–321.
5. Ceschel GC: In vitro permeation through porcine buccal mucosa of *Salvia desoleana* Atzei and Picci essential oil from topical formulation. *Int J Pharmaceut* 2000;195:171–177.
6. Price S, Price L: *Aromatherapy for Health Professionals*, 2nd Ed. London: Churchill Livingstone, 1999.
7. Battaglia S: *The Complete Guide to Aromatherapy.* Virginia, Australia: The Perfect Potion, Ltd., 1995.
8. Valnet J: *The Practice of Aromatherapy.* Safron Walden, UK: CW Daniel, 1982.
9. Gattefossé RM: *Gattefossé's Aromatherapy.* Translated by Tisserand RB. Saffron Walden, UK: C.W. Daniel, 1993.
10. Achterrath-Tuckerman U, et al: Pharmacological investigations with compounds of chamomile. V. Investigations on the spasmolytic effect of compounds of chamomile. *Planta Medica* 1980;39:38–50.
11. Roulier G: *Les Huiles Essentielles Pour Votre Sante.* St-Jean-de-Braye, France: Dangles, 1990.
12. Eremenko AE, et al: Volatile fractions of essential oil based phytoncides as a component of therapeutic-rehabilitative complexes in chronic bronchitis. *Tikhomirov AA Ter Arkh* 1987;59:126–130.
13. Boyd EM, Sheppard EP: The effect of steam inhalation of volatile oils on the output and composition of respiratory tract fluid. *J Pharmacol Exp Ther* 1968;163:250–256.
14. Parasuraman R: *Effects of fragrances on behavior, mood and physiology.* Paper presented at the annual meeting of the American Association for the Advancement of Science, Washington, DC, 1991.
15. Hiramoto RN, et al: Conditioning fever: A host defense reflex response. *Life Sci* 1991;49:93–99.
16. Miles C, Jenkins R: Recency and suffix effects with serial recall of odours. *Memory* 2000;8:195–206.
17. Macht DI, Ting GC: Experimental enquiry into the sedative properties of some aromatic drugs and fumes. *J Pharmacol Exp Ther* 1921;18:361–372.
18. Schnaubelt K: *Medical Aromatherapy: Healing with Essential Oils.* Berkeley, CA: Frog Ltd, 1999.
19. Redd WH, et al: Fragrance administration to reduce anxiety during MR imaging. *J Magn Reson Imaging* 1964;4:623–626.
20. Sense of Smell Institute: *Living Well with the Sense of Smell.* Available at http://www.senseofsmell.org
21. Nasel C, et al: Functional imagining of effects of fragrances on the human brain after prolonged inhalation. *Chem Senses* 1994;19:359–364.
22. Barker S, et al: Improved performance on clerical tasks associated with administration of peppermint odor. *Percept Motor Skills* 2003;97:1007–1010.
23. Fox K: *The Smell Report.* The Social Issues Research Centre. Available at http://www.sirc.org/publik/smell_contents.html.
24. Frawley D, Ranade S, Lele A: *Ayurveda and Marma Therapy.* WI: Lotus Press, 2003.

REVIEW QUESTIONS

Multiple Choice

1. These compounds present in essential oils can be toxic to the living plant and so must be stored in specialized structures such as glands, ducts, scales, and hairs. These compounds are:
   a. Mostly terpenes
   b. Not chemical in nature
   c. Only found in flowers
   d. Mostly aldehydes

2. Aromatherapy is said to affect the mind, body, and spirit. Essential oils have a physiological effect on the body. How do they affect the mind and spirit?
   a. Through their effect on the limbic system after inhalation
   b. Through absorption of the oil into the bloodstream
   c. Through olfactory effects but only when paired with hypnosis
   d. Through the ability of black pepper oil to break addictive behaviors

3. Volatility is best described as:
   a. The ability to scent an area for a given period
   b. The ability to turn from a liquid to a gas at room temperature
   c. The ability to attract useful and needed insects to the plant
   d. The ability to defend the plant against microbial infection

4. Essential oils are described as:
   a. Chemically complex with from 100 to 400 or more chemicals present in the oil
   b. Chemically simple with three to five chemicals found in the oil
   c. Not chemical when they are in a natural form
   d. Chemically dangerous unless they are adjusted in a laboratory before sale to the public

5. Distilled essential oils smell:
   a. Just like the plant from which they have been extracted
   b. Burnt—distillation should not be used to produce essential oils
   c. Slightly different than the natural plant because some chemical compounds are lost during the distillation process
   d. Sweeter than the plant in its natural form

Fill in the Blank

6. In the process of extraction known as _____, essential oils are placed in a still and steam is used to burst the essential oil storage sites.

7. The therapeutic value of essential oils decreases with age, even under ideal storage conditions, mostly because of oxidation and the resulting chemical changes this causes. Replace essential oils if they have not been used within _____. Citrus oils should be replaced every _____.

8. When the potential unwanted side effects of one compound are decreased or eliminated by one or more other compounds present in an essential oil, it is referred to as _____.

9. Many factors affect the chemical composition and, therefore, the therapeutic value of an essential oil. Three of these factors are _____, _____, and _____ _____.

10. The human body seems to respond differently to natural oils than it does to synthetic oils. Synthetic oils often cause _____, _____, and _____.

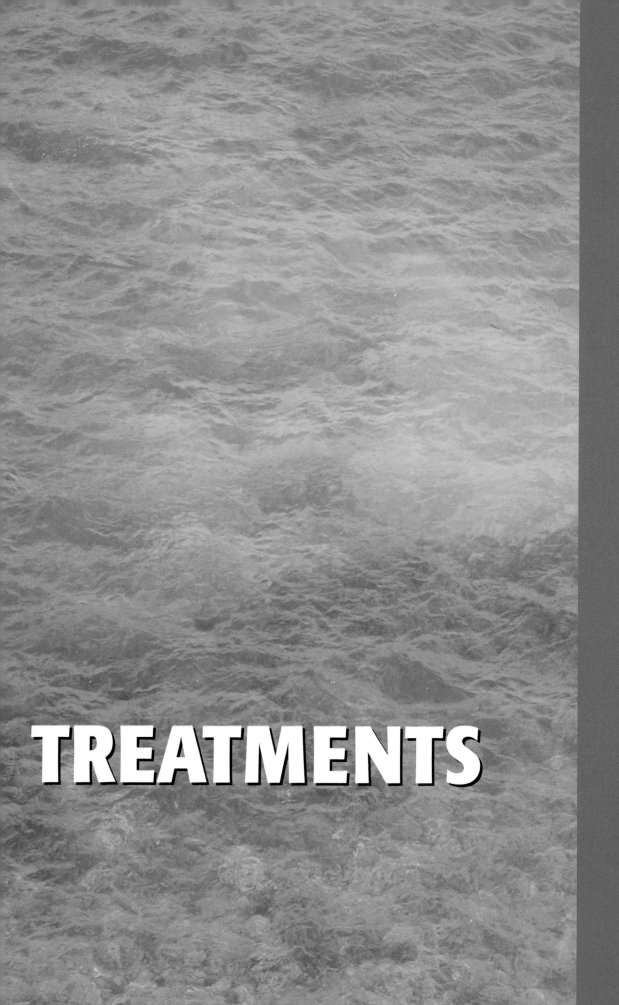

PART

two

TREATMENTS

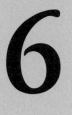

Exfoliation Treatments

Chapter Outline

Key Terms

Aura mist: An aromatherapy body mist that is used only at the very end of the treatment. It is misted in a high arch over the client from the head to the toes. It should be scented with an aroma that contrasts with the treatment products and fills the treatment room with a refreshing scent.

Dihydroxyacetone (DHA): The component in autotanning products that causes the skin cells to change color and appear tanned.

Dissolving exfoliants: Dissolving exfoliants are composed of alpha-hydroxy acids (AHAs) and beta-hydroxy acids (BHAs). AHAs include glycolic, citric, lactic, and malic acids. The most widely used BHA in cosmetics is salicylic acid or its related substances, sodium salicylate and willow extract.

Enzymatic exfoliation: Exfoliation that relies on biological action rather than physical abrasion. This type of exfoliation is applied to the skin and then rinsed off. The enzymes used dissolve keratin in the skin, thereby removing dead cells and supporting the natural process of exfoliation. Papain from papaya is an example of one of these enzymes.

Exfoliation: A process by which dead skin cells are removed to improve the skin texture and appearance. Benefits include increased circulation and lymph flow, increased immunity, and relaxation.

Mechanical exfoliation: A physical process in which the body is rubbed with an abrasive product or with a coarse handheld item such as a loofah.

Ultraviolet A (UVA) rays: Sometimes refered to as "aging rays," these rays from the sun penetrate deeper into the skin than ultraviolet B rays and cause photosensitivity reactions.

Ultraviolet B (UVB) rays: Also known as "burning rays, these rays from the sun are the primary rays associated with skin damage and cancer from the sun.

In a manual **exfoliation** treatment, the skin is polished, or scrubbed with a coarse-textured product that gently "sands" the skin's surface. This brightens the skin by removing the dull top layer of dead cells, deep cleanses the pores, and improves nutrient exchange. These actions are important for skin health and have other therapeutic benefits that work in synergy with massage. During an exfoliation treatment, blood and lymph flow are increased, immunity is enhanced, the vital energy of the body is improved, and the body is relaxed. This chapter describes the types of exfoliation treatments that are commonly used by massage therapists. It also provides a brief overview of other exfoliation treatments that are provided by estheticians and physicians in the spa industry.

Before delivering the treatments described in this chapter, the therapist may wish to review spa draping (see Chapter 3), herbal-infused towels (see Chapter 3), hot towel removal (see Chapter 3), and aromatherapy blending (see Chapter 5).

Types of Exfoliation Treatments

The two basic types of exfoliation are **mechanical exfoliation**, which is used by both massage therapists and estheticians, and **enzymatic** or **dissolving exfoliation**, which is used by estheticians or delivered only by physicians.

Mechanical exfoliants rely on the skin's being physically rubbed with a mildly abrasive exfoliation product or a coarse handheld item such as a loofah or cactus fiber cloth. Types of mechanical exfoliation include dry skin brushing, salt or sugar glows, body scrubs, friction, and body polish treatments.

Although the words *brush, scrub, glow, friction*, and *polish* are often used interchangeably, each of these words implies a type of product, implement, or the degree of abrasiveness in the treatment. The overview of manual exfoliation treatments provided in Table 6-1 helps spa therapists differentiate between these treatments.

The enzyme and dissolving exfoliants used by estheticians and physicians rely on their biological action

Table 6-1	Overview of Manual Exfoliation Treatments
Dry skin brushing	Dry skin brushing is a treatment in which the body is brushed to stimulate lymph and blood circulation, boost general immunity, increase the vital energy of the body, and desquamate dead skin cells. It is usually performed with natural bristle brushes, but rough hand mitts or terry cloths can also be used. This is a mild to moderate exfoliation treatment because only light pressure is used with the body brushes.
Wet skin brushing	Wet skin brushing is applied in the same manner as dry skin brushing except that the body is dampened with water, apple cider vinegar, or a foaming body shampoo before it is brushed.
Salt glow	In a salt glow treatment, a specialized salt is mixed with oil, body wash, water, apple cider vinegar, or other wet or oily product and applied to the body to stimulate circulation and lymph flow, smooth the skin, increase the vital energy of the body, or relax the body. The degree of vigor with which the therapist applies the strokes determines the abrasiveness of the treatment.
Sugar glow	A sugar glow treatment is less abrasive than a salt glow. Table sugar, brown sugar, or raw sugar is mixed with water, oil, milk, wine, or a body wash product and then applied to the body to increase circulation and lymph flow, relax the body, and smooth the skin.
Body polish	A body polish is different than a salt glow in that the exfoliation product is usually blended into an emollient base to protect the skin. A body polish often has a skin care focus, so the steps of the treatment follow those of a facial. This is the most relaxing and elegant of the manual exfoliation treatments, so stress reduction is often a primary treatment goal.
Body scrub or loofah scrub	As the name suggests, a body scrub is a vigorous and revitalizing treatment. A loofah mitt, rough hand mitts, or cactus fiber cloths are used with a foaming body wash to cleanse the skin, stimulate circulation and lymph flow, and rejuvenate the body.
Friction	In *Rational Hydrotherapy*, Kellogg[10] gives specific recommendations for the way that friction should be applied to a particular client for a specific physiological effect. For general purposes, a friction could best be described as a treatment in which the skin is rubbed in a back-and-forth motion with dry hands or with a wet lubricant such as apple cider vinegar or a body shampoo. Terry mitts or rough hand mitts may also be used with water at specific temperatures (e.g., cold mitt friction). The abrasiveness of a friction is based on the treatment goals of the individual service and the types of implements that are used.
Buff and bronze	A treatment that includes a full-body exfoliation, moisture massage, and the application of an autotanning product that leaves the client looking naturally tanned.

rather than simple physical abrasion. They are applied to the skin and then rinsed off. The enzymes used dissolve keratin in the skin, removing dead cells and supporting the natural process of exfoliation. These types of treatments are not described in this text because they are usually out of the scope of practice of massage therapists. Box 6-1 provides an overview of exfoliation treatments offered exclusively by estheticians or physicians in spas.

BOX 6-1
Broaden Your Understanding

Exfoliation Treatments Offered by Estheticians and Physicians in The Spa Industry

Ideally, all the therapists at a spa would have a working understanding of the different types of exfoliation treatments that are available. Massage therapists who understand the types of exfoliation treatments used by estheticians and physicians are better placed to advise clients on possible treatment options and can suggest appropriate providers for the client. The following exfoliation treatments are often seen in a spa but are not regularly performed by massage therapists.

Facial Exfoliation

A specially formulated product is used to exfoliate skin cells from delicate facial tissue. This treatment is usually part of a facial service.

Enzyme Exfoliation

An enzyme such as papain is applied to the skin, to dissolve keratin, and to remove dead and dulling skin cells. The product should not be rubbed in. Enzyme exfoliation treatments are most often used by estheticians in facial treatments but can also be used in full-body treatments.

Skin Peels

High concentrations of alpha hydroxy acids (AHAs), and beta hydroxy acids (BHAs) can be used to resurface the skin. Only estheticians with advanced training should use these products. Treatments should only be carried out under the supervision of a physician.

Chemical Peels

Chemical peel products include trichloroacetic acid or tretinoin (a vitamin A derivative) to decrease fine lines and wrinkles and "resurface" the skin. Chemical peels (known as chemo surgery) should be applied only by a physician.

Dermabrasion

Dermabrasion and dermaplaning help to "refinish" the skin's top layers. These treatments both involve a controlled surgical scraping and so should be performed only by a physician.

Microdermabrasion

Microdermabrasion is a nonsurgical procedure used by qualified estheticians. The skin is literally "sandblasted" with micro crystals of aluminum oxide to treat sun damage, wrinkles, hyperpigmentation, acne scarring, and stretch marks.

Laser Skin Treatments

Laser skin treatments use a carbon dioxide laser beam to remove layers of damaged skin. These treatments are commonly used for wrinkles, fine lines, scars, or uneven pigmentation. These treatments should only be performed by qualified, experienced physicians.

General Treatment Considerations

Therapists working in spas or massage clinics should check any scope of practice restrictions that may cover the exfoliation treatments that they wish to provide. They should also be aware of the individual client's overall skin condition and the dangers of overexfoliation.

SCOPE OF PRACTICE

Massage therapists in most (but not all) states must be careful not to encroach on the scope of practice for estheticians when they promote or deliver an exfoliation treatment. Massage therapists usually aim to increase circulation and lymph flow, decrease muscle tension, increase the vital energy of the body, and relax the body. A fair amount of soft tissue manipulation is usually included in the service to meet these treatment goals. To avoid problems, it is a good idea to highlight these body-oriented goals in the promotional description of the treatment rather than focus on the benefits of the treatment for the skin.

SKIN CONDITIONS

Exfoliation products should not be used on open wounds or broken skin, on clients with chronic skin conditions (unless recommended by a physician), on sunburned or inflamed skin, over varicose veins, or immediately after waxing or shaving. Using exfoliation products in these circumstances may cause irritation or complicate the condition.

OVEREXFOLIATION

The overuse of manual exfoliation products during a treatment can leave the skin sensitive and inflamed. If such products are used too frequently, the skin will start to thicken and grow leathery. Exfoliation treatments should not be given more than once a week for the best results.

Dry Skin Brushing

Dry skin brushing is a technique in which the skin and lymphatic system are stimulated with a natural bristle brush, rough hand mitts, or textured cloths. Dry skin brushing increases blood flow bringing fresh oxygen and nutrients to the skin, which helps the body to detoxify. The sebaceous glands are stimulated, and dead skin cells are removed to reveal the healthy new skin below. If dry skin brushes are used appropriately, lymphatic flow is increased to revitalize the body and boost immunity.

Dry brushing is a nice enhancer treatment before a full body massage. When the dry brushing is part of a spa treatment, each area can be brushed separately before applying the treatment product or the entire body can be brushed first before applying the spa product. When planning such a treatment, consider how many times the client will have to

turn over. The fewer times the client has to turn over, the more relaxing the treatment will be.

DRY SKIN BRUSHING TECHNIQUES

Use a natural fiber brush with very light pressure on dry skin, working from distal to proximal with rhythmic strokes. Although some claim that circular motions and figure eights are calming, dry brushing works best when it is done in brisk, straight lines with very light pressure directed toward the heart. Brushing techniques for each body area are described below and shown in Figure 6-1.

Posterior Legs

Undrape the first posterior leg and brush it with light, rhythmic strokes from the ankle to the knee. Overlap the strokes so that the entire area is covered. Brush from the knee to the hip across the top of the thigh with overlapping strokes. To brush the inner thigh, stand at the client's hip facing toward the foot of the table. Place both brushes on the medial aspect

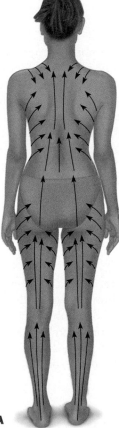

Back:
1. Side to center
2. Sacrum to mid-back
3. Mid-back to shoulders

Posterior leg:
1. Ankle to knee
2. Knee to hip
3. Medial thigh
4. Lateral thigh
5. Ankle to hip

A

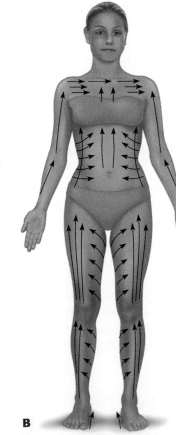

Chest area:
1. Navel to upper chest
2. Armpit to sternum
3. Upper chest

Anterior arms:
1. Fingers to elbow
2. Elbow to shoulder
3. Fingers to shoulder

Abdominal area:
1. Side to center
2. Hip to armpit

Anterior legs:
1. Medial leg
2. Ankle to knee
3. Knee to hip
4. Lateral leg
5. Ankle to hip

Feet:
1. Toes to heel

B

Figure 6-1 **Dry skin brushing techniques.**

of the thigh and pull them toward the outside of the leg in light, rhythmic strokes. To brush the lateral thigh, stand by the knee and run the brushes briskly up the iliotibial band to the hip. To finish dry brushing the posterior leg, brush from the ankle all the way up the leg with long, flushing strokes. Many therapists brush from the knee to the hip before they brush from the ankle to the knee. The reason for this is that they believe that brushing the proximal area first "clears and opens up" the lymph flow so that stagnation does not occur when the distal area is brushed.

The Back

Stand on one side of the client facing across the client's body. Place the brushes on the far side of the client and pull the brushes in light strokes toward the spine. Move around the table to the other side of the client in order to repeat the side brush. To dry brush the main area of the back, stand at the head of the table and begin the stroke at the sacrum, pulling the brush toward the client's head. To ensure that the strokes are rhythmic, only brush as far as the mid-back. Use a separate set of strokes from the mid-back to the shoulders.

Anterior Legs

When dry brushing the anterior legs, it is easiest to start with the medial leg by standing at the client's hip and facing toward the foot of the table. Start the strokes by the ankle and work up the leg. Each stroke runs from the medial side of the leg to the midline of the leg. To dry brush the top of the anterior leg, stand by the foot and brush upward toward the knee with light, overlapping strokes. The upper leg is brushed from the knee to the hip in straight, overlapping strokes. The lateral leg is brushed from the ankle to the knee along the peroneal muscles and from the knee to the hip along the iliotibial band. As with the posterior leg, some therapists prefer to brush from the knee to the hip before brushing from the ankle to the knee. To complete the anterior leg, brush from the ankle all the way to the hip with long, continuous strokes.

Abdominal Area

To brush the belly, stand to one side of the client and brush from the far side of the body toward the centerline. Brush the sides of the client from the hip into the armpit by standing at the head of the table and pulling the brushes upward in a straight line.

Chest

Stand at the head of the table and brush from below the navel, pulling in a straight line between the breasts with overlapping strokes. To avoid the breast drape, simply lift the brush and "jump" over it. Brush from the armpit up and around the breast, ending at the upper portion of the sternum. Again, "jump" the breast drape to keep the flow of the stroke. To finish the chest area, stand to one side of the massage table and brush across the upper chest from one shoulder to the other in a straight line.

Arms

Brush from the fingers to the elbow and from the elbow to the shoulder. Some therapists prefer to brush from the elbow to the shoulder before brushing from the fingers to the elbow. To complete the arms, use long strokes all the way from the fingers to the shoulder.

Feet

Brush the feet from the toes down to the heel. Brush firmly to avoid tickling the client, but if he or she is too ticklish to tolerate this, skip the feet and move on.

Sanitation

Before brushing the feet, check them carefully for fungal infections. If athlete's foot or any other contagious condition exists, skip the feet to avoid spreading the condition. When brushing the feet, wipe them first with a disposable antibacterial cloth such as a diaper wipe.

THE PROCEDURE

In the enhanced dry brushing treatment described below, an invigorating toning massage step, a herbal steam and the application of a lymphatic support lotion are added to the treatment. The addition of these simple enhancers creates a well-rounded and satisfying skin brushing service. For an overview of the treatment, review the dry skin brushing snapshot below and Figure 6-2.

Snapshot: Dry Skin Brushing

Indications
Sluggish circulation; poor lymph flow; low immunity; low energy; stress; to support a larger treatment aimed at detoxification; dull, congested skin; as preparation for application of a treatment product (the removal of dead skin cells supports product absorption)

Contraindications
Skin conditions, broken or inflamed skin, sunburn, high blood pressure, heart or circulatory conditions, illness or fever, lymphatic condition, cancer (except under the supervision of a physician), any condition contraindicated for massage

Supplies for the Treatment Table Setup
Massage sheet, blanket or bath sheet for warmth, bolster, warm packs as needed

Supplies for the Work Table Setup (for the Enhanced Procedure)
1) Dry brushes
2) Skin toner in a bottle with a flip-top lid
3) Soda cooler with nine herbal-infused towels
4) Lymphatic support lotion in a bottle with a flip-top lid or other finishing product
5) Aura mist

Basic Procedure
Dry brush the particular body area working from the distal area toward the heart. Begin on the posterior legs. Proceed to the gluteals and back; turn the client; and brush the anterior legs, belly, arms, and upper chest before brushing the feet.

Enhanced Procedure
1) Dry brush the particular body area working from the distal area toward the heart.
2) Apply a skin toner with a variety of massage strokes.
3) Steam the area with an herbal-infused towel.
4) Apply a lymphatic support lotion or seaweed gel to the area.
5) End the session with an aura mist of a contrasting scent.

Lymphatic Lotion Recipe
2 fl oz of plain unscented lotion, lavender essential oil (9 drops), grapefruit essential oil (15 drops), thyme essential oil (4 drops), juniper berry essential oil (2 drops)

Session Start

The client can begin the treatment in either a supine or a prone position because the order in which each area of the body is brushed is not fixed. In this particular procedure, the posterior legs, gluteals, back, and posterior arms are treated first. The client is then turned into the supine position so that his or her anterior legs, belly, upper chest, anterior arms, and feet are treated.

To start the service, place one hand on the client's sacrum and one hand on C7 and ask the client to take three slow, deep breaths. Deep breathing facilitates the flow of lymph. Next, undrape the first posterior leg and proceed with the treatment.

Step 1: Dry Brush the Area

Dry brush the particular area as described above under "Dry Skin Brushing Techniques." It is important to note that students learning dry skin brushing often make the mistake of brushing too hard. The lighter the brush strokes, the more effective the treatment in moving lymph and supporting detoxification.

Step 2: Toning Massage

Carefully pour skin toner into one hand from a bottle with a flip-top lid. Apply the toner to the client with massage strokes. Add more toner as needed until there is sufficient lubrication for massage. Most alcohol-free toners (avoid the use of products with alcohol because they dry the skin) contain glycerin, which makes them feel slippery and refreshing. Keep the toning massage brief because skin toners tend to be cooling, so the client may get cold if this step is carried on for too long.

Step 3: Application of a Steamy Herbal-Infused Towel

Remove a hot, moist, herbal-infused towel from the soda cooler and lay it over the body area that is being treated. Allow the towel to sit without touching it for up to 1 minute. To "activate" the towel and increase the client's perception of warmth, use compression strokes over the top of the towel. Remove the towel and blot the client dry with a soft hand towel.

Step 4: Application of a Finishing Product

In this treatment, a lymphatic support lotion is used as the finishing product, but seaweed gel, plain moisture lotion, or aloe vera gel may also be used. A lymphatic support lotion consists of a regular moisture lotion or gel product mixed with essential oils that support the lymphatic system (see the Snapshot for a recipe). Apply the lotion from the distal area to the proximal area with long, flushing strokes.

Session End

After each area of the body has been treated, end the service with a neck and face massage, a face steam, or a simple **aura mist**. Make sure to use an aroma that contrasts with the scent of the herbal towels and lymphatic lotion for the greatest olfactory impact.

Sanitation

At the end of the treatment, the dry skin brushes are washed in warm, soapy water and placed in alcohol for 20 minutes. They are allowed to air dry and then put back into a closed container. Because alcohol is very drying for the brushes, the brushes need to be replaced regularly.

The Salt or Sugar Glow

Salt and sugar glows are therapeutically useful because they increase circulation, stimulate lymph flow, increase the vital energy of the body, remove dead cells and impurities from the skin, and improve skin health. The role of minerals in

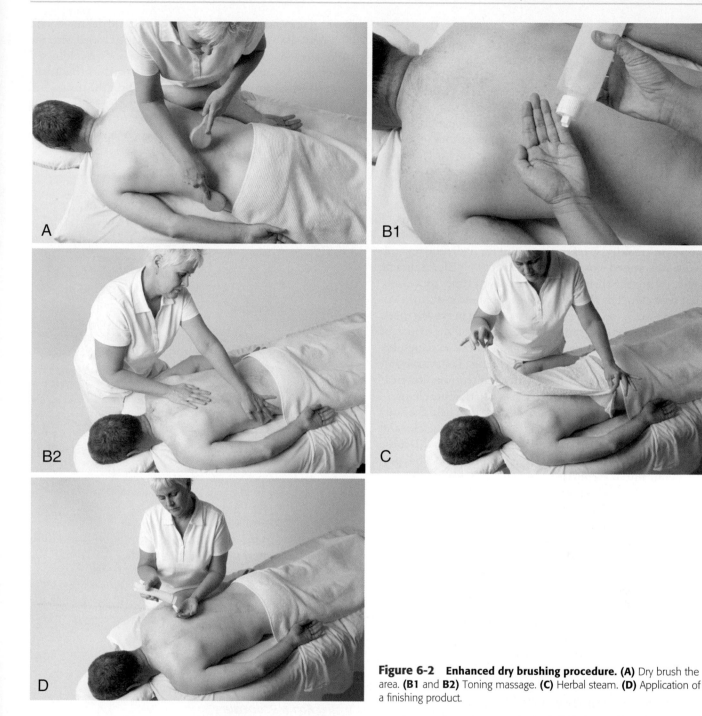

Figure 6-2 Enhanced dry brushing procedure. (A) Dry brush the area. **(B1** and **B2)** Toning massage. **(C)** Herbal steam. **(D)** Application of a finishing product.

healthy skin metabolism and body function is not fully understood. Minerals from Dead Sea salt and other salt deposits (e.g., Bearn salt from the Pyrenees Mountains in the South of France) are believed to help regulate some skin and certain body functions. In a study published in the International Journal of Cosmetic Science,[1] potassium from sea salt increased CO_2 transport, and calcium helped to regulate cell membrane permeability in the skin. Some minerals are hygroscopic (meaning that they attract water molecules), so they can be used to restore skin moisture, perhaps by increasing intercellular water capacity.

Of the many different types of salt that can be used for a salt glow, the least expensive and most readily available is ordinary sea salt, which is available at many local grocery stores. The most popular type of sea salt for spa treatments is Dead Sea salt.

The Dead Sea is an ancient landlocked sea whose water has been slowly evaporating over the centuries, producing a concentrated natural salt solution. After bathing in the Dead Sea, people often report a feeling of increased energy, well being, and special "baby-soft" skin. The main elements in Dead Sea water are chlorine, magnesium, sodium, calcium, potassium, and bromine.[1] These minerals are absorbed through the skin by bathing in the dissolved salts or by using a Dead Sea salt cosmetic preparation. In the study noted above, the skin smoothing effects of Dead Sea minerals in a cosmetic product were compared with the same cosmetic product containing no Dead Sea minerals. The control in the study, a plain gel with no active ingredients, showed an average decrease in skin roughness of only 10.4%, and the cosmetic product containing no Dead Sea minerals reduced roughness by 27.8%. The cosmetic product containing Dead Sea minerals reduced roughness by 40.7%.[1]

Bearn salt from springs in the Pyrenees Mountains of Southern France has well-known restorative and anti-stress properties, making it especially useful for hydrotherapy tub soaks. It is mined close to a small spa town called Salies de Bearn, where the thermal waters are seven times more salty than seawater. The thermal pool in the middle of town is a favorite place to soak tired feet after hiking in the Pyrenees. As early as the 16th century, the ladies of the court of Navarre would leave their chateaus to bathe in Salies, believing it would prevent premature aging. Today, the salt springs are still used to heal urinary infections, to treat arthritis, and for children with developmental problems.

Epson salts are inorganic mineral salts that help the body to detoxify. They are often used for sore, tired muscles and as a soaking agent for bruises, sprains, and strains. Because Epson salts are drying, they are best used on oily skin types.

Chemically, salt consists of 60.663% elemental chlorine (Cl^-) and 39.337% sodium (Na^+). Table salt is processed, so it contains higher levels of chlorine than other types of salt. The relatively high chlorine content of table salt can burn a client's skin, and this is the reason that it is not suitable for use in spa treatments. Sea salt and mineral salts are safer for spa use because they contain a wider range of minerals and proportionately less total chlorine; therefore, they are gentler, less irritating to the skin, and can be safely used in spa treatments.

Sugar is gentler than salt and has emollient and humectant (moisturizing) properties that leave the skin feeling soft and smooth. When dissolved, sugar can be applied to the skin as a "glaze" to soften, increase water content, and aid in healing. Brown sugar and table sugar are granular, so they can be used for exfoliation. Honey, molasses, and dissolved sugar are used as body glazes.

THE PROCEDURE

As with all spa treatments, there are a number of different delivery options for this service. Often a salt or sugar glow will be a quick 30-minute treatment that is used to prepare the body for another service. Sometimes the salt or sugar glow is given together with a Vichy shower to take advantage of the contrasting water temperatures, an equally important part of the treatment. The treatment described here is not traditional in its approach but will quickly gain popularity with clients. It is meant to be used in a dry room and delivered with a full-body massage. The massage step is intertwined with the salt or sugar step so that each part of the body is addressed separately. Because so much massage is used in this treatment, it takes from 60 to 90 minutes to deliver the treatment. For an overview of the treatment, review the salt or sugar glow snapshot and Figure 6-3. Table 6-2 describes different salt and sugar mixtures and various ways to apply the salt or sugar to the body.

 Snapshot: The Salt or Sugar Glow

Indications
Low energy; low immunity; sore muscles; sluggish circulation or lymph flow; stress; dull, rough skin; as preparation for the application of a treatment product in a larger service

Contraindications
Skin condition, inflamed skin, broken skin, high blood pressure, heart or circulatory condition, illness, fever, any condition contraindicated for massage

Supplies for the Treatment Table Setup (from the bottom to the top layer)
1) Plastic table protector
2) Bottom massage sheet
3) Bath towel (the weave of the bath towel will catch excess salt or sugar that falls off the client during the first half of the treatment; when the client turns over, the towel will prevent him or her from feeling the salt or sugar granules)
4) Top massage sheet
5) Blanket or bath sheet for warmth

Supplies for the Work Table Setup
1) Salt or sugar in a bowl or a cheese shaker
2) Massage oil or body wash gel for mixing up salt or sugar
3) Aroma mist or skin toner
4) Mist bottle or cosmetic sponges for applying aroma mist or toner
5) Finishing product (e.g., lotion, gel)
6) Soda cooler and hot moist towels
7) Bowl of warm water
8) Other items as needed for variations or enhancers (e.g., slippers, robe, foot soak, essential oils)

Dry Room Procedure
1) Massage the body area.
2) Apply salt or sugar and exfoliate the area.
3) Remove the salt or sugar with a hot towel.
4) Apply an aroma mist or skin toner.
5) Pat the area dry with a hand towel.
6) Apply a finishing lotion or gel.
7) Redrape the body area and move on to the next area.
8) At the end of the treatment, massage the neck and face then finish with an aura mist of a contrasting scent.

Wet Room Procedure
1) Begin on the posterior of the body.
2) Wet the body with warm water.

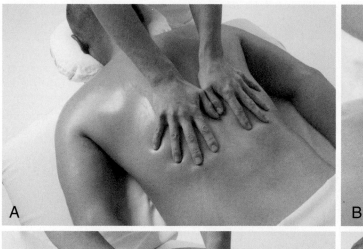

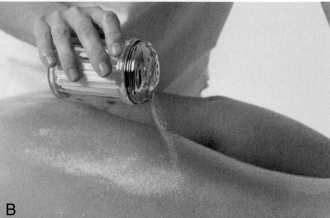

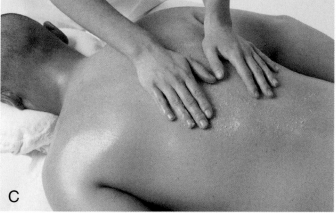

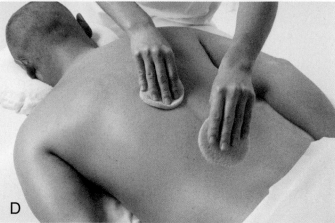

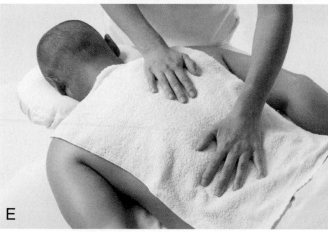

Figure 6-3   The salt or sugar glow. (A) Massage. Undrape the desired body area and apply massage oil with Swedish strokes. **(B)** Apply salt or sugar to the body with a shaker (the salt or sugar can be pre-mixed with oil or bath gel and applied by hand if preferred). **(C)** Exfoliation. Using gentle, superficial strokes rub the salt or sugar across the surface of the body. **(D)** Product removal. Remove the salt or sugar with a moist, hot towel and apply a skin toner to firm the skin and remove excess salt. **(E)** Redrape. Dry the area with a soft hand towel, redrape, move to the next body area, and repeat the same steps.

3) Apply salt or sugar in a bath gel.
4) Add warm water and exfoliate the posterior body.
5) Rinse the salt or sugar from the body.
6) Turn the client and repeat on the anterior body.
7) Dry the client and move him or her to a massage table.
8) Apply a finishing lotion or gel. Note: if a Vichy shower is used (instead of a handheld shower), the rinsing step can take up to 10 minutes.

Session Start

In a salt or sugar glow procedure, the client is bolstered in the same way as for a massage. The order in which each body area is addressed is not fixed, but it works well if the client starts in a prone position, beginning the treatment with the posterior legs and gluteals and progressing to the back. The client can then be turned into a supine position for the last half of the treatment while the anterior legs, feet, belly, upper chest, and arms are treated. The treatment ends with a neck and face massage.

Table 6-2	Salt and Sugar Mix Ups

SALT OR SUGAR SILK

Most often, salt or sugar is mixed with a fixed oil such as sunflower or sweet almond oil (a variety of fixed oils can be used) and then applied directly to the skin by hand. Therapists can choose from premixed products purchased through a spa supply outlet or can mix their own in house.

CREAM SILK	SWEET AND SILKY	SEA SILK
¼ cup Dead Sea salt, ¼ cup table sugar, 2 Tbsp milk powder, 1 Tbsp sweet almond or sunflower oil, and ¼ cup of body cream make a nice emollient salt or sugar glow mixture. Depending on the granule size of the salt, more or less lotion may be required.	½ cup table sugar, ¼ cup brown sugar, 1 Tbsp ground lavender powder, and 1 Tbsp aloe vera gel. Add sweet almond or sunflower oil to create a slightly runny paste or to achieve the consistency desired by the individual therapist.	½ cup Dead Sea salt, ¼ cup plain sea salt, 1 tsp seaweed powder, and 1 Tbsp aloe vera gel. Add sweet almond or sunflower oil to create a slightly runny paste or to achieve the consistency desired by the individual therapist.

SALT OR SUGAR FOAM

If the salt or sugar glow is delivered in a wet room with a Vichy, Swiss, standard, or handheld shower, a body wash gel makes a desirable base. The gel will turn to bubbles that are easily rinsed away, leaving the skin clean and smooth. The dry room option is to apply the salt or sugar with oil as noted above and then add foaming body wash over the top. The therapist places his or her hands in warm water and then uses the water to work the body wash into a lather. The therapist then removes the body wash, salt or sugar, and oil with one hot, moist towel and proceeds to the next body area.

FOAMY FLOWERS	FOAMY FRUITS	FOAMY AND FLIRTATIOUS
¼ cup plain body wash, ¼ cup brown sugar, 2 drops ylang ylang essential oil, 7 drops mandarin essential oil, and 5 drops lavender essential oil. The therapist may choose to add more or less sugar depending on the consistency desired.	¼ cup plain body wash, ¼ cup sea salt, 8 drops grapefruit, 6 drops lemon, and 1 drop peppermint essential oil. The therapist may choose to add more or less salt depending on the consistency desired.	¼ cup plain body wash, ¼ cup table sugar, 11 drops lime oil, 2 drops jasmine oil, and 2 drops rosemary oil. The therapist may choose to add more or less sugar depending on the consistency desired.

SALT OR SUGAR SHAKE-UP

Dry salt or sugar is stored in a cheese shaker and sprinkled on the body after it has been massaged generously with oil. This feels like cool raindrops falling onto the body. Extra oil is added as needed to provide adequate lubrication for the salt or sugar exfoliation.

SEA SHAKE	EARTH SHAKE	MILK SHAKE
Dead Sea salts mixed with 1 Tbsp seaweed powder stored in a cheese shaker	Table sugar with 1 Tbsp Sedona clay stored in a cheese shaker	Table sugar with ½ cup powdered milk stored in a cheese shaker

SALT OR SUGAR HAPPY HOUR

These mixtures are blended and applied directly to the skin as in the mixtures made with oil. The therapist first massages the client with a generous layer of oil so that there is sufficient lubrication for the exfoliation. The "happy hour" products are applied over the top of the oil, and then the entire mixture is removed with a hot moist towel.

SANGRIA	JAPANESE PLUMB	CHAMPAGNE SPARKLER
½ cup of table sugar, ¼ cup of red table wine, ¼ cup of orange juice, and 2 Tbsp of grapeseed oil. More sugar can be added at the discretion of the therapist.	½ cup of table sugar, ½ cup of Japanese plumb wine, and 2 Tbsp of sesame seed oil. More sugar can be added at the discretion of the therapist.	½ cup of table sugar, ½ cup of champagne, and 2 Tbsp of sunflower oil. More sugar can be added at the discretion of the therapist.

MARGARITA	CREAM DE COCO	SEA BREEZE
½ cup of finely granulated sea salt, 6 drops of lime essential oil, and sunflower oil to the consistency desired by the therapist	½ cup of table sugar, ½ cup of powdered cocoa, and sunflower oil to the consistency desired by the therapist	½ cup of finely granulated sea salt, ½ cup of cranberry juice, and 2 Tbsp of sunflower oil

Step 1: Massage

Undrape the desired body area and apply massage oil with Swedish strokes. The length of the massage step and the depth used will be determined by the therapist. Obviously a salt or sugar glow that is offered for 60 to 90 minutes will contain a longer massage, including a full range of strokes.

Step 2: Exfoliation

Be careful not to apply salt or sugar to a body area that is not well oiled because this may cause irritation to the skin and will feel abrasive to the client. After lubricating the area with massage oil, lightly sprinkle the salt or sugar onto the area with a cheese shaker or scoop it up from a bowl after it has been mixed with oil and apply it by hand. Avoid using too much salt or sugar because a very small amount gives good results. Also, be careful not to get the salt or sugar all over the massage table when sprinkling.

Work the salt or sugar across the top of the skin with gentle circular strokes to stimulate circulation and lymph flow and to remove dead skin cells. Massage therapists often overexfoliate because they tend to work into the muscle rather than keeping the strokes superficial. With coarse crystalline products such as salt, this can cause some discomfort to the client. It is advisable to check regularly if the client is happy with the depth of the application and the sensation of the exfoliation.

The salt or sugar often trickles off the client onto the bath towel underneath. Although this should be avoided as much as possible, there is no way to prevent some of the salt or sugar from falling off the client. If large amounts fall off the client, it may feel uncomfortable when the client is turned and has to lie on it. In this case, the therapist is probably using too much salt or sugar and not enough oil.

Step 3: Product Removal

Remove the salt or sugar mix with a hot towel. It should be possible to remove all of the salt or sugar using just one hand towel per body part.

Step 4: Aroma Mist or Skin Toner

Apply an aroma mist or skin toner to the area and then blot the skin dry with a soft, dry hand towel. Large facial sponges can also be used to apply skin toner directly to the skin.

Step 5: Application of a Finishing Product

Lotion, body cream, or a light gel product can be applied to the skin to lock in moisture and add to the overall effect of the treatment. Redrape the area and move on to the next body part.

Session End

After each area has been treated, massage the client's neck and face with a massage cream. This rounds out and completes the treatment. The session can end with an aura mist spritzed in a high arch above the client to fill the treatment room with a refreshing scent.

The Full-Body Polish

A full-body polish is usually delivered as a standalone service and involves an elegant four-step exfoliation process that focuses on skin care and deep relaxation. This treatment also increases circulation, stimulates lymph flow, removes dead skin cells, and cleanses and smoothes the skin's surface.

In a body polish, an exfoliation product, a cleanser, a toner, and a moisturizer are used separately in each step of the treatment to mimic the steps in a facial. Usually, the exfoliation product has a fine-textured ingredient such as mesh pumice that is suspended in a heavy emollient to protect the skin. This creates a softer sensation than a salt, sugar, or dry brush exfoliation. For this reason, a full-body polish is considered the more elegant and gentle of the exfoliation treatments.

The development of a well-considered treatment concept and smell-scape enhances the client's perception of this service and gives it a unique flare. For example, the Four Seasons Hotel and Spa[2] offers a crushed pearl and lavender polish, and the Ritz-Carlton Hotel and Spa[3] highlights the alpine berry body polish on their treatment menu. The sugar sand polish featured at the Beau Rivage Spa on the Mississippi's Gulf Coast uses the fine white sand found only on the Gulf's barrier islands.[4] Samasati Spa on the Caribbean Coast uses the refined sand from their beaches in an avocado and black sand body polish.[5] Each of these treatment names suggests a certain type of smell-scape that adds interest to the treatment. Matched products can be purchased from spa suppliers, or the therapist can create his or her own using essential oils.

THE PROCEDURE

As with the salt or sugar glow, the treatment described below was developed for massage therapists to use in a dry room. In a traditional body polish, massage would not normally be included as part of the treatment. This takes longer, but clients respond well to treatments that include an exceptional massage; therefore, aim to deliver this service in 60 to 75 minutes, depending on the length of the massage. It should be noted that in a traditional body polish, the cleanser step is always first (just as in a facial). In a dry room, it is helpful to exfoliate before using the cleanser because the cleanser helps to "lift" the fine-mesh exfoliant off the skin, leaving the skin smoother. The full-body polish snapshot and Figure 6-4 provide a quick overview of the service.

Snapshot: The Full-Body Polish

Indications

Dull, congested skin, stress, to facilitate relaxation, or as preparation for the application of a treatment product

Contraindications

Skin conditions, broken or inflamed skin, sunburn, high blood pressure, circulatory conditions, heart conditions, illness, fever, any condition contraindicated for massage

Supplies for the Treatment Table Setup (from the bottom to the top layer)

1) Plastic table protector
2) Bottom massage sheet
3) Bath towel (the bath towel will catch any excess moisture from the treatment, keeping the client drier)
4) Top massage sheet
5) Blanket or bath sheet for warmth

Supplies for the Work Table Setup

1) Bowl of warm water
2) Exfoliation gloves (optional)
3) Exfoliation product
4) Body wash product
5) Body mist or skin toner product
6) Rich moisture cream
7) Soda cooler
8) Hot, moist towels
9) Dry hand towel

Dry Room Procedure

For each body area:
1) Dampen the body area with warm water.
2) Apply the body polish product with bare hands or exfoliation gloves.
3) Apply the body wash product and work into a lather.
4) Remove the polish and body wash product with a hot, moist towel.
5) Apply aroma mist or skin toner.
6) Blot the area dry with a soft hand towel.
7) Apply rich body cream with massage strokes.
8) Redrape the area and move onto the next area.
9) Finish the service with a neck and face massage and an aura mist of a contrasting scent.

Wet Room Procedure

1) Wet the posterior body with the handheld shower and apply the body wash product.
2) Rinse off the cleanser with the handheld shower.
3) Apply body polish with the hands to the posterior body.
4) Rinse with the handheld shower (if a Vichy shower is used, the rinse step can be a 10-minute contrast shower).
5) Turn the client into the supine position and repeat steps 1 to 4 on the anterior body.
6) Move the client to a massage table covered with massage sheets.
7) Apply the toner to the posterior body and blot with a soft hand towel

8) Apply moisture lotion, cream, or gel with massage strokes to the posterior body.
9) Turn the client into the supine position.
10) Repeat steps 7 and 8 on the anterior body.
11) Provide a neck and face massage if desired.
12) Finish with an aura mist of a contrasting scent.

Session Start

In this procedure, each body area is treated in exactly the same way, so the sequence of body areas is not important. It works well to begin with the client in the prone position with the posterior legs, gluteals, and back and to then turn the client into the supine position for the anterior legs, feet, belly, upper chest, and arms. End the treatment with a neck and face massage and an aura mist to revitalize the client before he or she leaves the spa.

Step 1: Exfoliation

Wearing exfoliation gloves, the therapist places his or her hands in a bowl of warm water and lightly wets the body area that is being treated. Use the water sparingly. Do not allow droplets of water to roll down the sides of the client. Add a small amount of body polish to the gloves and use circular motions to manually exfoliate the area.

In a wet room setting, a Vichy or handheld shower would be used to rinse the product off. In a dry room, hot, moist towels are used to remove the product. To save on laundry, the exfoliation product is not removed before the cleansing step. Instead, the cleansing product is applied on top of the exfoliation product, and both products are removed with one towel.

Step 2: Cleansing

Apply a liquid or lotion-based cleanser to the body with the hands and work it into a gentle lather. Remove the product with a hot, moist towel. The body wash is used to "lift" exfoliant off the skin, leaving the skin smoother.

Step 3: Aroma Mist or Skin Toner

Apply an aroma mist with a spritz top or apply skin toner with large cotton pads or facial sponges. Blot the skin dry with a soft hand towel.

Step 4: Moisturize

If the moisturizing step is also the massage step, a heavy moisturizing cream works best. If massage is not part of the treatment, a light body milk, lotion, or gel product can be used.

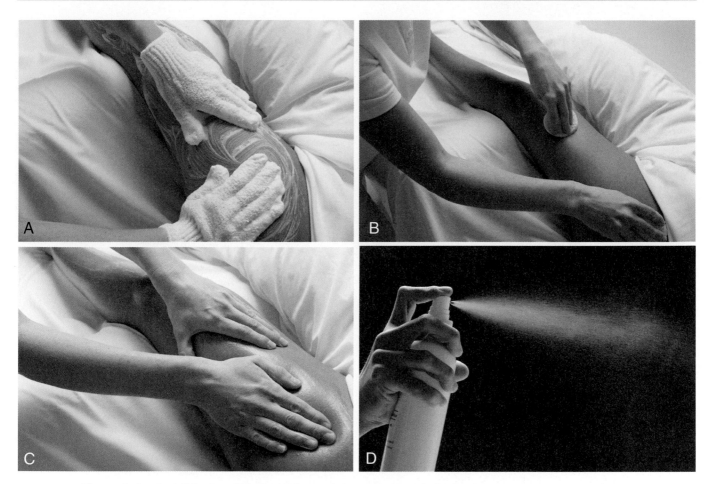

Figure 6-4   The full-body polish. (A) Exfoliate and cleanse. Dampen the body area with warm water and apply an emollient exfoliation cream. Textured exfoliation gloves can be worn if desired by the therapist. After the exfoliation is applied, cleanser helps to lift the exfoliation product off the skin, leaving the body feeling clean and smooth. Remove the cleanser and exfoliation product together in one step. **(B)** Tone. Apply a skin toner or aroma mist with cosmetic sponges or a mist bottle. Dry the skin with a soft, dry hand towel. **(C)** Moisturize. Use a heavy moisture cream if this will also be the massage step. If massage is not included a light lotion or gel can be used. **(D)** End the session with an aura mist.

Session End

If the treatment ends with the client in the supine position, a neck and face massage can be given as a closing step. End the session with an aura mist spritzed over the client in a high arch to fill the treatment room with a refreshing scent.

The Body or Loofah Scrub

The body or loofah scrub is the most invigorating and least formal of the exfoliation treatments. It is often paired with uplifting and refreshing smell-scapes such as eucalyptus or citrus and mint. Similar to the salt glow or body polish, the amount of massage that is provided with this service determines the amount of time required for delivery. Although this treatment is not described in step-by-step detail, the

loofah scrub snapshot and Figure 6-5 provide an overview of this service.

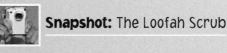

Snapshot: The Loofah Scrub

Indications

Low energy, to revitalize the body, to decrease stress, to smooth the skin and stimulate circulation and lymph flow, or as preparation for the application of a treatment product

Contraindications

Skin conditions, broken or inflamed skin, sunburn, high blood pressure, circulatory conditions, heart conditions, illness, fever, any condition contraindicated for massage

Supplies for the Treatment Table Setup (from the bottom to the top layer)

1) Plastic table protector
2) Bottom massage sheet

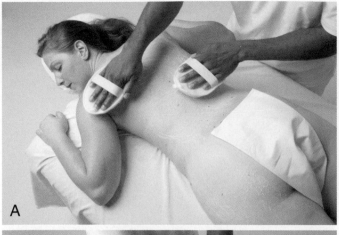

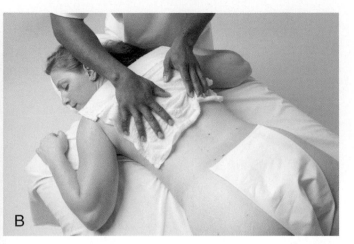

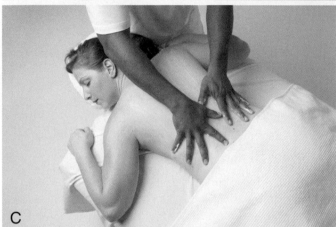

Figure 6-5   The loofah scrub. (A) Loofah scrub. Apply a foaming body wash with two handheld loofah mitts to the posterior body. Use a gluteal drape so that the entire area can be treated at once. **(B)** Remove. Use hot, moist towels to remove the foaming body wash from the posterior body and then dry the client with a hand towel. **(C)** Moisture massage. Redrape the posterior body with a sheet and massage moisture cream into each body area separately. Repeat the scrub on the anterior body using a breast drape and anterior pelvic drape.

3) Bath towel (the bath towel will catch any excess moisture from the treatment, keeping the client drier)
4) Top massage sheet
5) Blanket or bath sheet for warmth

Supplies for the Work Table Setup
1) Body wash product
2) Two loofah mitts
3) Bowl of warm water
3) Body mist or skin toner
4) Dry hand towel
5) Moisturizer

Dry Room Procedure
1) Use a gluteal drape so that the entire posterior body can be treated at one time.
2) Apply a foaming body wash with two handheld loofahs to the posterior body.
3) Apply a body mist or skin toner to each body area.
4) Redrape the body and massage each posterior area with a massage cream or moisturizing lotion.
5) Turn the client and repeat the steps on the anterior body.
6) Provide a neck and face massage if desired.
7) Finish with an aura mist of a contrasting scent.

Wet Room Procedure
1) Wet the posterior body with the handheld shower and apply the body wash product with two handheld loofahs.

2) Rinse the cleanser with the handheld shower (if a Vichy shower is used, the rinse step can be a 10-minute contrast shower).
5) Turn the client into the supine position and repeat steps 1 and 2 on the anterior body.
6) Move the client to a massage table set with massage sheets.
7) Apply the toner to the posterior body and blot with a soft hand towel.
8) Apply moisture lotion, cream, or gel with massage strokes to the posterior body.
9) Turn the client into the supine position.
10) Repeat steps 7 and 8 on the anterior body.
11) Provide a neck and face massage if desired.
12) Finish with an aura mist of a contrasting scent.

Sanitation

The handheld loofahs (approximately $2.00 each) should be thrown away or given to the client after each treatment. If facial sponges are used to apply the toner, these should also be discarded because they deteriorate when sanitized with alcohol.

The Buff and Bronze

As people became more aware of the dangers of natural tanning in the sun over the past few decades, tanning booths became popular because they were marketed as a healthier alternative. Tanning booths use mainly **ultraviolet A (UVA)** rays to cause pigment changes without burning. Because tanning booths are more or less **ultraviolet B (UVB)** free, it was thought that they were safe. As more research has been conducted, both UVA and UVB rays have been found to be implicated in skin damage, immune suppression,[6] premature aging,[7] and skin cancer.[8]

Artificial "sunless" tanning products provide an alternative to tanning booths. The professional products available through spa suppliers produce natural looking results that are safe for the skin and easy to maintain. Avoid over-the-counter products that are of lower quality and sometimes have an orange tint. Artificial tanning products can be applied in many different ways, including air brushing, buff and bronze spa treatments, and even in sunless tanning booths.

Although booths and air-brushing techniques are quick and effective, full-body buff and bronze treatments are effective and also relaxing and enjoyable to receive. All three types of application have linked home care products that help to generate more income for the spa or clinic. Buff and bronze treatments can also be used to attract male clientele, especially bodybuilders, who must look tan under the bright lights of the competition stage. Bodybuilders often shave their bodies, making application simple. With hairy men, the therapist should plan extra treatment time to work the product into the skin well.

Most of the sunless tanning products use the chemical interaction of **dihydroxyacetone (DHA)**, a sugar, with the amino acids in the dead skin cells in the upper layers of the skin. The chemical interaction causes the cells to change color, leaving the skin golden brown until the skin cells naturally slough off.[9] Although the rate at which skin cells slough off varies from person to person, sunless tans usually start to fade in about 3 days, and the product needs to be reapplied.

THE PROCEDURE

Clients should shave or remove unwanted hair from the body the evening before the treatment. Exfoliation is usually not performed on freshly shaved or waxed skin. For this reason, only a gentle, fine-mesh product should be used in this treatment. If shaving or waxing takes place after the treatment, it will streak the autotanner, even if the tan has already developed. Usually, an exfoliation product is sold with the autotanning product and a specific type of moisturizer to make product planning easy for the therapist.

Autotanning products stain clothing and the palms of the therapist's hands, so it is best to wear vinyl gloves. An apron and beige or dark-colored treatment sheets can be purchased to protect both bedding and clothing from staining. The buff and bronze snapshot and Figure 6-6 provides an overview of this service.

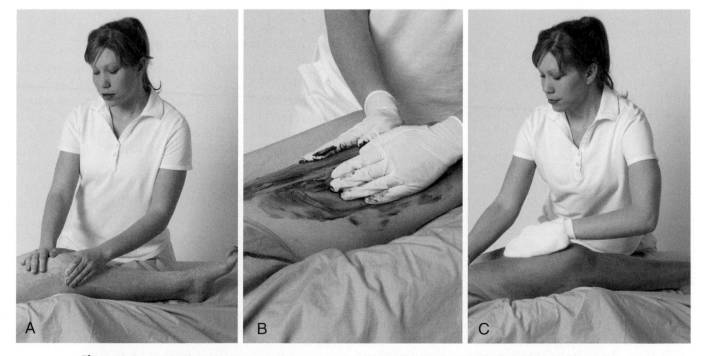

Figure 6-6   The buff and bronze. (A) Exfoliate, cleanse, and moisturize all anterior body areas and then turn the client to the pone position to repeat these steps on the posterior body. Apply moisturizer liberally to each area until the client is evenly moisturized. **(B)** Apply autotanning product to the posterior body areas, allow the client to air dry, and buff the posterior body. Turn the client and repeat these steps on the anterior body. **(C)** Buff. Lightly buff fleshy body areas such as the abdominal area. The knees, ankles, elbows, and wrists can be buffed more vigorously.

Snapshot: The Buff and Bronze

Indications

For cosmetic purposes to hide skin discolorations, to appear tan while protecting the skin from the sun, relaxation

Contraindications

Broken skin, inflamed skin, sunburned skin, allergies to DHA, heart or circulatory condition, illness, fever, any condition contraindicated for massage

Supplies for the Treatment Table Setup (from the bottom to the top layer)

1) Beige or dark massage sheet
2) Bath towel
3) Top massage sheet
4) A warming device such as a heat lamp because the client will air dry and may become cold if warming is not planned

Supplies for the Work Table Setup

1) Bowl of warm water
2) Exfoliation product
3) Body wash product
4) Moisturizing product
5) Autotanning product
6) Vinyl gloves
7) Buffing mitts
8) Soda cooler
9) Hot, moist towels

Dry Room Procedure

The client should be in the supine position. Each area is treated with the same series of steps before moving on to the next body area.

1) Exfoliate the area.
2) Cleanse the area.
3) Remove both products with a hot towel.
4) Apply moisturizer (do not apply autotanning product to the anterior body yet).
5) Turn the client prone and repeat steps 1 to 4 on the posterior body.
6) Apply the autotanning product to the posterior body areas.
7) Allow the product to air dry.
8) Buff the posterior body.
9) Turn the client back into the supine position.
10) Apply more moisture lotion if the skin feels dry.
11) Apply the autotanning product to the anterior body areas.
12) Allow the client to air dry.
13) Buff the anterior body.

Session Start

The client is positioned in the supine position. The anterior body is exfoliated, and then the client is turned for exfoliation of the posterior body. On the posterior side, the moisturizing and bronzing steps are carried out right after the exfoliation. The client is then turned over again so that the moisturizing and bronzing steps can be completed on the anterior side of the body. This prevents the wet exfoliation from streaking the bronzing product and allows the client to finish the treatment face up.

If the client has extremely dry or "patchy" skin with some very dry areas, apply a cold pressed oil such as sunflower or sweet almond oil to the body before the rest of the treatment. This conditions and softens the skin. When the exfoliation product and cleanser are used in their normal sequence, they will remove the excess oil and not affect the autotanner.

In some clinics, the therapist has the client perform the exfoliation step themselves. In this case, the therapist takes the client to the shower and shows the client how the product should be applied. After the shower, the client is moved to a treatment table and proceeds with the moisturizing and autotanning steps. When clients do the exfoliation themselves, this cuts the treatment time by about 20 minutes. Another option is for the therapist to apply the exfoliation product to the entire body, remove it with a Vichy or handheld shower, and then move the client to a massage table for the rest of the service.

Step 1: Exfoliate the Anterior Body

Bolster the client in the supine position and exfoliate the legs, belly, and arms by wetting the hands and applying a generous amount of exfoliant to the area. Pay special attention to the areas around the ankles, knees, elbows, and wrists. The arm can be lifted to expose the armpit and the side of the body. This area is often overlooked and should be carefully addressed with all of the products.

Step 2: Cleanse the Anterior Body

Apply a foaming cleanser over the top of the exfoliation product and work it into a lather with warm water. Remove both with a hot towel.

Step 3: Moisturize the Anterior Body

Apply the moisturizer to anterior areas, paying particular attention to the elbows, knees, ankles, and wrists. If the moisturizer soaks in quickly, apply the moisturizer a second time so that the skin is soft and evenly moisturized. Do not apply the autotanning product at this stage because water or moisture from the posterior exfoliation would streak it. Turn the client and bolster him or her in the prone position.

Step 4: Exfoliate the Posterior Body

Apply warm water and a generous amount of exfoliant to the posterior legs, gluteals, back, and posterior arms. Pay special attention to the wrists, elbows, ankles, and back of the neck.

Step 5: Cleanse the Posterior Body

Apply a foaming cleanser over the top of the exfoliation product and work it into lather with warm water. Remove both with a hot towel.

Step 6: Moisturize the Posterior Body

Apply the moisturizer to any dry areas first such as elbows, knees, ankles, and wrists. Use enough moisturizer to completely hydrate the area. If it absorbs into the skin quickly and dries out, apply a second coat so that the skin feels soft, silky, and evenly moisturized. Apply moisturizer in this way to the entire posterior body.

Step 7: Autotanning Application to the Posterior Body

Apply the autotanning product evenly over the posterior of the body. Rub it in a little, but not completely. Excessive rubbing when the product is first applied may rub away some of the tan. Leave the autotanning product in a slightly moist state and allow it to absorb into the skin.

It is a good idea to turn up the lights while the autotanning product is being applied. Most autotanning products have a brown tint added to make it easier to see where the product has been applied, but it is still difficult to see the product clearly in a dark treatment room.

Step 8: Buff the Posterior

The autotanning product should only be buffed after it has absorbed into the skin and had time to air dry. To "buff" an area, simply place a buffing mitt on each hand and use circular motions to gently smooth the product. The buffing should be light and even. It is important not to overbuff the client by rubbing too hard with the mitts. The mitts are meant to smooth out any areas where product may have absorbed unevenly. Pay particular attention to areas such as the elbows, knees, ankles, and wrists. When the posterior body has been buffed, turn the client and proceed with the moisturizing, autotanning, and buffing steps on the anterior body.

Step 9: Remoisturize the Anterior Body

If the body still feels moisturized, proceed with the autotanning step. If it has dried out, apply a second layer of moisturizer to the anterior body.

Step 10: Autotanning Application to the Anterior Body

Apply the autotanning product evenly over the anterior of the body and allow the product to air dry to prevent streaking during buffing.

Step 11: Buff the Anterior Body

Lightly buff the anterior body, making sure to buff across any lines where product application was overlapping. Buff into the elbows, knees, ankles, and wrists carefully to prevent streaking in these tricky areas.

Tricky Places

Feet and Hands   Do not apply autotanning product to the bottoms of the feet or the palms of the hands because it would look strange and out of place. Apply a small amount of product across the top of the feet (do not work it in between the toes) and the top of the hands (do not work it in between the fingers). Use a damp tissue to remove product from the nails and edges of the cuticles immediately after the feet and hands have been covered.

Ankles, Wrists, and Knees   If these areas have been adequately moisturized, they should tan evenly. Light applications of autotanning product are better than heavy applications. Heavy applications tend to discolor the area because dry patches turn darker. Buff the ankles, wrists, and knees into the surrounding tissues for the best results. Although the "fleshier" areas of the body such as the belly and arms should not be overbuffed, areas such as the ankles or knees, where the skin tends to be dry or wrinkled, need to be buffed well. This will create a smooth look and prevent these areas from absorbing excess product and appearing darker than the main areas of the body.

Underarms   Lift the arm and sweep the product across the underarm and smoothly down the sides of the body to avoid a white streak. Use the buffing mitts to smooth the transition zone between the anterior and posterior sides of the body. The underarms should have been shaved if necessary the evening before the treatment takes place. Autotanning product does not develop when it is applied over top of antiperspirants or deodorants, so the underarms should be cleansed before application.

Face   Apply a small amount of autotanning product to the face after the skin has been well moisturized. Work in upward strokes from under the chin to the forehead. Make sure to work the product into the earlobes and sides of the face down the neck to avoid uneven coverage. Make sure to apply product to the back of the neck and behind the ears to avoid uneven coverage if the client chooses to wear the hair up. Some products look streaky as they dry. This is normal, and they will look fine within 3 hours when the tan starts to emerge.

HOME CARE AND RETAIL

To keep the tan looking natural or to darken the tan to a deeper shade, clients can purchase home care tanning products from the clinic or spa. Instruct the client to moisturize daily to keep the tan looking smooth. Every 3 days, reapply autotanning product to maintain the desired color. The body should receive a gentle exfoliation before the moisturizer and autotanning product are applied. If the product tends to streak when the client applies it at home, tell him or her to exfoliate in the morning and apply the autotanning product in the evening before bed. Often clients exfoliate too aggressively, which causes the skin to absorb the product unevenly.

For a darker tan, the client should apply the autotanning product 3 nights in a row or until the tan is the desired shade. The client can apply the product as often as every 3 hours. The client should not exfoliate before each of these applications if they take place on the days after the initial treatment. If the client waits 2 to 3 days before using the home care product, he or she should exfoliate on the first day but not on the second and third days.

SAMPLE TREATMENTS

Ocean Pearl Polish

Promotional Description

Release yourself to the siren's song with this refreshing treatment that smoothes and purifies the body by using healing benefits from the sea. Your body is buffed to the translucency of a fine pearl with a combination of seaweed gel and sea salts. Next, bubbles fragrant as Atlantic air deeply cleanse and remove impurities before hydrating sea milk is applied with relaxing massage strokes. Your body shimmers and is renewed and balanced by this relaxing "journey to the deep."

Treatment Outline

Follow the treatment steps for a full-body polish.

Product Notes

Seaweed products are popular and easy to find through spa supply outlets. Check the resources at the end of the book for specific suppliers or review the sample treatment section of Chapter 10 for product ideas.

Zen Glow

Promotional Description

This lava luscious treatment combines heated volcanic stones, Chinese herbs, mineral salts, and the fragrant oils of mandarin, sweet ginger, ylang ylang, and lemon. The warmth of the stones releases muscle tension while the skin is polished to a radiant glow. Think tranquility!

Treatment Outline

Add 10 medium basalt stones to a heating unit and heat them in water to 120° to 135°F (the water is 120° to 135°F; the stones are cooler). Pull two hot stones from the heating unit and use them to warm the muscle tissue with effleurage strokes in the massage step of the salt or sugar glow procedure described above. Place the stones back in the roaster after use to reheat them for the next body area. Review Chapter 12 for more information. Products for in-house formulation are outlined below. Pre-blended products that are suitable for this treatment can be purchased from spa supply companies (see sources listed at the back of the book).

In-House Products for the Zen Glow

Zen Massage Oil

1 fl oz sunflower oil, mandarin essential oil (7 drops), lemon oil (5 drops), ylang ylang oil (2 drops) CO_2 ginger oil (1 drop). CO_2-produced ginger smells sweeter than steam distilled ginger and provides a better base note for this particular smell-scape.

Zen Body Mist

1 oz purified water in a spritz bottle, sandalwood oil (8 drops), gardenia (or ylang ylang) oil (2 drops), lemongrass oil (1 drop), turmeric oil (4 drops)

Zen Finishing Gel

2 fl oz of aloe vera gel, mandarin (8 drops), patchouli (1 drop), tagetes (1 drop), sandalwood (5 drops)

Wine and Roses

Promotional Description

Spoil yourself with an afternoon of wine and roses that leave your body replete with moisture and deeply relaxed. Cane sugar, red wine, and olive oil are slathered over the body to revitalize and to prepare the way for a dewy application of damask flower water. A light Swedish massage with Victorian rose cream completes the indulgence.

Treatment Outline

Treatment steps differ slightly from the basic salt or sugar glow steps.

1. Exfoliate (sugar, wine, and grapeseed oil are pre-mixed).

2. Remove with hot rosemary towels.

3. Mist with rose flower water.

4. Blot dry with a towel.

5. Massage with a heavy cream. Rosemary towels are discussed in Chapter 3.

In-House Products for the Wine and Roses Glow

Wine and Roses Scrub

1 cup cane sugar, 1/4 cup red wine, 1 Tbs extra virgin olive oil

Damask Flower Water

Purchase a damask rose (species *Rosa x damascena*) hydrosol (flower water) from an essential oil distributor and store it in the refrigerator between uses.

Victorian Rose Cream

2 fl oz unscented body cream or a professional vitamin C cream, rose oil (6 drops). Alternative blend: Rose oil (2 drops), violet leaf oil (8 drops), lavender oil (13 drops), clary sage oil (5 drops), black pepper oil (1 drop).

Solar Glow

Promotional Description

You want a glowing tan—AND you want to protect your skin from the sun. The solar glow body treatment is the answer. Your skin is polished to satiny smoothness and drenched in moisture-rich creams before an expert application of a professional autobronzing product. No orange finish here. This treatment will leave you shimmering in radiant gold.

Treatment Outline

Follow the buff and bronze procedure.

Summary

In an exfoliation treatment, the skin is polished manually or by using an enzymatic or dissolving product. Mechanical exfoliation can be performed by a massage therapist to stimulate lymph flow, increase circulation, boost immunity, address low energy, and relax the body. Enzymatic or dissolving exfoliants are used by either an esthetician or physician to dissolve keratin in the skin, which removes dead skin cells and decreases the appearance of fine lines and wrinkles.

Massage therapists often deliver exfoliation treatments, including dry skin brushing, salt or sugar glows, body polishes, body scrubs, and buff and bronze treatments. The most appropriate choice of exfoliation treatment depends on the particular set of treatment goals. Salt glows and body scrubs are more vigorous than body polish or dry skin brushing treatments. Some treatments aim to revitalize and energize the body, and others aim to help the body relax. Exfoliation treatments can be viewed as standalone treatments or as the first step in another treatment such as a body wrap.

REFERENCES

1. Ma'or Z, Yehuda S: Skin smoothing effects of Dead Sea minerals: comparative profilometric evaluation of skin surface. *International Journal of Cosmetic Science* 1997;19:105–110.
2. The Crushed Pearl and Lavender Polish at the Four Seasons Hotel and Spa. Available at http://www.fourseasons.com
3. The Alpine Berry Body Polish at the Ritz-Carlton Hotel and Spa. Available at http://www.ritzcarlton.com
4. The Sugar Sand Polish and Magnolia Massage at the Beau Rivage Spa. Available at http://www.veaurivage.com
5. The Avocado and Black Sand Body Polish at the Samasati Spa. Available at http://www.samasati.com
6. Ullrich SE, Kripke ML, Ananthaswamy HN: Mechanisms underlying UV-induced immune suppression: implications for sunscreen design. *Exp Dermatol* 2002;11:13–16.
7. Wang SQ, et al: Ultraviolet A and melanoma: a review. *J Am Acad Dermatol* 2003;48:464–465.
8. Krutmann J: Ultraviolet A radiation-induced biological effects in human skin: Relevance for photoaging and photodermatosis. *J Dermatol Sci* 2000;23(suppl):22–26.
9. Kunin A: *Sunless tanners. Derma doctor.* Available at http://www.dermadoctor.com/pages/newsletter239.asp?WID=57BA13B66D0-C4E8-4E24
10. Kellogg JH: *Rational Hydrotherapy*, 2nd ed. Philadelphia, F.A. Davis Company, 1903.

REVIEW QUESTIONS

Multiple Choice

1. There are two basic types of exfoliation. These are:
   a. Assisted and releasing
   b. Cleansing and scraping
   c. Mechanical and enzymatic or dissolving
   d. Biological and assisted

2. Because of scope of practice restrictions in most states, massage therapists cannot generally:
   a. Cleanse the face or feet.
   b. Cleanse, exfoliate, or mask the face.
   c. Use salt or sugar.
   d. Apply any exfoliation treatment.

3. Exfoliation treatments are indicated for the following situations:
   a. Skin disorders
   b. Freshly shaved skin
   c. Increased lymph flow and circulation
   d. Sunburn

4. When using salt or sugar as the exfoliation product, the massage therapist should:
   a. Use light pressure and not work into the muscle tissue.
   b. Use deep pressure and work into the muscle tissue.
   c. Use only circular compressions.
   d. Use only those strokes that are directed proximal to distal.

Fill in the Blank

5. Name three conditions that are contraindicated for an exfoliation treatment: _____, _____, _____

6. _____ salt should not be used in spa treatments because it will burn the client, cause skin irritation, and lead to extreme dryness. Sea salt and Epson salt are much safer.

7. The overuse of exfoliation products can leave the skin sensitive and inflamed. Over time, they can make the skin look _____.

8. Chemical peels can only be applied by a _____.

9. Microdermabrasion is a nonsurgical procedure used by qualified _____. The skin in literally "sandblasted" with micro crystals to treat skin conditions.

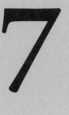

Body Wraps

Chapter Outline

Key Terms

Claustrophobia: The fear of being enclosed in narrow spaces.

Cryogenic products: A product that cools the body area to which it is applied.

Emollient: A substance that softens the skin by slowing the evaporation of water.

Fomentek: A type of water bottle that is designed to lie flat on the massage table.

Interferons: Proteins secreted by some cells that protects them (and other cells) from viral infection.

Poultice: Usually a cloth filled with heated herbs, clay, or a medicated product spread on a cloth and applied to wounds or an injury.

Body wraps could be considered as the earliest known "spa treatment." The ancient Egyptians used body wraps when they embalmed bodies using herbs, resins, and spices. This practice preserved body tissues and prevented degradation and decay. Emollient wraps in modern-day spas have the same aim: to fortify the skin and prevent premature aging. Many soft tissue conditions can benefit from wraps aimed at decreasing chronic holding patterns, stimulating circulation and lymphatic flow, or by simply relaxing the body and providing time for reflection. Today, a wide variety of body wraps are used for cosmetic purposes or to treat conditions such as rheumatism, low immunity, fatigue, and muscular aches and pains.

There are numerous ways to perform a body wrap, and as with any spa treatment, the therapist can mix and match methods to best meet treatment goals. It is helpful to understand three different wrapping procedures: the hot sheet wrap, the "cocoon," and the tension wrap. It is important to point out that the words *hot sheet wrap* and *cocoon* are used to differentiate two distinct procedures. This is a device to provide clarity and not meant to suggest that the word *wrap* always means a hot sheet wrap and the word *cocoon* always means that the product is applied directly to the body. The words *wrap*, *cocoon*, *swathe*, *envelopment*, and *envelope* can all be used freely at the discretion of the therapist to describe any type of wrap.

The types of products that can be used in hot sheet wraps and cocoons are limited only by the imagination. Table 7-1 gives a brief description of some different treatments that are currently offered in the spa industry. Table 7-2 provides an overview of some of the products that can be used with each type of wrap. As the reader can see, the products are often the same. The difference is in the way the product is prepared and the method that is used to wrap the client.

Before delivering the treatments described in this chapter, the therapist may wish to review basic dry room equipment (Chapter 2), spa draping (Chapter 3), client positioning for product application (Chapter 3), dry room and wet room removal techniques (Chapter 3), and exfoliation techniques (Chapter 6).

General Treatment Considerations

Before delivering any type of body wrap, a careful pretreatment health interview must be carried out with the client to make sure that there are no contraindications for the

Table 7-1	Sample Body Wrap Treatments	
SPA	**TREATMENT NAME**	**TREATMENT DESCRIPTION**
Double Eagle Resort and Spa, June Lake, CA[5]	DeVine Grapeseed Mud Therm	In this treatment, the body is dry brushed before grape seed enriched–mud is layered on the skin. This spa uses a piece of equipment called a Hydro Therm, a combined steam cabinet and Vichy shower, to enhance their service. The mud is steamed to facilitate product absorption, and then the Vichy shower rinses the mud away. The treatment concludes with the application of a grapeseed lotion.
Sonnenalp Resort, Vail, CO[6]	Swiss Paraffin Dip	This service begins with a dry brush treatment and is followed by the application of body milk (light lotion). The paraffin is layered over the body milk, and then the client is wrapped in thermal blankets.
Chateau Elan at St. Andrews Bay, Scotland[7]	Papaya A Peel	The Papaya A Peel begins with an exfoliation that uses Caribbean Sea sand and freshly mashed papaya. The body is then wrapped in a combination of coconut and yogurt.
Grand Geneva Resort and Spa, Lake Geneva, WI[8]	Ocean Essence Body Wrap	This wrap uses a seawater gel that is warmed and mixed with essential oils of lavender, ylang ylang, sandalwood, basil, and sage. The service ends with a 30-minute massage.
Lake Austin Spa Resort, Austin, TX[9]	Babassu Butter Wrap	In this 40-minute treatment, the client receives an aromatherapy steam followed by a sugar exfoliation. Babassu butter (*Orbignya phalerata*) from the Amazon is applied to the skin before the body is wrapped. A face and scalp massage complete the service.
Lake Tahoe Resort and Spa, Incline Village, NV[10]	Mountain Rain Herbal Wrap	This treatment consists of a classic herbal hot sheet wrap and aromatherapy massage.

| Table 7-2 | Hot Sheet Wraps and Cocoons |

HOT SHEET WRAPS			COCOONS		
Herbal	Coffee	Seaweed	Emollient	Aloe	Essential oil
Mud	Clay	Peat	Paraffin	Vitamin	Seaweed
Milk	Honey	Cider	Mud	Clay	Peat
Juice	Other		Mint	Cryogenic	Other
INDICATIONS FOR HOT SHEET WRAPS			**INDICATIONS FOR COCOONS**		
Detoxifying	Slimming	Firming	Detoxifying	Slimming	Firming
Cellulite	Skin focus	Sore muscle	Cellulite	Skin focus	Sore muscle
Revitalizing	Immune boosting	Weight loss	Relaxing	Revitalizing	Immune boosting

treatment. The therapist should also be aware of problems that might arise during this particular type of spa treatment.

CONTRAINDICATED INDIVIDUALS

Very hot wraps, very cold wraps, and wraps that result in an aggressive detoxification should not be used on children, elderly individuals, pregnant women, or those with a heart condition or high blood pressure. Hot wraps are contraindicated for those who have recently been in a car accident, suffered a soft tissue injury, have rheumatoid arthritis, have a fever (unless under the supervision of a medical doctor), or are contraindicated for massage. With wraps that use hot or cold temperature extremes, check that the client does not have any nerve damage that may interfere with his or her ability to sense hot or cold. These types of wraps increase the load on the cardiovascular system and kidneys and may aggravate an existing condition. For example, clients with impaired circulation or those with advanced or poorly treated diabetes should not receive hot or cold wraps. Tension wraps are contraindicated for individuals with spider veins, varicose veins or weakened veins or arteries, and poor circulation.

HEALING CRISIS

Wraps may trigger a rapid detoxification of the body, which may result in a headache and nausea. It is normal for a client to experience mild detoxification symptoms. However, if the symptoms are intense or if they occur during the wrap itself, remove the client from the wrap and encourage him or her to drink water and to rest at a comfortable temperature. If the client's symptoms persist after he or she is unwrapped or if the symptoms get worse rapidly, the client could be in danger, and the therapist should consult a physician or call the emergency services.

ALLERGIES OR SENSITIVE SKIN

Carefully check for allergies to herbs, essential oils, iodine (which is present in seaweed), and other ingredients in the products being used, especially with hot sheet wraps. Heat increases the irritation potential of any product being applied. Individuals with sensitive or thin skin often experience skin irritation with hot sheet wraps and are better treated with cooler cocoons.

MODESTY

In a hot sheet wrap, the client should be wearing disposable undergarments or an old swimsuit so that they are always covered. During the wrap procedure, the client will need to lie down on top of the hot sheet quickly after it has been unfolded by the therapist. To maintain modesty, the client will wear the robe over the undergarments up until the moment they get onto the treatment table.

WHEN THE WRAP GOES WRONG

Like any spa treatment, hot sheet wraps, cocoons, and tension wraps require practice, but even experienced therapists have days when the wrap goes wrong. For example, if the therapist cuts the plastic sheeting too short, while trying to wrap it around the client, there may be a gap. The best practice in this case is to cover the gap with two bath towels and keep going with the treatment. If the hot sheet wrap turns cold before the client is wrapped, continue to wrap the client and then place a hot pack under the feet and turn up the heat in the room as high as possible. If the hot sheet wrap is so cold that the client is uncomfortable, the therapist has two options. The first is to start again by reheating the wrap sheet and the client. The second is to offer an alternative treatment and give the client a gift certificate.

CLAUSTROPHOBIA

Even clients who have no previous experience with **claustrophobia** can become anxious or panic stricken when wrapped up as tightly as they are in a hot wrap. It is recommended that the therapist remains with the client at all times in order to remove the wrapping if the client becomes anxious. Watch for signs of distress such as rapid breathing or a concerned expression on the client's face. As a compromise, the client can be wrapped with their arms outside the sheets and blankets, but this will result in heat loss, which may reduce the effectiveness of the wrap.

WRAPPING MATERIALS

In a hot sheet wrap, the therapist can choose to use two wrap sheets (both cotton, cotton and linen, cotton and muslin, or cotton and fleece) or a wrap sheet and a bath towel. A bath towel is handy because it can be unfolded very quickly, so it does not get cold before the client is wrapped. The only concern with the bath towel is that it is difficult to wring out completely, so it may have very hot pockets that could potentially burn the client. If a towel is used for the hot wrap, the therapist should purchase cheap, very thin towels rather than thick, plush towels. Thinner towels wring out more easily, so they are safer. Flannel sheets are also difficult to wring out completely, so their use is not advised.

The Hot Sheet Wrap

In a hot sheet wrap, the treatment product (e.g., herbs, coffee, milk, honey, seaweed, mud) is dissolved in hot water. Two sheets (or a sheet and a bath towel) are steeped in the dissolved product and then wrapped around the client. This method is often used for detoxification treatments or when the goal is to stimulate metabolism as part of a weight loss program, to decrease water retention, or to boost immunity.

Hot sheet wraps elevate body temperature, creating an "artificial fever" that accelerates detoxification and decreases water retention through perspiration. Fevers commonly occur during infection and inflammation. They are part of a natural healing response that intensifies the production of **interferons**, inhibits the growth of some microbes, and speeds up chemical reactions involved in cell and tissue repair. Fever also increases the heart rate, which speeds up the delivery of white blood cells and oxygen to body tissues. At the same time, antibody production and T-cell proliferation increase, further boosting immunity. Despite the name, cold sheet wraps are hot wraps, and they create the same response in the body as hot wraps. The cold sheet "shocks" the body, which tries to quickly warm itself. This burst of warming body heat gets trapped inside the heavy wrap materials, causing increased perspiration and detoxification. In a cold sheet wrap, the client should already be perspiring when wrapped in the ice-cold sheet. The client is "preheated" in a sauna, hot shower, hot bath, hydrotherapy tub, steam cabinet, steam room, or by carrying out some sort of aerobic activity. If the client is not hot enough when wrapped in the cold sheet, the body cannot usually get warm enough to perspire, so the purpose of the wrap will not be achieved.

TYPES

There are many different types of products that can be used in a hot sheet wrap procedure. Common hot sheet wraps include herbal body wraps; coffee wraps; seaweed, mud, clay, or peat wraps; milk and honey wraps; and cider or juice wraps.

The Herbal Body Wrap

The herbal body wrap dates back to early medical practices in which herbs were applied to the body in a **poultice** to heal disease. Many ancient healing traditions, including those of the Romans, Chinese, Native Americans, and Indians, used herbs as medicine to decrease "toxins" or "evil humors" in the body. Today, these treatments are marketed to jump start a diet, support an internal cleansing regimen, decrease pain and stiffness in muscles, decrease water retention, aid in a weight loss program, slim the contours of the body, or to rid the body of specific chemicals while breaking an addiction (e.g., to nicotine).

In preparation for this service, the appropriate herbs are placed in a muslin bag and soaked in hot water (165°F) to make a strong "tea." Usually, about 1 cup of dried herbs is used per treatment (steeped in approximately 16 quarts of water). Table 7-3 provides some combinations of herbs for different treatment goals. Premixed herbs are available from spa suppliers.

The Coffee Wrap

Coffee wraps have been used for some time in spa treatments to firm tissue and decrease water retention. Coffee has the same pH as the skin and is useful for evening out the skin's texture and tone. A recent study conducted at Rutgers University by Conney[1] found that caffeine lowers the risk of skin cancer in mice when it is applied topically. A second compound (EGCG) found in green tea was also tested. This study has prompted the use of coffee and green tea as ingredients in after-sun products.

In preparation for a coffee hot wrap, 3/4 cup of finely ground coffee is placed in a muslin bag and soaked in approximately 17 quarts of hot water for 20 minutes. For a coffee and green tea wrap, 1/2 cup finely ground coffee and 1/2 cup of green tea leaves give good results.

Table 7-3	Herbal Combinations for Hot Sheet Wraps		
DETOXIFICATION	**SORE MUSCLES AND JOINTS**	**SKIN SOOTHING**	**SLIMMING**
Rosemary	Eucalyptus	Red clover	Juniper
Juniper	Juniper	Lavender	Lemon peel
Clove	Peppermint	Chamomile	Thyme
Allspice	Ginger root	Calendula petal	Fennel seeds
Ginger root	Clove	Oatmeal (powdered)	Ginger root
Echinacea	Agrimony	Borage	Dulse
Goldenrod	Bay laurel leaves	Chickweed	Horsetail
Lemon peel	Nettle	Comfrey	Kelp powder
Nettle	Pine needles	Elder flower	Parsley
Parsley	Thyme	Rose petal	Raspberry leaf
Sage	Wintergreen	Feverfew	Yarrow
	Yarrow		

The Seaweed, Mud, Clay, or Peat Hot Sheet Wrap

Seaweed powder, mud, clay, or peat can be dissolved in hot water and then used in a hot wrap. Add 1 Tbsp of powdered seaweed to approximately 17 quarts of hot water during the setup for a hot wrap. If mud, clay, or peat is used as the hot wrap product, 1 cup is dissolved in approximately 17 quarts of hot water (stronger concentrations can be used if desired). Before delivering a seaweed or mud treatment, it is helpful to review the contraindications for these products in Chapters 9 and 10.

Sanitation

Used herbs, coffee, clay, or mud should not be put down a standard drain after the treatment. Over time, these items can block the drain or damage the pipes. Filter the water out using a strainer and throw the solid matter away separately.

The Milk and Honey Hot Sheet Wrap

Milk, buttermilk, full-fat milk, and honey can also be used as a hot wrap product. This fragrant mix is deeply relaxing and softens and smoothes the skin. One to 2 cups of honey and 2 to 4 cups of powdered milk or regular milk are dissolved in approximately 15 to 16 quarts of water for this hot wrap (the concentration of the mix is up to the therapist).

The Cider or Juice Hot Wrap

Hot cider or juices such as orange, cranberry, or pineapple can be used in a hot wrap to brighten the skin's appearance, firm tissue, stimulate circulation, relax the body, and stimulate lymph flow. At Christmas time, cider and honey mixed with wine mulling spices make a deliciously aromatic seasonal hot wrap. One gallon of either juice or cider is mixed with one gallon of water and heated to 165°F.

THE PROCEDURE

Dissolve the products chosen for the hot wrap in hot water (165°F) in either an 18-quart roaster oven or a hydrocollator. Fold the wrap sheets into tight squares (directions for folding are given in Fig. 7-1) and place them in the product solution (while it is heating in the roaster oven or hydrocollator) for 20 minutes. A stone or weight placed on top of the sheets keeps them submerged completely. The water must be hot enough for the sheets to be pulled out of the heating unit, wrung out, stored in a cooler, and then unfolded on the treatment table without becoming cold. If a cold sheet wrap is being used, place the sheet and towel in a bucket of ice water for 10 minutes.

It is helpful to set up the massage table at a lower height so that it is easy for the client to climb onto the table and lie down on top of the hot sheet. If the therapist is going to deliver a full-body massage after the wrap, the table should be higher to minimize physical stress. In this case, the client should get onto the table using a small step stool.

A basic hot sheet wrap takes approximately 20 to 30 minutes to deliver. This does not include the preheating phase,

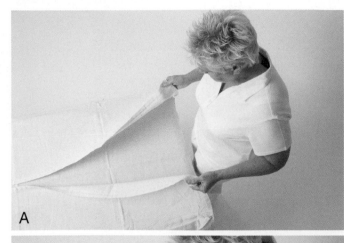

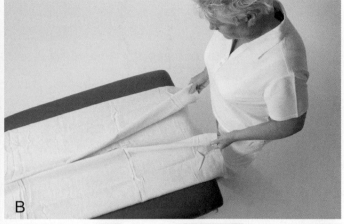

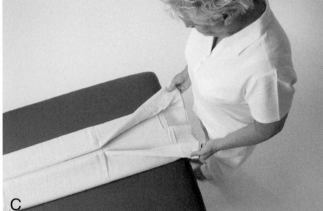

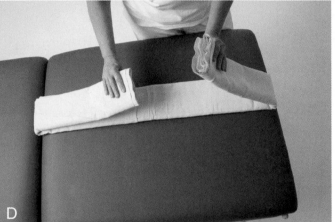

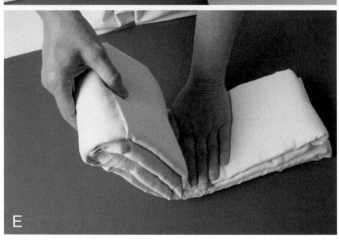

Figure 7-1   Folding a wrap sheet. (A) Open the sheet lengthwise across the width of the massage table and fold the long sides into the center. **(B** and **C)** Fold the two new sides into the center until the sheet is long and narrow. **(D** and **E)** Fold the ends of the long, narrow strip into the middle until the sheet is square.

which takes up to 20 minutes beforehand. For this reason, a hot wrap is often given together with other treatments or enhancers to create a more rounded and fulfilling service. To enhance the treatment, depending on the equipment available, the client could be dry brushed on a wet table and a Vichy shower could be used as the heating phase just before the client is wrapped. Another idea is to give the client a refreshing body scrub at the end of the wrap to help him or her cool down and to remove the impurities released during the wrap. A toning massage (delivered with skin toner and not oil) could be given before the wrap or a moisture massage could be given after the wrap. For an overview of

the basic treatment, see the hot sheet wrap snapshot and Figure 7-3.

 Snapshot: Hot Sheet Wrap

Indications
Detoxification; internal cleansing regimens; slimming; low immunity; low energy; water retention; to help with the treatment of an addiction (e.g., nicotine, sugar, soda); sore, tight muscles; certain skin conditions; to promote weight loss

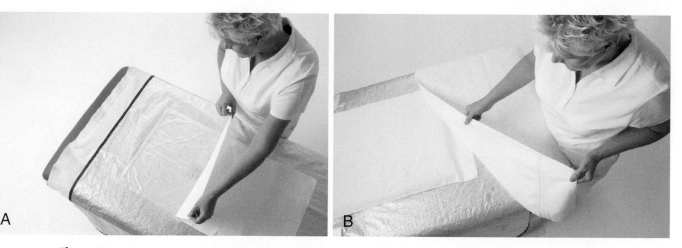

Figure 7-2   Massage table setup for a hot wrap. (A) The massage table is set from outermost layer to innermost layer as follows: wool blanket, thermal space blanket (shiny side up), and Fomentek (covered by a pillowcase). The hot sheet will be unfolded on top of the thermal space blanket (and Fomentek) directly before the client gets on the table and is wrapped up. **(B)** A bath towel is placed lengthwise over the edges of the blankets on each end of the table. One of these bath towels will be used to wrap up the head and the other to wrap up the feet.

Contraindications

Heart condition, high blood pressure, pregnancy, vascular condition, neurological condition, illness or fever, acute condition, inflammatory condition, weakened condition, children, elderly individuals

Supplies for the Treatment Table Setup (from the bottom to the top layer)

1) Wool blanket placed horizontally so that the long edges fall off either side of the treatment table
2) Thermal space blanket placed horizontally
3) **Fomentek** hot water bottle
4) Pillow case to cover the Fomentek
5) One bath towel placed horizontally at the top of the treatment table
6) One bath towel placed horizontally at the bottom of the treatment table.

The table setup is shown in Figure 7-2.

Supplies Needed for a Dry Room Treatment

1) Insulated gloves
2) Soda cooler
3) Wrap sheets soaking in dissolved product in a heating unit
4) Foot soak container filled with warm water
5) Comfortable chair
6) Warm neck pillow (optional)
7) Warm pack for the feet
8) Robe and washable slippers
9) Warm herbal tea
10) Glass of water with a flexible straw
11) Disposable undergarments
12) Aroma mist

Dry Room Procedure

1) Foot soak and warm herbal tea
2) Hot sheet wrap
3) Process in the wrap

4) Unwrap
5) Session end (massage, body scrub, cool shower, and so on)

Facility with Sauna or Soaking Tub Procedure

1) Sauna or hot immersion for 15 minutes
2) Hot sheet wrap
3) Process in the wrap
4) Unwrap
5) Session end (massage, body scrub, cool shower, and so on)

Session Start

Ask the client to change into a robe, slippers, and disposable undergarments in the room where the treatment will end (so that the clothing is close by). The robe and slippers allow the client to move about the spa in comfort. Escort the client to a sauna, steam room, or wet room for step 1 of the service if such facilities are available. If step 1 (i.e., increased core body temperature) takes place in a dry room with a foot bath, the robe makes it easy for the client to soak his or her feet and still keep warm.

Sanitation

It is important for clients to wear disposable or washable slippers when they move about the spa or clinic to avoid cross-contamination with fungal infections. Robes and washable slippers must be freshly washed and dried (with heat) for each client.

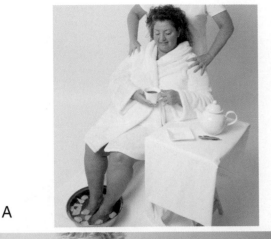

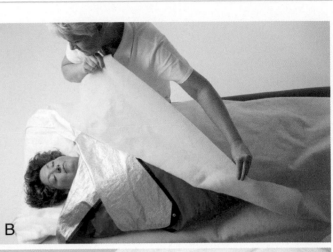

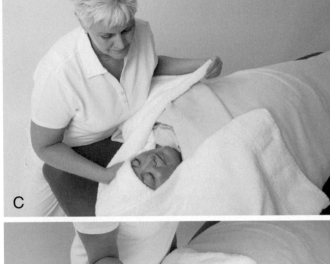

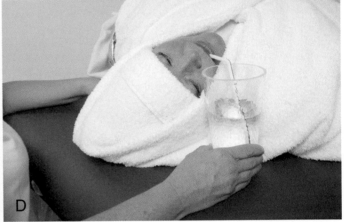

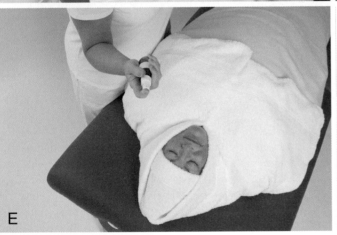

Figure 7-3   The hot sheet wrap. (A) Increase core body temperature. In a dry room setting, a warm foot bath and cup of herbal tea are used to increase the client's core body temperature. A sauna, steam room, warm bath, or hot shower can also be used. **(B)** The wrap. The sheet is wrapped around the client, and the infused bath towel is placed on top of the sheet before the thermal blanket and wool blanket are brought up and around the client. The therapist must work quickly to trap the maximum amount of heat. **(C)** The wrap. The towel at the top of the table is brought up around the client's head. The second bath towel is wrapped around the feet, and a hot water bottle or hydrotherapy pack is placed under the feet for additional warmth. **(D)** The processing phase. Water is offered through a straw during the processing phase of the wrap. **(E)** Aroma mist. The client is regularly misted with a soft, refreshing scent during the wrap phase of the treatment.

Step 1: Increase Core Body Temperature

The therapist can elevate the client's core body temperature in a number of ways. For example, the client can sit in a sauna or steam cabinet; soak in a warm hydrotherapy or standard soaking tub; receive a Vichy, Swiss, or Scotch hose treatment; take a hot shower; or rest sipping warm tea while soaking his or her feet in a tub of warm water. If a foot soak is used as the preheating method, it is helpful to ask the client to drink a cup of warm (not hot) herbal tea while relaxing. Hot tea must cool down, so the client will often leave it instead of drinking it. Warm flax seed

packs or corn packs can be placed around the client's shoulders, and a heat lamp can be used to further heat the body. The goal is to get the client to perspire slightly before being wrapped, especially if the goal of the treatment is detoxification.

It is important to note that some clients will not perspire. They will feel warm throughout the treatment but never hot. This can happen even if the therapist does every step of the wrap correctly and efficiently. The hot sheet wrap is still relaxing, even if perspiration and, therefore, detoxification are minimal.

Step 2: Final Preparation for the Wrap

The table is set up with the wrap blankets and a Fomentek hot water bottle before the treatment. While the client is soaking his or her feet, remove the sheets from the hot water solution. Using heavy, insulated gloves, wring out the sheets (or sheet and bath towel) as quickly as possible and place them in the cooler. If possible, the client should not see the therapist wring out the sheets with thermal gloves. The use of thermal gloves makes clients think that the sheet will be too hot, so they hesitate when they get on the treatment table. This hesitation results in a loss of valuable heat.

Take the client's feet out of the foot bath and dry with a towel. The client should stand on one side of the treatment table, and the therapist should stand on the other side. It is a good idea to describe the procedure to the client so that he or she knows what to do at each stage of the treatment. When both the client and therapist are ready, the hot sheet is removed from the cooler and unfolded as quickly as possible on the massage table. It is placed horizontally so that the long edges can be brought up around the client.

Step 3: The Wrap

The client removes the robe (the client is also wearing disposable undergarments) and places him- or herself in the supine position on the massage table while the therapist, holding the sheet on one side, looks away to preserve the client's modesty. Clients often find that the sheet feels too hot on their gluteals, so it is a good idea to put a hand towel on the sheet where the gluteals will rest before the client gets on the treatment table. Men often find that the sheet is too hot on their genitals (disposable undergarments are very thin). To solve this problem, the male client can hold a hand towel in front of his genitals so that this area is insulated when the sheet is wrapped over him.

The therapist quickly wraps the first hot sheet around the client and then pulls the second hot sheet (or towel) from the cooler and lays this on top of the first hot sheet. The second sheet is only unfolded as much as needed to completely cover the top of the client. Next, the space blanket and then the wool blanket are tucked around the client. This wrap works best if it is fairly tight and snug. The towel at the top of the table is brought up around the client's head in a "turban drape" to lock body heat inside the wrap. The second bath towel is wrapped around the feet, and a hot pack (e.g., flax seed, hydrocollator, rice, hot water bottle) is placed under the feet for additional warmth. After the client has been wrapped, a bolster can be placed under the knees (outside the wrap blanket). Throughout the wrapping process, the therapist needs to move quickly and efficiently to trap the maximum amount of body heat.

Step 4: Process

The client usually starts to perspire within 5 minutes of being wrapped up. The client may continue to perspire freely throughout the treatment. An aroma mist can be spritzed high over the client's face at various points during the wrap. This cools and calms the client. The face can also be dabbed with a cool cloth if desired. Water is offered through a flexible straw every 3 to 5 minutes during the wrap. The flexible straw allows the client to sip water without lifting the head. It is important that the therapist stays with the client at all times to provide support and remove the client immediately from the wrap if he or she becomes claustrophobic.

Step 5: Unwrap

At the end of the wrap (the standard wrap time is between 20 and 30 minutes), the outer blankets and towels are removed, leaving one sheet loosely draped around the client. When the client is ready, he or she can sit up and slip back into the robe. Help the client from the table and offer a seat. Once seated, the client can sip cool water and dry off with a hand towel. With most infused or dissolved wrap products, the client will not feel sticky or unclean after the treatment.

Session End

The treatment can end in a number of different ways. In the dry room option described above, the client is moved to a chair to sip water and cool down. While the client is cooling down, put clean massage sheets on the treatment table. After the client is back on the table, massage him or her with a light cream or gel. A gel-based product works well because it feels velvety and cooling to the client, who may still be hot and perspiring slightly. Alternatively, a refreshing body scrub or body shampoo can be offered to remove the impurities released during the wrap. If a wet room is available, a graduated shower or cold plunge can be used to end the service. In all cases, the client is asked to drink plenty of water for the rest of the day to rehydrate and ensure that the detoxification continues.

Sanitation

The thermal space blanket is often overlooked in the clean-up process. Perspiration can soak through the wrap sheet and contaminate the space blanket. Spritz the inside of the space blanket with alcohol and let it air dry before it is folded and returned to a closed cabinet.

The Cocoon

In a cocoon, the wrap product is not dissolved in water but is applied directly to the client before the client is wrapped in plastic and a blanket. Although this type of wrap might still be used for detoxification and slimming treatments (e.g., seaweed, paraffin), the client does not need to perspire for the wrap to work well. Sometimes this wrap procedure is used with a product that aims to cool the body tissues (e.g., a sunburn wrap). In this case, the body is wrapped lightly in plastic to allow air to circulate around the client.

In a cocoon procedure, the body is almost always exfoliated before the treatment product is applied (except in a sunburn wrap because exfoliation is contraindicated for sunburned skin). The removal of dead skin cells increases the absorption of the product into the skin.

TYPES

Many different types of product are used in cocoons. Cocoons can be based on an emollient product, aromatherapy products, paraffin or Parafango, cellulite or firming products, vitamins, aloe vera, cryogenic products, seaweed, mud, clay, peat, or other natural elements. Some cocoon products are shown in Figure 7-4.

Treatment outlines for cocoons based on each of these products are given below. Unlike the hot sheet wrap there is a wide degree of variability in the way a cocoon might be delivered or enhanced. These outlines are just samples and are not meant to suggest that this is the only way to do a particular treatment.

Emollient Cocoon

Emollient cocoons make use of the healing qualities of medium to heavy lipids such as shea butter, almond butter, evening primrose, wheat germ, jojoba, hemp seed, and borage oil to revitalize the skin, increase the skin's moisture content, and provide a moisture barrier. Emollient cocoons are often enhanced by adding essential oils that give the treatment a wider range of benefits. Hemp seed oil (*Cannabis sativa* L.) is of special interest to massage therapists because of its anti-inflammatory and pain-relieving qualities. When used in a cocoon, it is good for sore muscles and soft tissue conditions such as fibromyalgia and chronic pain. It degrades easily, so it must be stored in a refrigerator at all times.

Shea butter comes from the nut of *Vitellaria paradoxa* (synonym: *Butyrospermum parkii*), a tree found only in the semi-arid Sahel region of West Africa and Cameroon. Shea nuts have traditionally been processed and used by women in West Africa to protect their skin from drying out in the hot African sun. As the demand for shea butter increases, international and local nongovernmental organizations are starting to provide funding for modern processing equipment, which has led to the availability of high quality shea butter in the United States.

Pure shea butter has a firm texture and must be slowly warmed in a double boiler until it is a liquid before it is applied to the body with a brush and left to absorb. Excess shea can be massaged into the skin at the end of the service. Alternatively, the shea is warmed until it is a liquid and then

essential oils and a small amount of a fixed oil such as wheat germ are added. The warm shea mixture is then whipped in a blender as it cools so that it has a frothy texture when applied to the body. Shea butter is composed mainly of triglycerides and linoleic acid. It is high in vitamins A, E, and F. It has antioxidant, anti-inflammatory, anti-arthritic, skin soothing, skin healing, and skin moisturizing properties, and it is believed to bring relief from chronic skin diseases, scarring, and stretch marks. It is finding its way into many hair care products because a small amount revitalizes dry, damaged hair.

An emollient cocoon using shea butter might be delivered as follows:

1. Exfoliate.
2. Brush warm melted shea onto the body.
3. Cocoon.
4. Unwrap.
5. Perform a full-body massage using excess shea as the lubricant.

If the spa or clinic has a steam canopy, the shea emollient cocoon can be delivered as:

1. Exfoliate.
2. Perform a full-body massage with whipped shea butter and essential oils.
3. Place a steam canopy over the client and steam the shea for 15 minutes.
4. Blot the client dry with a hand towel.

Aromatherapy Cocoon

An aromatherapy cocoon can be offered as a standalone service using premade blends or as a more comprehensive service that includes a professional aromatherapy consultation, custom blending session, massage, and wrap. The oils may be chosen for their physiological effects (i.e., detoxify the body, stimulate lymph flow, warm muscle tissue) or for their effects on the mind and spirit. The goal is to provide a space where the body and mind can rest, be still, and reflect while surrounded by inspiring and uplifting fragrances. Essential oils can be mixed into a number of different carrier products, including seaweed, clay, shea butter, and aloe vera gel. Aromatherapy and blending are covered in detail in Chapter 5. A sample aromatherapy cocoon outline might be delivered as follows:

1. Aromatherapy consultation
2. Custom blend
3. Dry brush exfoliation
4. Massage with essential oils in a massage cream
5. Application of steamy aroma-infused towels to the anterior body
6. Cocoon
7. Firming face massage while the client is cocooned
8. Unwrap
9. Aura mist to end the session

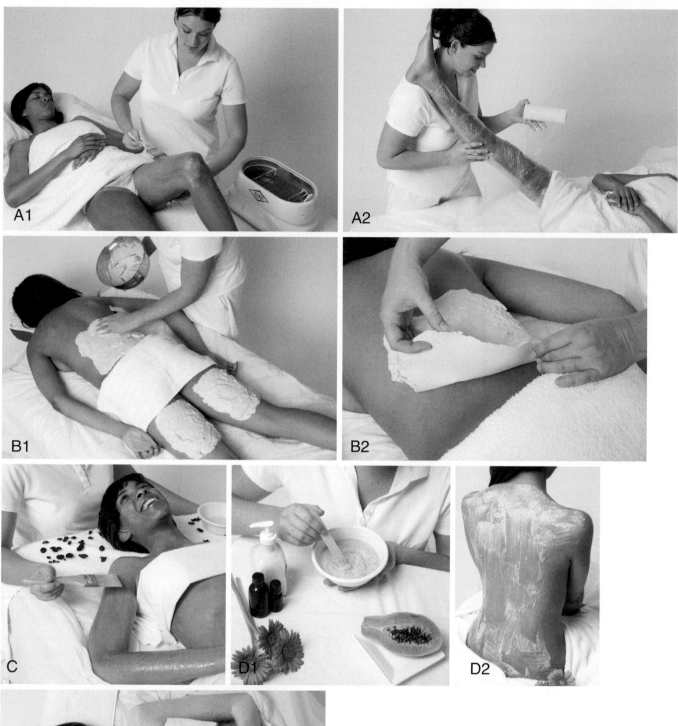

Figure 7-4   Types of cocoons. (A1 and **A2)** Parafango. In a Parafango wrap, a tension wrap is often used on target areas for slimming before the entire body is cocooned. **(B1)** Cryogenic. Cryogenic products can make the client cold, so they are often used for spot treatments. **(B2)** Some cocoon products such as this cryogenic product are made with a component that causes them to rubberize after a short time. They are pulled off the client in one piece, making cleanup easy. **(C)** Emollient (shea). Shea; honey; and other heavy butters, creams, or oils are used in a cocoon to relax the body and rejuvenate the skin. In this particular wrap, essential oils have been added to the shea butter, so it could also be considered an aromatherapy wrap. **(D1** and **D2)** Natural elements (papaya and yogurt). **(E)** Seaweed or fango.

Paraffin or Parafango Cocoon

Paraffin provides deeply penetrating warmth to the area where it is applied. It traps heat and moisture at the skin's surface, which increases circulation and helps with product absorption (sometimes a product such as a cellulite cream is applied under the paraffin). It is an effective treatment for clients with chronic arthritis and painful joints. It also leaves the skin feeling soft and supple.

Parafango is a combination of fango (mud) and paraffin with different melting points. It is heated and applied with a brush or is poured into forms to make large body packs. Parafango has been used successfully as a means of thermotherapy for such conditions as osteoarthritis, chronic conditions, muscular spasms, and scleroderma. The superior heat retention properties of Parafango have led to its use in the United States for the reduction of cellulite and inch loss in target areas. The flow of heat from Parafango is continuous and long lasting. Traditional hydrotherapy packs cool within 30 minutes, but Parafango packs remain warm for up to 60 minutes. Parafango is different than peat or mud in that it is designed for heat delivery, and there is little or no absorption of minerals through the skin. The heat it delivers increases circulation and lymph flow, facilitates perspiration, helps with product absorption, decreases hypertonicities of muscular tissue, decreases pain, and increases relaxation.

In a full-body paraffin or Parafango cocoon, the product is applied with a large application brush (large paintbrush size) and then covered in plastic using the sit-up method described in Chapter 3. Sometimes gauze strips are dipped in the paraffin or Parafango and then layered on the body. Because these two products are often used in cellulite treatments, a cellulite cocoon outline is described here:

1. Perform a full-body exfoliation.
2. Apply cellulite cream to target areas.
3. Apply paraffin or Parafango over the cellulite cream in target areas.
4. Cocoon.
5. Massage face or feet.
6. Remove the paraffin or Parafango.
7. Massage firming cream into target areas.

A treatment designed for sore back pain and using Parafango might consist of the following steps:

1. With the client prone, apply Parafango to the back.
2. Massage the legs.
3. Remove Parafango from the back and massage the back.
4. Apply a cooling, pain-relieving aroma support lotion to the back.
5. Turn the client supine.
6. Massage the neck and shoulders to complete the session.

Aloe Vera Cocoon

At tropical and resort spas, it is common to see an aloe sunburn relief wrap included in the menu of services. Guests often overexpose themselves to the sun during the first few days of their vacation. Research has supported the use of aloe for dry skin, ulceration, acne, chapped skin, and to soothe the inflammation and itching in conditions such as eczema, poison ivy, and allergic reactions.[2] A combination of aloe and essential oils that works well for sunburn is 1½ cup of aloe vera gel, 20 drops of German chamomile essential oil, 10 drops of lavender essential oil, and 2 drops of peppermint essential oil. Mix well and apply this blend to the skin in a heavy layer (do not exfoliate sunburned skin). A treatment outline might look like this:

1. Apply aloe vera blend or an aloe-based treatment product with a brush.
2. Cocoon in plastic and a light blanket for 20 minutes.
3. Massage the feet while the aloe absorbs (as long as the tops of the feet are not sunburned).
4. Unwrap the client and apply cool coffee- or green tea–infused towels to the body and allow them to sit for 5 minutes.
4. Apply an after-sun lotion with gentle hands or with a brush without removing the aloe vera.

Cryogenic Cocoon

Cryogenic products are often composed of a kaolin clay base with menthol as the active ingredient. Menthol increases the peripheral circulation and affects cold receptors in the skin, resulting in a cooling sensation. Besides the cooling effect, menthol has a numbing, pain-relieving action that is indicated for use on stiff or sore muscles. It alleviates itching from skin conditions and stimulates circulation and lymph flow.

The problem with cryogenic products is that they may make the client cold—really cold. For this reason, cryogenic applications work best as spot treatments. For a sports application, the therapist can apply the cryogenic product to areas of particular stiffness such as the lower back, hamstrings, and gluteals. The rest of the body is warmed with blankets, heat lamps, or hot water bottles. A cryogenic sports outline might progress as follows:

1. Massage the back.
2. Apply a cryogenic product to sore areas of the back. Avoid covering the entire back because this would be too cold. Focus on one area of particular stiffness such as the upper back and shoulders, directly down the spine, or on the low back.
3. Massage the legs.
4. Apply the cryogenic product to the hamstrings or lower legs.

5. Remove the cryogenic product from the back and apply a pain-relieving finishing lotion.
6. Remove the cryogenic product from the legs and apply a pain-relieving finishing lotion.
7. Turn the client to the supine position and massage the neck and shoulders to finish the treatment.

The cryogenic product used in Figure 7-4 can be removed without water and hot towels. A component of this mask rubberizes shortly after it is mixed up. A number of different products are currently being formulated to rubberize so they can be removed easily without a shower or even hot, moist towels.

Seaweed Cocoon

Seaweed has a number of positive benefits for the body when it is applied topically. It has been used successfully to promote endocrine balance, to reduce the symptoms of fibromyalgia, for detoxification, to decrease pain from sore muscles, and to stimulate circulation and lymph flow. It is a popular choice for slimming and firming treatments because it increases skin tone and makes the body appear smoother and more contoured. Seaweed is discussed in detail in Chapter 10. A general seaweed cocoon might progress in this manner:

1. Exfoliation
2. Application of seaweed
3. Cocoon for 20 minutes (massage the face and feet)
4. Removal of seaweed
5. Full-body massage

Fango Cocoon (Mud, Clay, or Peat)

Mud, clay, and peat are therapeutically different, so they are each used for different reasons in a treatment. Each of these substances is discussed in depth in Chapter 9. In general, these substances can be used for musculoskeletal injury and health or to refine the texture of the skin. A general fango cocoon outline might progress as follows:

1. Exfoliation
2. Application of fango
3. Cocoon for 20-30 minutes (massage the face and feet)
4. Removal of fango
5. Full-body massage

Natural Elements Cocoon

Some spas specialize in using natural food elements such as papaya, pumpkin, avocado, honey, yogurt, oatmeal, or cucumber in cocoons. Often, the food item is mashed and spread on the body in the same manner as seaweed or mud. Many natural food items are beneficial for the skin and have pleasing fragrances. However, they do tend to be more messy and time consuming than premixed, prepackaged items. Similar to the seaweed and fango cocoon, a natural elements cocoon will follow the standard cocoon progression:

BOX 7-1
Broaden Your Understanding

The Vitamin Cocoon

Vitamin cocoons use products that are high in vitamins A, C, B, and E to nourish the skin. Vitamin A helps to balance and normalize (in terms of pH and sebaceous output) dry skin or skin that has been overexposed to the sun. High levels of vitamin A (Retinol) are used to decrease fine lines and wrinkles. Vitamin B5 (panthenol) functions as a moisturizer and skin conditioner, and vitamin B3 (niacinamide) speeds the turnover of surface skin cells to clarify the skin and improve its texture.[3] Vitamin E is a well-known antioxidant that acts as a natural preservative, helping to decrease the development of wrinkles and discolorations. With age, the number of papillae in the epidermal–dermal junction in human skin is reduced, restricting the supply of nutrients to the epidermis and contributing to skin aging. Vitamin C (ascorbic acid) decreases the oxidative stress on the skin and increases the number of papillae in the dermis.[4]

Vitamin facials are currently a popular treatment performed by estheticians, which has recently led to the availability of full-body vitamin products. Because the main goal of vitamin treatments is to improve the health of the skin, they are not usually within the scope of practice for massage therapists in most states. Vitamin products also tend to be a little expensive but usually have linked home care products that generate a greater income for the spa or clinic.

1. Exfoliation
2. Application of natural element
3. Cocoon
4. Removal
5. Massage

THE PROCEDURE

The procedure described here is a basic cocoon that can be used with a variety of products. As mentioned earlier, there are many ways to deliver this type of body wrap, so therapists are encouraged to explore other options or to modify techniques as they deem appropriate. For example, if a steam canopy is available the therapist can "steam" the product instead of using wrap blankets. The procedure here ends with a massage but could just as easily end with a Vichy shower or a hydrotherapy tub soak.

Snapshot: The Cocoon

Indications

Indications depend on the product that is chosen for the treatment.

Contraindications

Contraindications depend on the product that is chosen for the treatment. For example, seaweed is contraindicated for pregnant clients and clients with thyroid disorders. A shea butter cocoon is suitable for such individuals.

Supplies for the Treatment Table Setup (from the bottom to the top layer)

1) Blanket (wool or cotton) set horizontally so that the long edges fall on either side of the table
2) Thermal space blanket turned horizontally (optional)
3) A plain flat sheet turned in its normal orientation on the table (if the product needs to be removed in a dry room)
4) A plastic sheet turned horizontally
5) One bath towel placed horizontally at the top of the table
6) One bath towel placed horizontally at the bottom of the table
7) A drape

A Fomentek bottle might be used under the massage sheet if additional warmth is needed. The table setup for a cocoon is shown in Figure 7-5.

Supplies for the Work Table Setup

1) Exfoliation product
2) Treatment product
3) Application brush or vinyl gloves
4) Finishing product
5) Aroma or aura mist
6) Soda cooler
7) Hot, moist towels
8) Dry hand towels
9) Disposable undergarments

Procedure

1) Exfoliation
2) Treatment product application
3) Cocoon
4) Processing time when the feet or face could be massaged
5) Unwrap
6) Application of finishing product

The therapist can ask the client to wear disposable undergarments, use standard draping practices, or use a combination of both. With a very messy product such as seaweed or mud, standard draping can be challenging. The product invariably gets all over the drape and from the drape onto the floor, on the therapist, and so on. In a wet room, this is not so much of a problem as it is in a dry room. The simplest method is to start with the client wearing disposable undergarments, drape the client as much as possible with a bath towel, and have a heat lamp available for extra warmth. The cocoon snapshot and Figure 7-6 provide an overview of this service.

Session Start

Because the client needs to be in a supine position for the wrapping up phase of the treatment, he or she must begin the service fully draped in the prone position.

Step 1: Exfoliation of the Posterior and Anterior Body

A number of different types of exfoliation can be given at the beginning of a cocoon treatment. Choose the technique that best supports the overall treatment goal. For a dry skin brush, exfoliation will probably be given with a cocoon that

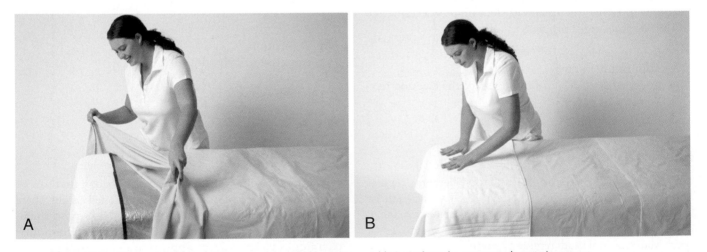

Figure 7-5   Massage table setup for a cocoon. (A) The massage table is set from the outermost layer to innermost layer as follows: blanket (wool or cotton), thermal space blanket (optional), and a plain flat sheet in its normal orientation on the massage table (for dry room removal only). On top of this, place a plastic sheet turned sideways on the table so that it covers the blanket. **(B)** A bath towel is placed across the top and bottom of the plastic sheet at either end of the table to anchor the plastic wrap sheet.

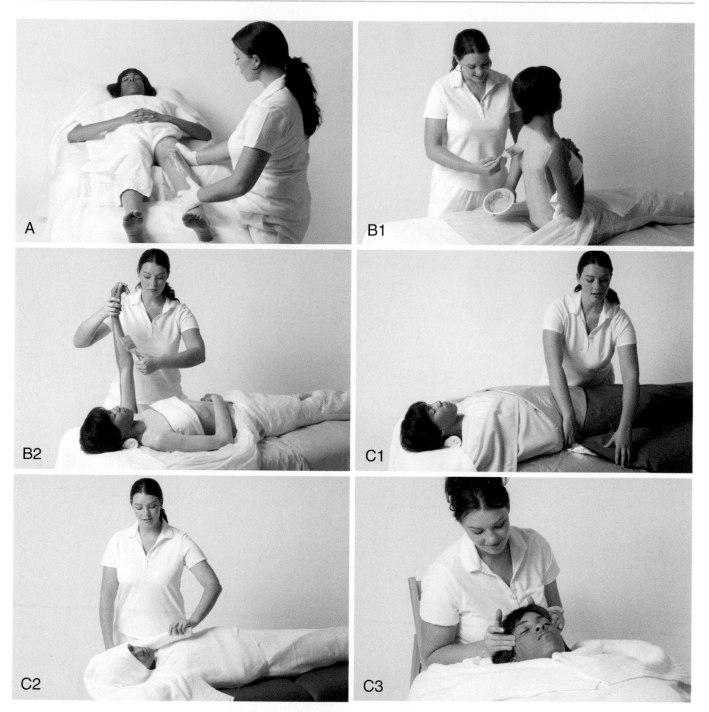

Figure 7-6   The cocoon. (A) Exfoliation. Exfoliate the client in the prone position and then turn the client to the supine position. This way, the client is face up for the cocoon. **(B1** and **B2)** Product application. Apply the treatment product to the newly exfoliated body areas with massage strokes or with a large application brush. In these pictures, the legs have already been treated and wrapped up in the plastic. **(C1** to **C3)** Cocoon. The plastic wrap and blankets are pulled up and around the client. The towel at the top of the table is wrapped around the head in a turban drape, and the towel at the bottom of the table is wrapped around the feet. Massage the feet or face. Notice that a light cotton blanket is used instead of a heavy wool blanket. A client does not need to perspire in a cocoon, so lighter wrap materials are used. **(D1** to **D5)** Removal from the cocoon. If the cocoon product (e.g., shea butter) does not need to be removed from the client, the client is left on the plastic for the remainder of the treatment (massage or application of a finishing product). If the product is messy (like this marine clay), it will need to be removed from the client, and the plastic will need to be removed from the treatment table before the massage or application of a finishing product. These images were also used in Chapter 3 with step-by-step instructions for moving a client from plastic to a massage sheet.

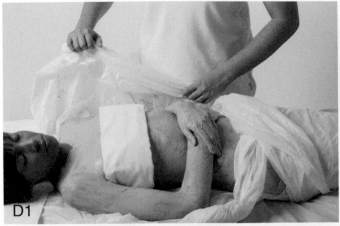

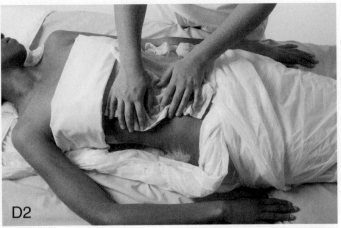

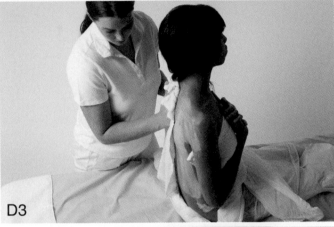

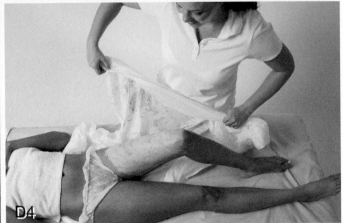

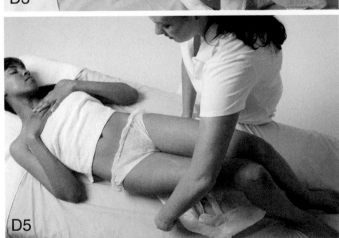

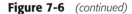

Figure 7-6   *(continued)*

aims to stimulate detoxification. A body polish might be given when the cocoon aims to relax the client. A salt glow would be most appropriate for cocoons that energize the body. Step-by-step directions for each of these techniques are discussed in Chapter 6.

The way the exfoliation is conducted will be determined by the method of product application (discussed in Chapter 3): For example:

- **The sit-up method:** 1. Client prone, 2. exfoliate the posterior body, 3. turn the client supine, 4. exfoliate the anterior body, and 5. apply product using the sit-up method.
- **The flip-over method:** 1. Client prone, 2. exfoliate the posterior body, 3. apply product to the posterior body, 3. the client flips over, 4. exfoliate the anterior body, and 5. apply product to the anterior body.
- **The side-lying method:** 1. Client supine, 2. exfoliate the anterior body, 3. position the client in a side-lying position and exfoliate the posterior body, 4. apply product, 5. roll client to the other side, and 6. apply product.

Step 2: Product Application

The product application method shown in Figure 7-5 is the sit-up method (other methods are described in Chapter 3). It is therefore assumed that both the posterior body and anterior body have been exfoliated, and the client is now in the supine position. The knees are bent, and the treatment product is applied to both the anterior and posterior sides of the legs. The legs are flattened against the plastic body wrap, and the client is asked to sit up (remove the bolster first). The treatment product is applied to the back and gluteals, and the client is asked to lie back down. Finally the belly, upper chest, and arms are treated, and the client is wrapped in the plastic.

If the treatment product is applied using massage, the therapist will exfoliate the posterior body and then apply the treatment product as in the flip-over method. It is a good idea for the therapist to wear gloves so that the hands do not need to be cleaned. The treatment product is massaged in from the posterior legs to the gluteals and then on the back. Depending on the product, a full range of strokes might be used. The client is "flipped," and the anterior body is exfoliated and then massaged with the treatment product. The client is now in the supine position and ready for the cocoon.

Step 3: Cocoon

The plastic wrap is pulled up around the client and tucked in loosely. Next the outer wrapping materials are pulled up and around the client. The bath towel at the top of the massage table can be used around the client's head in a turban drape or tucked into the top of the cocoon. The feet are wrapped with the towel at the bottom of the massage table. Hot water bottles, heat lamps, or warm packs can be used for additional warmth if they are needed.

Step 4: Process

While the client is "processing" in the wrap, a relaxing face massage can be given using a face cream. Offer the client a sip of water or herbal iced tea through a flexible straw and mist the client with an aroma mist or spring water. After the face massage has been completed, the feet can be massaged. In a hot sheet wrap, the client is perspiring freely and will not appreciate either a face or foot massage. In a cocoon, enhancers such as a face massage, hot stone foot massage, reflexology, a scalp treatment, or other special extras will help to make the treatment exceptional for the client.

Step 5: Unwrap

To remove the wrap, the blankets are pulled off the client. At this point, the client is still wrapped in plastic. The therapist now has two options based on the equipment available.

Option 1 If a shower is available, the therapist can leave the client wrapped loosely in the plastic and move the client to the shower. If the client has to go outside the treatment room to get to the shower, he or she will need to be draped over the top of the plastic with a bathrobe or sheet. As the client steps into the shower, the plastic is handed back to the therapist, who throws it away. While the client showers, the therapist changes the treatment table to massage sheets. The treatment can end with a full-body massage or with a quick application of a finishing lotion, cream, or gel.

Option 2 If the product is messy and a shower is not available, the plastic sheeting will need to be removed completely from underneath the client as he or she is cleaned off with hot towels. With certain products that are not messy (e.g., aloe vera, shea butter), removal of the plastic or product is not necessary. To remove a plastic sheet, a clean sheet will need to have been placed under the plastic when the table was made up. This procedure is described in Chapter 3 but is repeated here for convenience.

The product is removed from the client's arms, upper chest, and abdominal area, and the client is asked to hold onto the breast drape and sit up. The product is removed from the back and the posterior arm. The plastic sheet is rolled up until it sits as close as possible to the gluteals. The feet are wiped with a hot towel, and the client is asked to bend the knees and hold the feet up. The plastic that is underneath the client's feet is rolled so that the dirty side is rolled up. The client's clean feet are placed on the massage sheet, which was placed beneath the plastic earlier (the client's knees are still bent). The product is removed from both legs with hot towels and then plastic is rolled up as high as possible under the gluteals. The clean legs are placed flat on the massage sheet and covered with a sheet or towel for warmth. The client lies back down on the massage sheet and slightly lifts up the hips for the plastic to be removed completely. The client is now draped with a massage sheet for the rest of the treatment.

Session End

The treatment can end in different ways, as already mentioned. Some treatment products absorb completely, so the finishing product is simply applied over top of the first product. The therapist may choose to provide a full-body massage at the end of the cocoon. Alternatively, a full-body massage may have been given before the wrapping-up phase. With some treatment products (e.g., emollient products), the skin does not need a finishing lotion or cream. With others, it does. An aura mist may be spritzed high over the client to signal the end of the session and fill the treatment room with a refreshing scent.

Sanitation

After every treatment, product bottles and equipment should be sanitized with alcohol. This is important to prevent cross-contamination. For example, if the therapist massages the client's feet, does not sanitize his or her hands, and then picks up the bottle of finishing lotion, the bottle is now contaminated. If it is used on another client without being sanitized, the second client has potentially been exposed to an infectious pathogen.

Tension Wraps

A tension wrap is used in combination with a treatment product (e.g., cellulite cream) with the aim of "pushing" excess fluid out of a limb (e.g., thigh) or to compress tissue so that it appears slimmer when unwrapped. Tension wraps also increase heat in a body area so that the area perspires and so detoxifies. The tension wrap is either made of terry cloth strips that are soaked in a treatment product (e.g., herbal infusion, dissolved seaweed) or of heavy cellophane on a small roll. The wrap strip or roll is "circled" up the limb or torso, either with the treatment product on it or over top of a treatment product that has already been applied to the area.

Tension wraps are controversial. Some therapists believe that treatments featuring tension wraps mislead clients into believing that these wraps can make them lose inches and weight. In fact, the results experienced with tension wraps are usually temporary. Other therapists swear by tension wraps and point to their popularity with clients. Tension wraps are offered in many spas, so spa therapists should know the methods that are used in this type of body wrap so that they can make their own decision about this treatment's viability.

It is important to note that tension wraps are potentially dangerous and can cause damage to blood vessels if a limb is wrapped too tightly. Overtight wrapping most often occurs with the heavy cellophane wraps that are easy to pull tightly and twist to flatness against the skin. In one case of overtight tension wrapping, the client developed a varicose vein as a result of the treatment. The need for caution cannot be stressed enough. Do not apply a tension wrap to a client with poor circulation, diabetes, circulatory conditions, high blood pressure, spider veins, or varicose veins.

The therapist may choose to measure the size of target areas before and after the application. Usually the mid-calf, mid-thigh, hips, waist, and sometimes the upper arm are measured and treated. A session that includes the use of a tension wrap might progress as follows:

1. The client is measured
2. Full-body exfoliation
3. Application of a specialized cellulite cream or firming product to target areas
4. Tension wrap
5. The body is cocooned in warm blankets to process
6. Removal of the blankets and tension wrap
7. Application of a finishing product to target areas
8. Remeasure the client

TECHNIQUES

If terry strip tension wraps are used, they are rolled up and then placed in a crock pot or roaster oven full of dissolved treatment product similar to the hot sheet wrap. The terry strips are then removed and wrung out before being placed in a soda cooler to keep them hot. The strips are wrapped around the area that is being treated. Sometimes a treatment product such as a cellulite cream is applied underneath the wet tension wrap.

If a cellophane wrap is used, the treatment product is applied directly to the client, and then the area is wrapped. Sometimes more than one product is applied, as in the case of a Parafango cellulite treatment. In this treatment, a specialized cream is massaged into target areas and then covered by hot Parafango, which activates the specialized cream. The tension wrap is applied on top of the Parafango.

The wrapping techniques are described using the cellophane wrap, but wrapping with terry strips is carried out in the same way. Cellophane is a bit easier to work with because it sticks to itself, so the therapist does not have to worry about it slipping. Terry strips loosen and slip easily. The reader may notice that for some of the techniques described here, the client is standing up. This is not the ideal because the client cannot fully relax during the session. In many cases, a good wrap and noticeable results are more important to the client than relaxation, so the client will not mind this positioning. Tension wrapping techniques are shown in Figure 7-7.

Tension Wrapping the Legs: Client on the Table

With the client supine, unwrap a small bit of plastic from the cellophane roll and hold it in place on the client's foot as you lift their leg at a straight angle onto your shoulder. While one hand holds the plastic wrap onto the foot, the other brings the wrap roll around the ankle to begin wrapping the client's leg. Work distal to proximal, twisting the wrap with each turn to keep it flat against the client's skin. The aim of the wrap is to encourage tissue fluid to move from the distal area of the leg toward the heart.

As you reach the knee, lift the leg up from your shoulder and move your body weight forward as you continue to wrap the plastic. When you reach the client's hip, anchor the plastic under the client and repeat the process on the opposite leg.

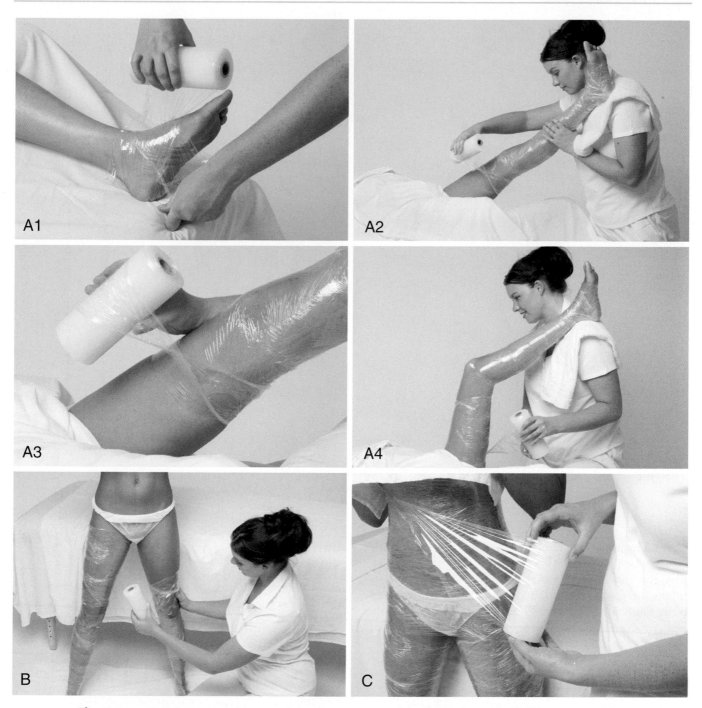

Figure 7-7 **Techniques for tension wraps.** **(A1** to **A4)** Tension wrap of the legs on the table. Start on the foot and wrap up the leg. Move forward as you work higher. Twist the wrap to keep it flat against the client's leg. **(B)** Tension wrap of the legs: standing. **(C)** Tension wrap of the hips and belly. **(D)** Tension wrap of the arms. **(E1** to **E3)** Removal of tension wrap.

Tension Wrapping the Legs: Client Standing

This is the easiest way to get a good wrap. The client stands with the legs apart. The therapist anchors the strip of plastic under the client's heel and wraps from the ankle up the leg, twisting the plastic to keep it flat against the client's leg. After both legs have been wrapped, move onto the waist and hips.

Tension Wrapping the Hips and Belly

It is very difficult to get a good wrap on the hips and belly with the client supine on the table. If the client is sitting up, this does not work well either because the client's belly will pouch, so the wrap becomes loose when the client lies down. It is easiest to get a good wrap with the client stand-

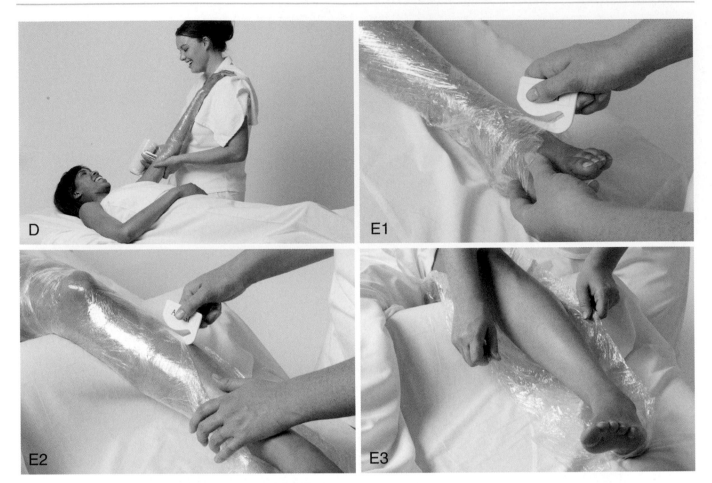

Figure 7-7 *continued*

ing up. This way, the therapist can move directly from the last leg wrapped to the hips and then from the belly up to the top of the waist. The wrap is simply circled around the client's torso and pulled tight. If the client is standing next to the table, he or she simply leans back and swings onto the table to relax during the processing time.

Tension Wrapping the Arms

Usually the lower body is treated and allowed to "process" while the upper body is treated. The arm is wrapped from the wrist up to the deltoid even though the lower arm is not usually covered in treatment product.

Unwrap

To remove terry strip wraps, simply unwind them from the client's body. Cellophane wraps are cut in a straight line up the front of the wrap using a specially designed safe cutter.

Sanitation

The terry wraps should be stored in a closed, ventilated container after they are removed from the client. Right after the session, the wraps should be laundered in hot water with a commercial-grade laundry detergent and dried with heat. They are then rerolled and stored in a closed cabinet.

SAMPLE TREATMENTS

Herbal Diet Right Wrap

Promotional Description

This detoxification wrap is the perfect way to jump start a diet or fuel a diet that has hit a plateau. The session begins with a Roman dry brush that stimulates circulation and lymph flow. Next, the body is warmed with a soothing foot bath and hot herbal tea. Linen sheets steeped in rosemary, juniper, ginger, clove, and sage are wrapped snugly around the body to facilitate detoxification. The session ends with a relaxing application of seaweed firming lotion. Looking great never felt so good!

Treatment Outline

The Roman dry brush is simply a dry brush with the word "Roman" added for marketing purposes. Spas also use the words "Celtic dry brush" for the same reason. Follow the directions for the hot sheet wrap using an herbal infusion for the treatment product. A list of spa suppliers is given in the resources section at the back of the book. There are many types of seaweed gel that can be used as a finishing product. It should be noted that inch loss and weight loss with herbal wraps is temporary only because of water reduction in superficial tissues. Herbal wraps do help to stimulate metabolism.

Café Cocoon

Promotional Description

Don't drink coffee—be wrapped in it! Coffee stimulates circulation; decreases water retention; and tones, firms, and conditions the skin. Coffee culture begins with a revitalizing body buff and foot soak. Linen sheets steeped in a steaming French roast envelop the body to slim and soften. As a finishing touch, moisturizing lotion with green tea and caffeine are smoothed on to protect the skin from damaging sunlight.

Treatment Outline

Begin the treatment with an exfoliation and then follow it with a hot sheet wrap using coffee as the treatment product.

Desert Nectar Honey Glaze

Promotional Description

A relaxing body polish prepares the skin for the luxury of pure Arizona honey and rich buttermilk spun to a golden glaze. While enveloped in this nectar of the desert, enjoy a firming face massage and soothing foot rub. Steamy rosemary towels and a cooling mist of chamomile water leave the body drenched and radiant.

Treatment Outline

Follow the directions for a cocoon using honey and warm buttermilk as the treatment product. For the body glaze, mix 1/2 cup honey with 1/2 cup hot water until it is dissolved. Add 1/2 cup buttermilk and brush on the body with a large application brush. Chamomile hydrolate (flower water) can be bought from an aromatherapy supplier, or the therapist can add 2 drops of German chamomile essential oil to 1 oz of purified water.

Athlete Muscle Aid

Promotional Description

If muscle pain and stiffness are slowing down your workouts, this treatment is right for you. A deep tissue massage with sweet birch and bay laurel (essential oils that are well known to decrease muscle pain) is enhanced with the latest in spa technology—a cryogenic sports mask. This tingly mask helps to detoxify the body, leaving muscles refreshed and ready for action.

Treatment Outline

This treatment does not follow the normal procedure.

1. Massage the back.
2. Apply cryogenic product to back.
3. Massage the legs.
4. Apply cryogenic product to the legs.
5. Massage the arms while the client is prone.
6. Remove the product from the back and legs.
7. Turn the client.
8. Treat the anterior areas or massage the neck to finish.

For the deep tissue massage oil, add 4 drops of sweet marjoram, 6 drops of bay laurel, and 5 drops of sweet birch essential oil to 1 fl oz of carrier oil (a mix of hemp seed and sunflower give good results).

Summary

In a body wrap, the body is enclosed in sheets or plastic and insulating blankets to trap heat. This stimulates detoxification through perspiration and helps the skin to absorb any products that are applied. Today, a wide variety of body wraps is used for cosmetic purposes or to treat conditions such as rheumatism, low immunity, fatigue, and muscular aches and pain or simply for relaxation.

There are numerous ways to give a body wrap, but two procedures that work well are the hot sheet wrap and the cocoon. In a hot sheet wrap, the treatment product (e.g., herbs, coffee, milk, honey, seaweed) is dissolved in hot water. Two sheets are steeped in the dissolved product and wrapped around the client. In the second procedure, which is called a cocoon, the product is not dissolved in water but is applied directly to the body. The indications and contraindications depend on which products are used. Hot sheet wraps tend to be more aggressive and, therefore, are more likely to be contraindicated for certain individuals.

In some treatments, a tension wrap is used. Tension wraps are made of terry strips or heavy cellophane. They are wrapped around target areas to compress the tissue and make the area appear slimmer. Care must be taken to not wrap an area too tightly because damage to veins is possible.

REFERENCES

1. Conney AH, et al: Inhibitory effects of tea and caffeine on UV-induced carcinogenesis: relationship to enhanced apoptosis and decreased tissue fat. *Eur J Cancer Prev* 2002;11(suppl):28–36.
2. Syed TA, et al: Management of psoriasis with aloe vera extract in a hydrophilic cream: A placebo-controlled, double-blind study. *Trop Med Int Health* 1996;1:505–509.
3. Draclos ZD: Topical vitamins for the skin. Available at http://www.olay.com/dematology/arch_topical_vitamins.htm.
4. Raschke T, et al: Topical activity of ascorbic acid: From in vitro optimization to in vivo efficiency. *Skin Pharmacol Physiology* 2004;17:200–206.
5. The Double Eagle Resort and Spa. Available at http://www.doubleeaglerosort.com
6. The Sonnenalp Resort of Vail. Available at http://www.sonnenalp.com/activities/spa/tretments.html
7. St Andrews Bay Chateau Elan Spa. Available at http://www.standrewsbay.com/Spa/treatments.htm
8. The Grand Geneva Resort and Spa. Available at http://www.grandgeneva.com/recreation/spa/spa_treatments.asp
9. The Lake House Spa at Lake Austin Resort. Available at http://www.lakeaustin.com/lakehousespa.php
10. The Lake Tahoe Resort, Spa and Casino. Available at http://www.laketahoe.hyatt.com/property/sportsrelax/spa/body_treatment.jhtml

REVIEW QUESTIONS

Multiple Choice

1. A cold sheet wrap is a form of this type of wrap:
   a. Detoxification and immune boosting wrap
   b. Cryogenic wrap
   c. French hydrotherapy wrap
   d. Skin care wrap

2. Hot wraps elevate body temperature and create an artificial fever, which:
   a. Dehydrates the body and causes brain damage.
   b. Accelerates the elimination of toxins through perspiration.
   c. Causes a temporary reduction in immunity.
   d. Causes antibody production and T-cell proliferation to decrease.

3. In a cold sheet wrap:
   a. The body experiences a vascular flush effect.
   b. The body shivers, which tones muscles.
   c. The skin is cooled, which softens its texture.
   d. The muscles contract, which forces excess water from the tissues.

4. The client does not need to perspire in this type of wrap:
   a. Coffee slimming wrap
   b. Emollient cocoon
   c. Herbal hot sheet wrap
   d. Seaweed detoxification wrap

Fill in the Blank

5. Many ancient healing traditions used _____ as a medicine to decrease toxic buildup in the body.
   a. Aloe vera
   b. Shea butter
   c. Massage oil
   d. Herbs

Matching

Match the client to the most appropriate treatment option:

A. Herbal detox wrap

B. Cryogenic wrap

C. Lavender and rose petal wrap

D. Aloe vera wrap

E. Shea butter wrap

6. _____ Elderly client who is in good health but has minor circulatory insufficiency

7. _____ Healthy client who is about to start a diet

8. _____ Client with chronically dry skin

9. _____ Athlete who has sore and stiff muscles

10. _____ Sunburned client

Spa Foot Treatments

Chapter Outline

Key Terms

Arch: The bones in the foot are actually arranged to form three strong arches (medial longitudinal arch, lateral longitudinal arch, and transverse arch) that are commonly referred to as the arch of the foot. The arch provides the foot with the strength to support the body while remaining flexible and mobile.

Callus: A small area of thickened skin that is caused by continued friction or pressure. The epidermis becomes more active in response to mild, repetitive irritation. This causes a localized increase in the thickened tissue at the surface of the skin.

Cuticle: A fold of skin that partly covers the border of the nail. In a pedicure (or manicure of the hands), the cuticle is pushed back so the surface of the nail appears cleaner and smoother.

Dorsiflexion: Bending the top of the foot (the dorsal surface) toward the shin.

Nail technician: A certified or licensed practitioner who provides care of the nails or applies, repairs, or decorates gel nails or acrylic nails.

Pedicure: A treatment in which the foot is soaked, calluses are reduced, the nails are trimmed and filed, the cuticles are pushed back and trimmed, and the nails are buffed or polish is applied to the nails. Nail care is provided only by certified nail technicians or cosmetologists (depending on the laws of the particular state).

Plantar flexion: Bending the bottom of the foot (plantar surface) downward (as in pointing the toes).

Reflexology: A holistic therapy that is based on the belief that specific points on the hands, ears, and feet correspond to specific areas of the body, including the organs and glands.

Treatments that focus on the feet are well liked by clients, so these treatments are regularly offered on spa menus. **Pedicure** treatments, which are intended to beautify the skin and nails, are delivered by cosmetologists, estheticians, and **nail technicians** depending on the laws in the individual state. Massage therapists provide foot treatments that decrease foot pain, revitalize tired feet, enhance or promote relaxation, and support the balance of the body. Although in most states massage therapists cannot provide nail care or services aimed at improving the appearance of the feet, they can mix and match different treatment elements to create enjoyable services that quickly gain popularity with clients.

A foot treatment consists of basic steps that can be modified to fit the goal and concept of the service being provided. Most foot treatments include a general foot assessment, soaking and cleaning, exfoliation, application of a treatment product (e.g., mud, paraffin), and basic massage. These fundamental steps can be enhanced with massage, **reflexology** techniques, aromatherapy smell-scapes, and enhancers that tie in other areas of the body such as the hands and face. The goal of this chapter is to describe each element of a foot treatment and suggest some options for each step. Some specific massage and reflexology techniques are also discussed so that the therapist has the necessary building blocks in place to create unique foot treatments.

Before giving any of the treatments discussed in this chapter, readers may want to review Chapter 3 ("Foundation Skills for Spa Treatment Delivery"), Chapter 5 ("Introduction to Aromatherapy for Spa"), and Chapter 6 ("Exfoliation Treatments"). Chapter 13 ("Treatment Design and the Signature Spa Treatment") provides ideas for the creation of individual services.

General Treatment Considerations

Before giving spa foot treatments to a client, it is important to be aware of the possible contraindications, the types of reaction that clients may have to the treatment, and the regulations on reflexology certification. It is also useful to be aware of the positioning techniques that make reflexology less stressful on the therapist's body.

CONTRAINDICATIONS

If a client has pitted edema, broken bones or fractures, advanced or poorly treated diabetes, neuropathy, deep vein thrombosis, infections, ingrown toenails, painful corns, gout, warts, or athlete's foot in the area of the lower leg and foot, they should not receive a foot treatment. Caution should be used when working with elderly individuals, clients on multiple medications, and clients who have compromised circulatory systems. Reflexology techniques should only be used on such individuals with a light pressure to avoid overstimulation or accelerated elimination symptoms such as nausea, diarrhea, or headache.

REFLEXOLOGY CERTIFICATION

The foot spa treatments described in this chapter include reflexology techniques. To become a certified reflexologist requires specialized training. In some states, a specific license is required to practice as a reflexologist, but in other states, reflexologists must also be qualified as massage therapists before they can practice. Massage therapists who are not reflexologists can use "reflexology techniques" during their treatments but should not claim to be reflexologists. The American Reflexology Certification Board (ARCB) is an independent testing agency that requires students to take a hands-on reflexology course of no less than 110 hours and complete 90 postgraduate treatment sessions that have been properly documented using ARCB forms. To obtain the certification, students then have to take a 300-question test and a practical examination. The contact details for the ARCB and other reflexology organizations are provided in the back of the book.

POSSIBLE REACTIONS TO REFLEXOLOGY

Although negative responses are rare, clients may experience a variety of reactions to reflexology techniques. During the session, the client may have muscle cramping in the legs and feet, their feet and hands may perspire, and they may feel mildly nauseous or headachy. Some clients respond to reflexology by falling into a deep sleep during the session. Others will experience involuntary jerks of the arms and legs as the nervous system unwinds. In all cases, the therapist should monitor the client's comfort level and make necessary adjustments to the degree of pressure that is used in the treatment.

THERAPIST AND CLIENT COMFORT DURING REFLEXOLOGY

The massage table should be set up high enough so that the therapist does not have to hunch over the table while delivering the treatment. The client can use a step stool at the side of the massage table to get on and off the table safely. This is not the only way to position a client for reflexology. Some therapists place the client's feet on a stool in front of them. Others place the feet on a pillow to lift them up off the massage table. In this case, the client should be bolstered so that elevating the feet does not place unnecessary stress on the knees.

Elements of a Spa Foot Treatment

In the following section, different elements of a foot treatment are described along with techniques, variations in products, and alternative delivery steps. When each of these elements is understood, the therapist can mix and match options to create unique services. The sample treatment at the end of the chapter gives one example of how the different elements, products, and delivery steps can be combined. Table 8-1 provides an overview of the basic elements of a foot treatment, and Box 8-1 describes the steps in a classic pedicure.

A QUICK FOOT ASSESSMENT

When assessing the feet before a session, the therapist begins by looking for any obvious contraindications such as a fungal infection or pronounced edema. Corns, calluses, and areas of discoloration or dryness are not contraindicated but help the therapist to determine where extra stress is being placed on the foot or the body. In reflexology, for example, a callus on the medial side of the big toe might correspond to a client's chronic neck pain and stiffness. Eliminating the cause of the callus (often ill-fitting shoes) and specifically stimulating the area during the treatment may help to decrease the severity of the neck stiffness while relaxing and revitalizing the feet at the same time.

Table 8-1	Elements of a Spa Foot Treatment
TREATMENT ELEMENT	**DESCRIPTION**
Foot assessment	The foot is evaluated to rule out contraindications and identify areas of particular stress. The shoes of the client might also be appraised so that the therapist can describe to the client how the shoes might be contributing to foot pain or to hip, knee, and lower back conditions.
Soaking or cleansing	The feet are soaked in water, usually with a product to soften and clean the skin and to relax the muscles. Sometimes the feet are not soaked but are washed while the client relaxes on the treatment table.
Exfoliation	A granulated product (estheticians can also use an enzyme or dissolving exfoliant) is rubbed on the feet to remove dead skin cells, smooth the skin's surface, stimulate lymph flow, and increase local circulation.
Callus care	A heavy, specially formulated cream may be massaged into the callus to help reduce it, or a callus file or pumice stone may be rubbed across the callus to remove dead skin (in some states, this is prohibited for massage therapists).
Massage	The lower legs and feet may be massaged to relax muscles, stimulate lymph and blood flow, decrease pain, and revitalize the feet. A variety of techniques can be used, including hot stone massage, trigger point therapy, and lengthening and strengthening techniques such as active isolated stretching (AIS) and post-isometric relaxation (PIR).
Reflexology	Reflexology techniques may be used to decrease foot pain, increase the flexibility and pliability of the feet, relax the body, revitalize the feet, and balance the body.
Hydrotherapy	Foot soaks at specific temperatures, whirlpool baths, or affusions may be used to treat a specific condition, decrease inflammation, increase blood and lymph flow, and revitalize the feet. See Chapter 4.
Treatment product	A treatment product such as mud, seaweed, cocoa butter, or essential oils is applied to the feet and sometimes the lower leg to achieve a specific result (e.g., decrease foot pain, decrease of inflammation, stimulation of circulation, revitalization).
Foot cocoon	The feet and lower leg may be wrapped in a cloth soaked in herbs, heated towels, or thermal booties to warm the tissues or to activate a specific treatment product that has previously been applied to the area.
Finishing product	To end the treatment, a light gel or lotion may be applied to the feet, the feet might be misted with a toner, or a powder might be applied. Often, peppermint lotions are used because they leave the feet feeling tingly and refreshed.

BOX 8-1
Broaden Your Understanding

A Classic Pedicure

In a pedicure, the toenails are groomed, the skin is beautified, and the appearance of the foot is enhanced. This treatment can only be delivered by a professional licensed or certified to provide nail care (a cosmetologist, nail technician, or esthetician, depending on the laws in the particular state). In a classic pedicure, the therapist first removes old polish with acetone (nail polish remover) and then soaks, cleanses, and exfoliates the feet. A heavy, specially formulated cream may be massaged into **calluses** *to help remove them. Alternatively a callus file or pumice stone may be rubbed across the callus to remove the dead skin. Nail technicians can use a callus shaver to shave off layers of dead skin. This is a potentially dangerous piece of equipment and should only be used by a trained professional. The* **cuticles** *are treated with a cuticle cream, which softens the cuticle so that it can be pushed back off the nail. The nail is trimmed and then shaped with an emery board. A foot mask may be applied to soften and purify the skin, and then a light massage is provided. Finally, the nails are polished with a base coat, two coats of color, and a top coat to protect against chipping.*

The most common cause of foot pain and dysfunction is ill-fitting shoes.[1] Clients often wear shoes that are one or two sizes too small for their feet. This miss-sizing usually occurs because clients try on new shoes while they are sitting down (non–weight bearing), lace the shoes tightly around their feet, and then stand up and walk around. The shoes hold the foot in a cramped position so that the bones cannot lengthen out into a strong **arch**. Over time this may lead to foot pain and may contribute to knee, hip, and lower back conditions. It is a good idea to try on shoes in the afternoon when the feet are at their largest because of normal swelling. People's feet get wider as they age, so they should expect their foot size to increase over the years.[2]

The quick foot size test described below is an effective way to determine if a client is wearing a shoe that is too small for his or her feet (method taken from Runquist[3]). To perform the test, the client sits on a chair with the bare feet placed a shoulder's width apart. Pieces of cardboard are then placed under each of the client's feet, and the client is asked to stand up. The therapist then traces around each foot onto the pieces of cardboard. Because the client's weight is on the feet and he or she is barefoot, the imprints will indicate the true foot size for which shoes are required.

The therapist then cuts out the impressions of the feet and attempts to slip them into the client's shoes. If the cardboard impressions do not fit into the client's shoes, the shoes are too small. Ideally, the client would then throw away any shoes that do not fit the cardboard impressions. When clients first wear shoes that fit the cardboard impressions, they often make the comment that the shoes feel too large. This is because it takes some time for the foot to relax back into its natural lengthened position.

Although this is an oversimplified assessment of what can be a very complex situation, this easy "test" illustrates for clients the importance of purchasing shoes that are big enough. Clients with persistent foot pain, knee, hip, or lower back pain should be referred to a physician for professional medical assessment and treatment.

SOAKING AND CLEANSING THE FEET

Cleansing is required before any foot treatment for hygienic reasons. Different cleansing and soaking methods and equipment are shown in Figure 8-1. In the simplest cleansing method, the therapist wipes off the client's feet before massage with a disposable cleansing wipe such as a diaper wipe. Another simple method is to wet the hands in a bowl of warm water and apply a foaming cleanser to the feet while the client relaxes on the treatment table. The cleanser is removed with hot towels.

A more elegant cleansing might take place in a soaking container with warm water and a soaking additive. The client's feet are soaked for 5 to 10 minutes to soften the muscle tissue, increase circulation, and relax the body. The feet are pulled out of the water one after the other and washed with a cleanser. A nail brush can be used to clean under the nails if desired by the therapist. The feet are dried with a hand towel before the client is moved to a treatment table for the rest of the service.

Some spas have expensive pedicure equipment with a reclining chair attached to a multi-jet hydrotherapy foot tub. The client's feet remain immersed in the tub for much of the treatment and are pulled out and placed on a foot rest when necessary during the service. This type of equipment is ideal for a pedicure, but it is not strictly necessary for a foot treatment delivered by a massage therapist. A cheaper option is to use a foot soak basin and purchase a pedicure chair with an attached foot rest. This allows the therapist to work on the client's feet from a seated position rather than being down on the knees when cleansing and drying the client's feet during the soaking and cleansing step.

The presentation and style of the foot soak is important. Large decorative basins with whole flower petals or leaves floating on the surface of the water create an attractive display and add a sensation of luxury and indulgence. A cup of herbal tea on a side table, relaxing lighting, and soothing music add to the experience. The client might also be offered a shoulder and neck massage while his or her feet are soaking.

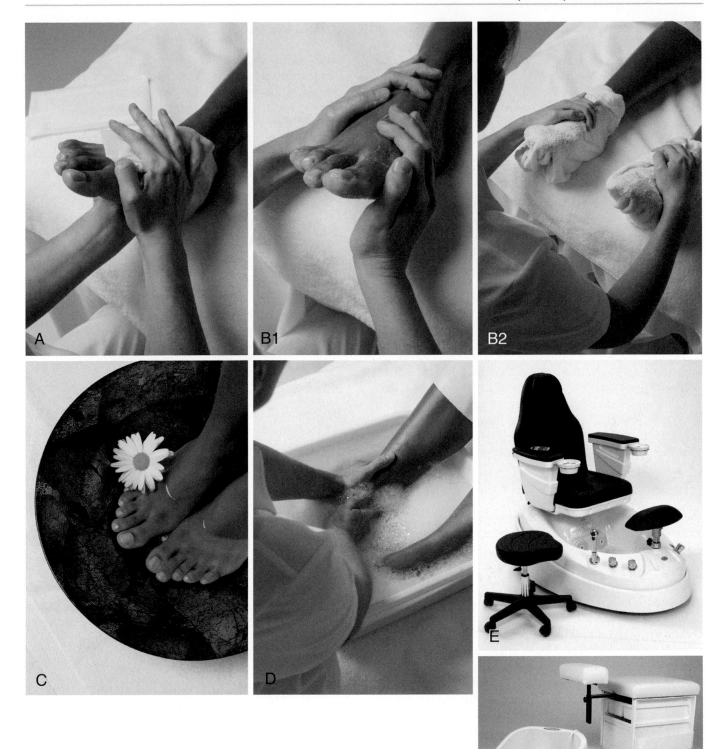

Figure 8-1   Cleansing and soaking the feet. (A) Cleansing with a disposable diaper wipe.
(B1 and **B2)** Cleaning with a cleanser and hot, moist towels. **(C)** Soaking in a decorative tub while
seated. **(D)** Soaking while positioned on the treatment table. **(E)** Professional multi-jet foot soak.
(F) Foot soak basin and pedicure chair.

In a third method, the foot soak is delivered while the client relaxes on the massage table. The client's legs are propped up with a large wedge or bolster. The foot-soaking basin is placed at the end of the table on top of a bath towel and a hand towel. The client places his or her feet into the bowl for the treatment and then lifts them out at the end of the soak. The therapist removes the container of water and places the client's feet on top of a preset hand towel to be dried. In this case, a plastic dish bowl is ideal for the soaking container. Large decorative containers are difficult for the therapist to lift and maneuver in this type of a soak.

Additives such as Epson salt, seaweed powder, and essential oils can increase the therapeutic benefits of a foot soak while helping to cleanse the feet of impurities. Table 8-2 provides an overview of some of the additives that might be used in the foot soak or cleansing step.

Sanitation

Any soaking basin that contains jets must be flushed with a small amount of bleach or an approved sanitation product between clients. This is also true for decorative items such as marbles or polished stones added to the soaking basin. Basins without jets should be washed with hot, soapy water; dried and sprayed with alcohol; and then left to air dry. Careful sanitation of foot-soaking containers is very important because this is often an area where bacteria can grow and spread between clients.[4]

EXFOLIATION

The feet can be buffed during the soaking process by lifting one foot out of the tub at a time, and applying an exfoliant cream or loofah mitt to the sole of the foot and the heel. This stimulates circulation and lymph flow, which supports the overall treatment goals of the service. A callus file or pumice stone can be rubbed across calluses while the feet are wet in some states. In most states, the use of a callus file or pumice stone is out of the scope of practice for massage practitioners. If the client is positioned on the massage table, the therapist can wet his or her hands in warm water and apply the exfoliation product directly to the feet and then remove it with a hot towel.

Sanitation

Callus-reducing files and other implements used on the feet should be washed in hot, soapy water at the end of the treatment; soaked for 20 minutes in alcohol; and left to air dry before being returned to a closed cabinet.

FOOT MASSAGE

One of the things that sets a massage therapist apart from other therapists delivering services at a spa is the depth and variety of the massage strokes that they use in a treatment. Few treatments are more relaxing and satisfying than an exceptional foot massage. Most massage therapists have a well-thought-out foot routine already, but students developing their skills may find the techniques offered below helpful (Fig. 8-2). Many of the strokes outlined here are taught by Geraldine Thompson and Lisa Hensel at the Seattle School of Reflexology.

The Sandwich Slide

The therapist laces his or her fingers and stands on the lateral side of the foot facing toward the table. The interlaced fingers slide down the medial edge of the client's foot to the heel and then back up to the starting position. The emphasis is on the downward stroke. This technique can be repeated up to 15 times.

Folded Hands Glide

Place one hand on top of the other with thumbs to the outside and hold the elbows close to the body so that body weight can be used to facilitate the stroke. With the edge of the hands contacting the ball of the foot (directly over the metatarsal heads), push the foot into **dorsiflexion**. After the foot is dorsiflexed, run the edge of the hands down the plantar surface of the foot and around the heel, pulling the foot into **plantar flexion** at the end of the stroke. This stroke can be repeated eight to 10 times. The therapist may notice that this stroke is difficult to perform with good body mechanics because it causes a pronounced wrist deviation. Holding the elbows close to the body and using body weight to facilitate this stroke is important. Although this stroke is very popular with clients, therapists must determine if they can provide it without injury to themselves or undue stress on their bodies.

Circular Thumbs on Top of the Foot

Starting at the distal part of the foot, use circular motions with the thumbs down the dorsal surface of the foot. This stroke can be repeated three to six times.

Circular Palms Around the Ankle

Apply moderate pressure in circular motions around the ankle with the palms of the hands.

Achilles Stroke

Run one hand up the anterior surface of the lower leg and the other down the posterior surface of the lower leg. Traction the ankle at the end of the posterior leg stroke.

Table 8-2   Additives for a Foot Soak

ADDITIVE	GENERAL PROPERTIES	HOW MUCH TO USE
Epson salt	Traditionally used as a soaking agent for sprained or bruised muscles and to decrease muscular pain and stiffness.	½ cup to 1 cup depending on the size of the soaking unit
Sea salt	Sea salts are skin softening and relaxing. Dead Sea salts aid psoriasis, eczema, and arthritis and are pain relieving.	½ cup to 1 cup depending on the size of the soaking unit
Seaweed	Seaweed powder is stimulating for blood and lymph flow, detoxifying, and revitalizing.	1 tsp is dissolved in hot water, and the mixture is poured into the tub
Clay	Clay is soothing, softening, and relaxing. Certain clays such as those derived from sea sediments or volcanic areas may remineralize through absorption.	The amount used is at the discretion of the therapist. Whereas 1 Tbsp softens and colors the water, larger amounts can create a runny but enjoyable "soup."
Mud or peat	Mud or peat can be added in moderate amounts to cool water temperatures to support the decrease of inflammatory conditions and refresh the feet.	1 cup or more. Some treatments may call for the feet to be soaked in undiluted mud or peat (although this is expensive).
Foamy soaking product	Spa suppliers carry a variety of scented foaming soaking products for the feet. Sometimes these products contain dyes that color the water. Clients who are sensitive to synthetic fragrances may prefer a more natural additive such as clay or sea salt.	Usually, 1 Tbsp is added and then frothed up with the hands. Follow the product directions if they are provided.
Fizzy soaking product	Fizzy soaking products are placed in the water and fizz when they dissolve like an Alka-Seltzer. They are often scented and contain dyes to color the water.	Read the product directions to determine how much product to add to a soaking tub.
Herbal infusions	Herbal infusions can be added to the foot bath to refresh the feet and senses. The same herbal mixture that is used for the herbal body wrap can be used in the foot bath. Eucalyptus leaf, juniper berry, clove buds, calendula, and rosemary leaf make a nice combination.	To make an herbal infusion, place ½ cup of dried herbs in a muslin bag or metal tea ball and cover with a quart of boiling water. Allow the mixture to steep for 15 minutes before adding it to the foot bath.
Essential oils	Essential oils have numerous properties that can be used in a foot soak.	Cover the client's feet with essential oils diluted in a fixed oil and then place them into a foot soak basin of warm water.
Powdered milk and honey	Powdered milk, buttermilk, full-fat milk, and honey make a soothing, softening, and relaxing foot soak.	Add ½ cup of powdered milk or one cup of regular or buttermilk and ½ cup of honey to the foot soak basin of warm water.
Other	A variety of other professional soaking products with different properties are available through spa suppliers.	Follow product directions.

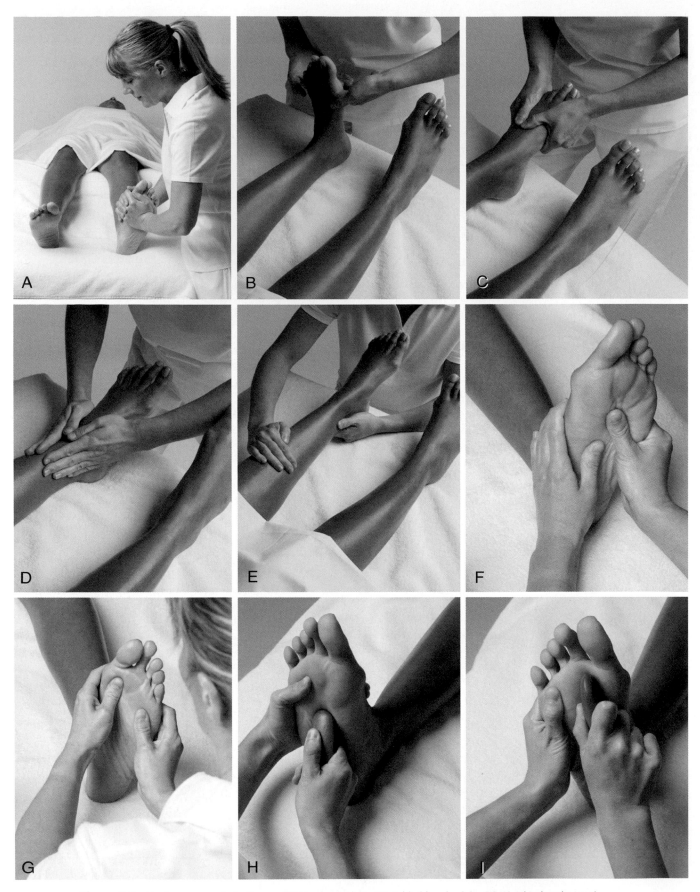

Figure 8-2 Foot massage techniques. (A) Sandwich slide. **(B)** Folded hands glide. **(C)** Circular thumbs on the top of the foot. **(D)** Circular palms around the ankle. **(E)** Achilles stroke. **(F)** Circular thumbs on the bottom of the foot. **(G)** Metatarsal pull. **(H)** Stone scrape. **(I)** Metatarsal stone roll. **(J)** Transverse thumb slide. **(K)** Rotation of all toes. **(L)** Circular finger friction. **(M)** Spinal twist. **(N)** Lung press. **(O)** Solar plexus hold. **(P)** Laced fingers hold. **(Q1** and **Q2)** Bounce–bounce–traction. Lift the legs and bounce them on the massage table three times. Lean back while holding the ankles and swing the legs right and left.

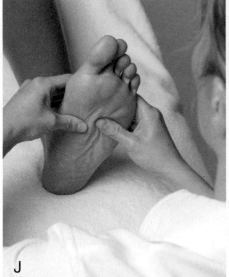

J

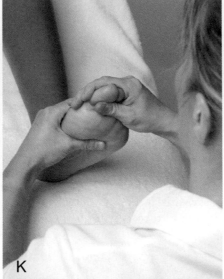

K

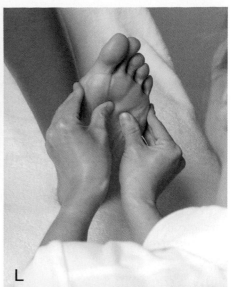

L

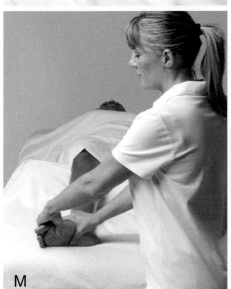

M

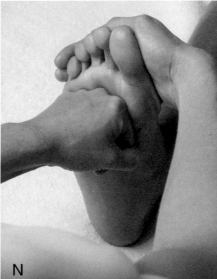

N

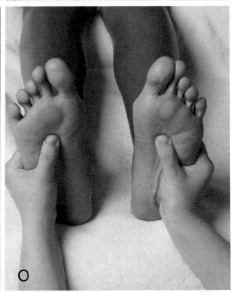

O

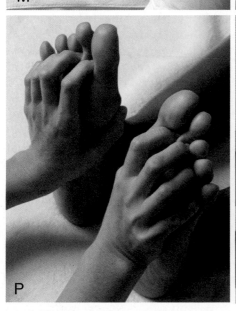

P

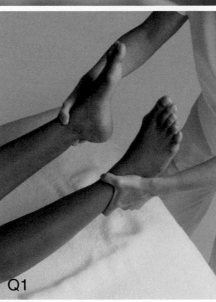

Q1

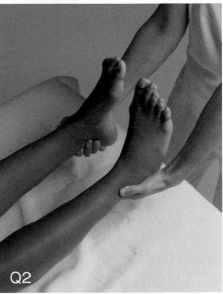

Q2

Figure 8-2 *(continued)*

Circular Thumbs on the Bottom of the Foot

Apply circular friction with the thumbs from the heel to the toes. This stroke can be repeated three to six times or combined with the metatarsal pull described below.

Metatarsal Pull

As the therapist approaches the top of the foot with circular thumbs, he or she gently grabs around the first metatarsal head with one hand and around the fifth metatarsal head with the other. The fingers fall into the groves created by the metatarsals. Loosen the foot in a sea-saw motion to complete this stroke.

Stone Scrape

Using the flat edge of a warm stone, scrape from the solar plexus point (the point directly beneath the ball of the foot) to the heel in a straight, even motion and repeat six to 10 times.

Metatarsal Stone Roll

Place the edge of the warm stone in between the fifth and fourth metatarsals and roll upward three or four times. Repeat this stroke between each of the metatarsals.

Transverse Thumb Slide

Thumb friction is applied in a crossing pattern from the bottom of the toes to the heel. When the heel is reached, the therapist begins again at the top of the foot or uses circular thumb friction to create a smooth transition. This stroke is repeated three to six times.

Rotation of All the Toes

Stabilize the foot with one hand while the other rotates all of the toes in a circle. Repeat, rotating the toes in the opposite direction. This stroke is followed by a toe twist in which each toe is lightly twisted back and forth while gentle traction is applied. The therapist will want to be careful not to pull too hard on the toes, which may cause the client discomfort.

Circular Finger Friction

With the thumbs on the plantar surface of the foot, circle the fingers down the sides of the foot using firm pressure. This stroke can be repeated three to six times.

Spinal Twist

The therapist stands at the end of the table in the center, facing out over the foot that he or she is working on. The therapist then places the hand closest to the table on the base of the client's ankle and stabilizes the foot. The outer hand twists the distal tarsals, metatarsals, and phalanges outward, moving the outer hand up the foot but leaving the lower hand firmly in place.

Lung Press

The therapist makes a fist with their outside hand and places it against the ball of the foot. The inside hand stabilizes the foot on the dorsal surface. Using a rhythmic motion, the therapist plantar flexes and dorsiflexes the foot to facilitate lymph flow.

To end a massage session, one or all of the following techniques might be used.

Solar Plexus Hold

The therapist sits while holding one foot in each hand. The thumb is positioned so that it rests on the point directly below the ball of the foot known as the solar plexus point. This is associated with deep breathing and calm. The therapist asks the client to take three deep breaths while the therapist applies firm pressure to this point on both feet at the same time.

Laced Fingers Hold

The fingertips of each hand are placed on the plantar surface of the foot, lacing them almost but not actually in between each toe. The therapist then hangs onto the foot as if hanging onto a ledge with just the fingertips. This position is held while the client is asked to take three deep breaths.

Bounce–Bounce–Traction

Standing at the end of the table in the center, hold each leg just above the foot. Lift the legs and bounce them on the massage table three times. The hands are then brought around the leg so that the therapist can lean backward and traction at the ankle while swinging the legs right and left. This releases the sacroiliac joint and relaxes the lower back. This sequence is repeated three to four times. It is important that this technique is not used with a client who has lower back, hip, pelvic, knee, or ankle problems.

The foot massage can be followed by reflexology techniques that help the body to balance and further relax and revitalize sore, tired feet.

REFLEXOLOGY

Reflexology is a therapy based on the belief that there are points on the feet, hands, and ears that stimulate the function of different parts of the body, including the glands and organs. Reflexology is most often used as a preventative therapy that aims to soothe the nervous system, reduce stress, improve circulation, and create the optimum internal environment for balanced energy, rest, and recovery. In this way, the body can draw on its natural ability to heal itself.

Although the hands, ears, and feet can all be manipulated to improve health and well being, the feet receive the most attention. The feet are considered to be very important because of their rich supply of superficial nerve endings (7000 in each foot). The feet connect us to the earth and support our bodies with an intricate structure that consists of 26 bones, 33 joints, 19 muscles, and 107 ligaments. In addition, circulation tends to stagnate in the feet because they are farthest from the heart. Inorganic waste materials such as uric acid and calcium turn to crystalline deposits that can build up in the bottom of the feet. Reflexologists focus on working every surface of the foot to decrease muscle tension and pain, increase circulation, loosen the foot so that it is more flexible and mobile, and stimulate the flow of energy through the body.

Modern reflexology owes its development to an American doctor named William Fitzgerald, who developed a comprehensive method for working the feet in the early 20th century. Dr. Fitzgerald discovered that when he applied gentle pressure to the feet, other areas of the body were affected. He called his work zone therapy and mapped out 10 zones in the body that could be accessed by "massaging" the feet or hands. When a zone on the feet or hands is worked, any gland or organ falling in the path of that zone is positively affected. Although "reflex zones" can be compared to meridians, it should be understood that although the two systems are based on similar ideas, the underlying philosophy is different.

Eunice Ingham, an American physical therapist, became interested in Fitzgerald's methods while working with Dr. Riley. She worked on a variety of patients over a number of years and kept detailed notes on her findings. She charted each body area on the foot, and through trial and error, she created an intricate map that shows the placement of reflex points for each gland and organ in the body. She is credited by many as being the first person to create an "anatomical" model of foot reflexes in which the feet are a mirror image of the body.

Ingham published her work in 1938 in a book entitled *Stories the Feet Can Tell Through Reflexology* and toured the country teaching her methods until the age of 80.[5] Her nephew, Dwight C. Byers, currently runs the International Institute of Reflexology, which counts its membership in the thousands.[6] The Ingham Method of Reflexology is a registered trademark of Dwight Byers and the International Institute of Reflexology.

Techniques

The most common technique used in reflexology is "thumb walking" (Fig. 8-3. To thumb walk, the therapist uses the edge of the thumb in an inchworm motion to take small "bites" out of the area he or she is working. The pressure is steady and firm. To practice the technique, the therapist can walk the thumb up his or her own forearm. Finger walking is similar to the thumb walk except that the edge of the index finger is used and the pressure is usually gentler. The

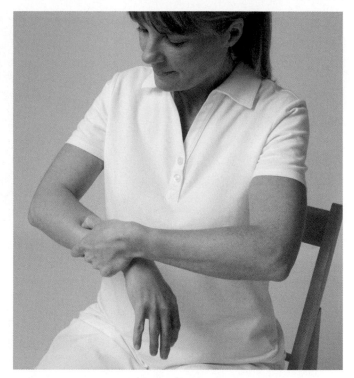

Figure 8-3   Thumb-walking technique.

hook and back-up technique is used to stimulate a specific point. The thumb is used to apply direct pressure to the point and is then pulled back slightly to hook the point (think of taking slack out of fascia). The point is then "reactivated" with direct pressure again. Sometimes a therapist will rotate his or her thumb on a point as a way of stimulating the point.

In general, when a tender area is revealed, it is noted and is given focused attention. Although the pressure used is firm, it should not feel unbearable. Areas of tenderness relate to what is considered "congestion" in the corresponding glands and organs of the body. It is important for the therapist to remember that the foot is a complex structure, prone to adhesions, hypertonicities, and inflammations, just as the rest of the body is. Congestion in an area does not necessarily indicate pathology, and the therapist should be careful not to alarm the client by relating tenderness specifically to an organ or gland.

A Stress Reduction Reflexology Routine

The amount of reflexology that is used in a spa foot treatment is left to the discretion of the therapist or the treatment designer. The routine described below takes approximately 25 minutes and works nicely when preceded by a 10-minute foot massage. This treatment focuses on "clearing the zones" and working on specific reflex points that can be activated to decrease stress and balance the body. An overview of the routine is provided in the reflexology snapshot and shown in Figure 8-4.

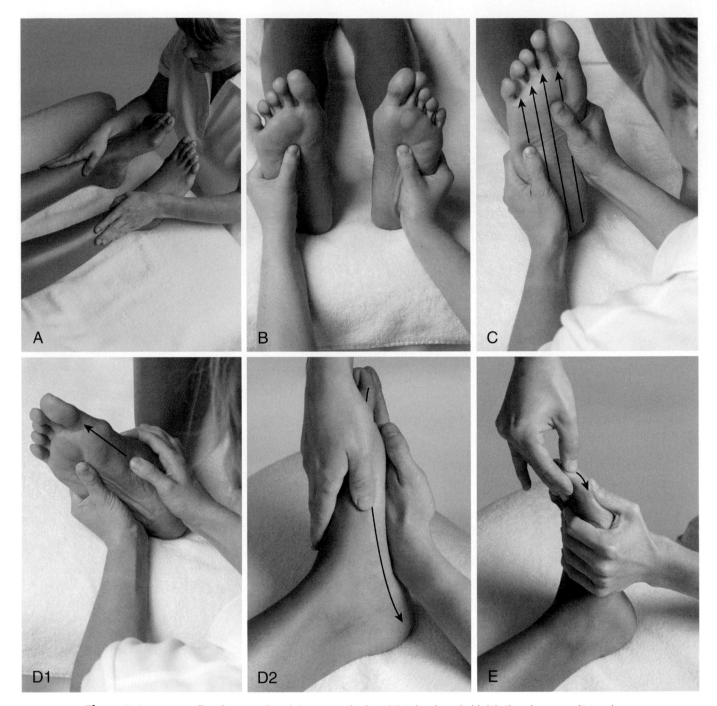

Figure 8-4   A core reflexology routine. (A) Massage the feet. **(B)** Solar plexus hold. **(C)** Clear the zones. **(D1** and **D2)** Spinal walk. Walk the spinal reflexes from the bottom up and then from the top down. **(E)** Thumb-walk the toes. **(F)** Pituitary press. **(G)** Thumb walk the horizontal lines. Thumb walk each horizontal line from zone 5 to zone 1. For longer sessions, walk the spaces in between the lines, working horizontally across the plantar surface of the foot. **(H)** Thyroid press. **(I)** Adrenal gland press. **(J)** Thumb walk the lung reflexes. **(K)** Solar plexus hold. Transition to the other foot.

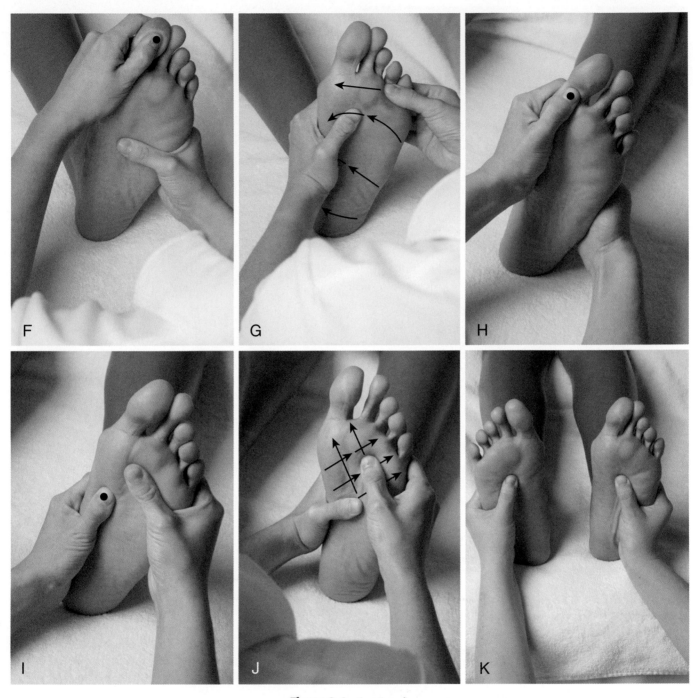

Figure 8-4   *(continued)*

Snapshot: A Reflexology Routine

Indications
Stress; for general relaxation; low energy; sore, tired feet

Contraindications
Pitted edema, broken bones or fractures, advanced or poorly treated diabetes, infections, ingrown toenails, painful corns, gout, warts, athlete's foot

Supplies for the Treatment Table Setup (from the bottom to the top layer)
1) Massage sheet
2) Bath towel situated horizontally at the bottom of the treatment table where the client's feet will sit
3) Top massage sheet
4) Blanket or bath sheet for warmth
5) Pillow for the client's head
6) Bolster

Supplies for the Work Table Setup
1) Antiseptic wipe such as a diaper wipe
2) Two hot, moist towels
3) Soda cooler
4) Massage cream
5) Dry hand towel
6) Aroma mist
7) Essential oils (optional)

Procedure
1) Cleanse the feet with a diaper wipe or cleanser and hot towels.
2) Massage.
3) Remove the massage cream from the feet.
4) Clear the zones.
5) Reflex specific points associated with relaxation.
6) Dot essential oils on reflex points (optional).
7) Aura mist to finish.

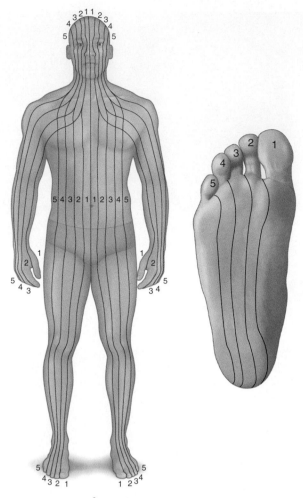

Figure 8-5 The 10 zones.

Session Start The client is supine on the treatment table with the feet at the very end of the table. The client is covered by a massage sheet and blanket for warmth. A pillow is placed under the client's head to facilitate relaxation, and the client's knees are bolstered. The therapist may choose to place a pillow under the feet to elevate them. The feet are cleansed with a disposable wipe such as a diaper wipe or with foaming cleanser and hot, moist towels.

Step 1: Massage the Feet A foot massage is used to warm up the tissue before the reflexology treatment. When the foot massage is complete, remove the lubricant from the feet with a hot, moist towel or diaper wipe. The feet need to be dry or the thumb will slip over the reflex points instead of grabbing them.

Step 2: Solar Plexus Hold The therapist sits down and places the hands in the correct position for the solar plexus hold, as described above. When it feels appropriate to move to the next step of the treatment, release and cover one foot.

Step 3: Clear the Zones When clearing the zones, make certain that the entire plantar surface of the foot has been stimulated. Figure 8-5 shows 10 zones on the bottom of the feet and the areas of the body to which they correspond. To clear the zones, thumb walk each zone from the heel to the top of the toe in that zone. It may take two or three passes over a zone before the therapist starts to feel the tissue soften. When an area of particular tension is felt, thumb walk it repeatedly to increase circulation.

Step 4: Spinal Walk Using Figure 8-6, identify the spinal reflexes. They are on the inside of both feet at the medial edge of zone 1. Thumb walk from the heel to the base of the big toe. Turn over the hand and support the plantar surface of the foot. Thumb walk from the base of the big toe to the heel. Repeat the stimulation of the spinal reflexes until the tissue softens.

Step 5: Thumb Walk the Toes Support the foot with one hand and thumb walk the toes with the other hand in a technique sometimes referred to as "biting." "Bite" the big toe first (five passes with 15 bites a pass) and work down to the little toe (three passes with 10 bites a pass). To finish the toes, roll the knuckle of a finger over each of the brain reflexes at the top of each toe.

Step 6: Pituitary Press Hook and back up on the pituitary reflex point (see Fig. 8-6 A). This point can be held with direct pressure for up to 2 minutes. A dot of lemon, pine, or myrrh essential oil (all reputed to balance the pituitary gland) can be placed on this point.

Step 7: Thumb Walk the Horizontal Lines Using Figure 8-7, identify the horizontal lines on the plantar surface of the foot. These lines include the shoulder line, diaphragm line, waist line, and pelvic line. Thumb walk each line horizontally from zone 5 to zone 1 and then again from zone 1 to zone 5. In a longer reflexology session, the areas in between each line can also be thumb walked in a cross pattern so that the entire plantar surface of the foot has again been stimulated.

Step 8: Thyroid Press Thumb walk the area associated with the thyroid point. Hook and back up on the area at the base of the big toe (see Fig. 8-4H). This point can be held with direct pressure for up to 2 minutes. A dot of pine oil or seaweed essential oil can be placed on this point after it has been stimulated.

Step 9: Adrenal Gland Apply direct pressure for up to 2 minutes to the adrenal gland reflex, which is located below the solar plexus, above the kidney, and toward the medial side of the foot (see Fig. 8-4I). A drop of rose, pine, or rosemary essential oil can be placed on this point after it has been stimulated.

Step 10: Thumb Walk the Lungs Beginning at the diaphragm line in zone 5, thumb walk diagonally across the lung reflexes to the base of the big toe. Next, thumb walk from the diaphragm line in zone 1 to the base of the little toe. Thumb walk from the diaphragm line in zone 4, diagonally across the lung reflexes to the base of the second toe. Thumb walk from the diaphragm line in zone 2 diagonally, across the lung reflexes to the base of the fourth toe (see Fig. 8-4J). The hand that is not thumb walking is always supporting the foot and holding it upright and open.

Step 11: Solar Plexus Hold and Transition to the Other Foot Take hold of the solar plexus point on both feet and take three deep breaths together with the client. Cover the foot that was just worked on, and repeat the routine on the other foot. At the end of the reflexology session, take hold of the solar plexus point and "balance the energy" between both feet with focused intent before moving onto the next section of the treatment or ending the session.

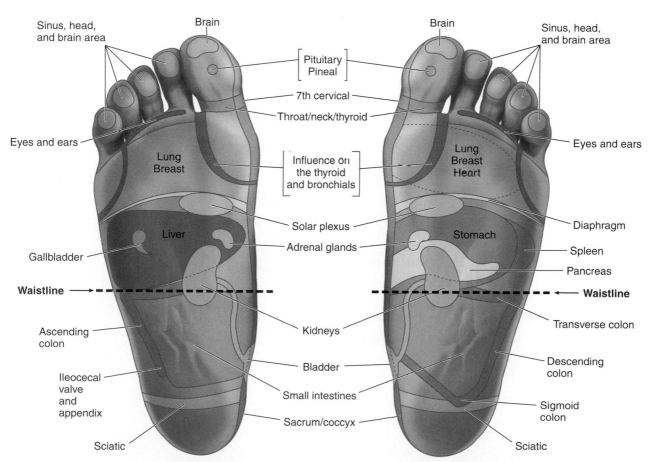

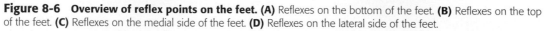

Figure 8-6 Overview of reflex points on the feet. (A) Reflexes on the bottom of the feet. **(B)** Reflexes on the top of the feet. **(C)** Reflexes on the medial side of the feet. **(D)** Reflexes on the lateral side of the feet.

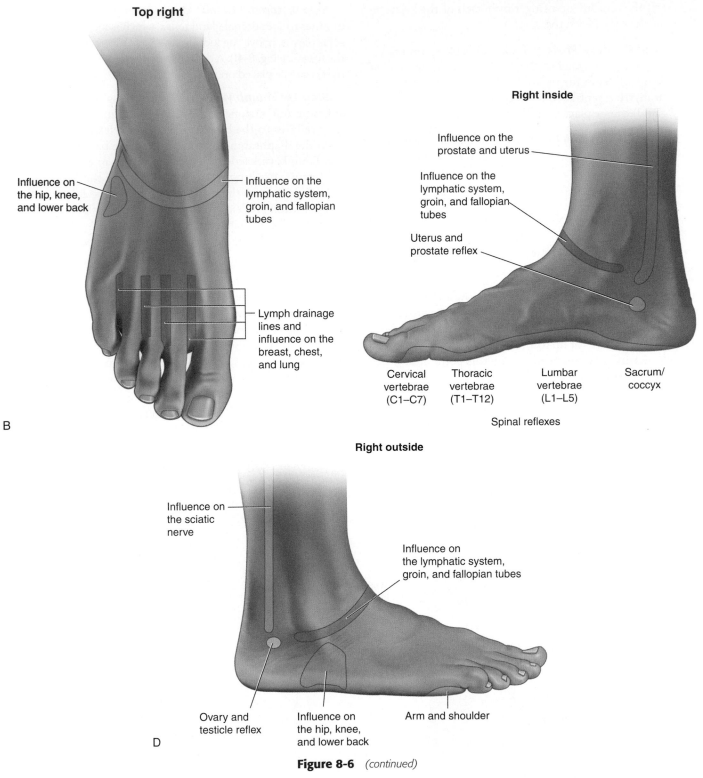

Top right

Influence on the hip, knee, and lower back

Influence on the lymphatic system, groin, and fallopian tubes

Lymph drainage lines and influence on the breast, chest, and lung

B

Right inside

Influence on the prostate and uterus

Influence on the lymphatic system, groin, and fallopian tubes

Uterus and prostate reflex

Cervical vertebrae (C1–C7)   Thoracic vertebrae (T1–T12)   Lumbar vertebrae (L1–L5)   Sacrum/ coccyx

Spinal reflexes

C

Right outside

Influence on the sciatic nerve

Influence on the lymphatic system, groin, and fallopian tubes

Ovary and testicle reflex   Influence on the hip, knee, and lower back   Arm and shoulder

D

Figure 8-6   *(continued)*

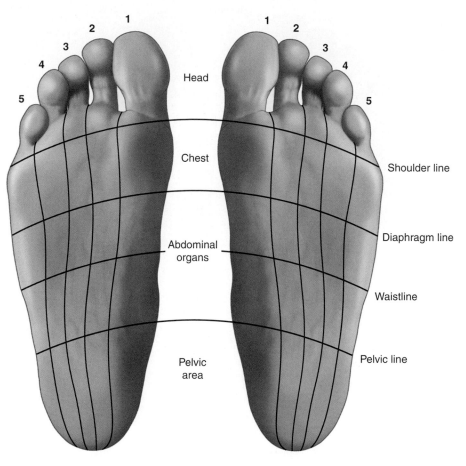

Figure 8-7   The horizontal lines on the bottom of the feet.

Designing a Reflexology Routine

By starting with steps 1 to 7 and then focusing on specific points in a systematic manner, a reflexology routine can be designed to suit most clients. For example, if a detoxification routine was indicated, steps 1 to 7 would be used and then the therapist would thumb walk or use direct pressure on the kidney, spleen, stomach, and colon points on the left foot and the kidney, liver, gallbladder, and colon points on the right foot (see Fig. 8-6A). Figure 8-8 shows some of the essential oils that are believed to have an affinity for each point.

TREATMENT PRODUCTS

Treatment products are sometimes applied as a mask to the feet and lower leg to further stimulate circulation and lymph flow, warm the feet, or soften the tissue. The physiological effect of the mask is based on the type of product used. Table 8-3 provides an overview of different masking products that might be used in a foot treatment. Before the treatment, unless the treatment product is designed to be applied cold, a sufficient amount is removed from its original container and put into a covered holding container, which is kept warm in a suitable heater (e.g., a lo-tion warmer, a roaster oven in warm water, a double boiler).

A small amount of petroleum jelly or thick, waxy cream is then applied to the cuticle and nail, covering the gap between the nail and the flesh on the tips of the toes completely. This prevents the treatment product from entering that gap and making the nail appear dirty or stained.

A piece of cellophane wrap or an open plastic bag is placed under each foot before the treatment product is applied (Fig. 8-9). This prevents messy treatment product from getting on the treatment table. After the product has been applied, the cellophane wrap or plastic bag is used to cover the foot, keep the product moist, and prevent the product from getting all over the place.

The treatment product can be applied with a gloved hand, a brush, or a fabric or a gauze strip, or the foot can be dipped into the product. To apply the product by hand, wear vinyl gloves, dip the fingers into the warm product, and smooth it evenly over the entire foot.

If a brush is used to apply the product, each clean foot is lifted by the metatarsal heads, and the heel is covered first. The heel is then placed down on top of a piece of cellophane or into the opening of the plastic bag. The top of the foot is now covered with the product, and the plastic or cellophane is brought up and around the foot.

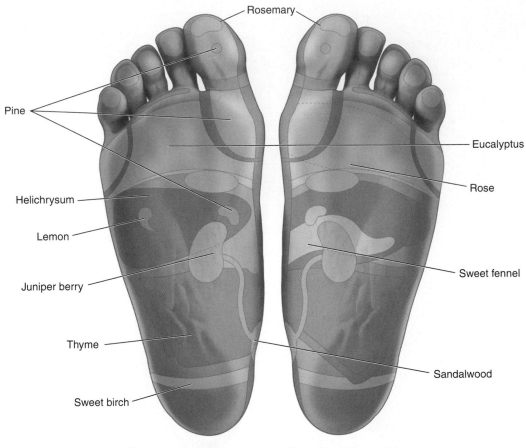

Rosemary

Pine

Eucalyptus

Rose

Helichrysum

Lemon

Sweet fennel

Juniper berry

Thyme

Sandalwood

Sweet birch

Figure 8-8 Sample essential oils for the reflex points.

Gauze strips can be dipped into the product and then wrapped around the foot. In this case, the product must be thick enough to cling to the gauze and not drip all over the floor and treatment table.

Sometimes the client's foot is dipped straight into a container of the product. This is often done with paraffin. This works best if the client is in a seated position so that the product container can be held directly under the client's foot. Dipping can also be used if the client is in a supine position, but this can be a bit tricky. The therapist brings the client's knee up toward the chest and then places the leg down along the side of the table controlling the lower leg. The therapist then brings the product container up underneath the foot. If the client is not very flexible, he or she may need to be moved to the edge of the table so that the leg is not overstretched as it is dropped over the side. All the shuffling from side to side feels a bit ungraceful and does not allow the client to relax completely.

 Sanitation

If the foot is dipped (e.g., for a paraffin dip), it should be misted with alcohol before it is dipped to prevent cross-contamination between clients.

After the product has been applied, the foot is wrapped up in cellophane or a plastic bag before being placed inside thermal booties (electric booties or microwavable booties) or being wrapped up in warm towels.

While the product is processing on the feet, the hands can be bathed and exfoliated and then dipped in paraffin. The neck, shoulders, and face can also be massaged, or the scalp can be treated.

Sanitation

After working with the feet, the therapist should always wash and sanitize his or her hands before touching any other part of the body to minimize the spread of an undetected fungal or bacterial infection.

There are two main ways to remove the product in a dry room setting. The feet can either be resoaked by placing them back into a fresh foot bath, or the product can be removed with hot towels. With heavy mud and thick seaweed, a second foot bath works well. With easy-to-remove masks such as shea butter or light clay, hot towels are quicker and easier. Special care should be taken to

Table 8-3	Foot Treatment Products

PRODUCT	BASIC THERAPEUTIC PROPERTIES
Lightening serum	Lightening serums are used to decrease skin discoloration, decrease age spots, and smooth the skin's surface. In most states, they can only be used by an esthetician or cosmetologist. Lightening serums make an excellent retail item for the gift shop.
Seaweed	Powdered seaweed can be mixed with a number of ingredients to make stimulating, detoxifying, and toning foot masks. Massage oil, water, kaolin clay, aloe gel, lotion, and essential oils can all be mixed with seaweed powders.
Fitness gels	Fitness gels are usually sold for use on the body. They often contain menthol or eucalyptus, which is pain relieving and refreshing. These products make revitalizing foot masks. The gels can be mixed up with kaolin clay to give them additional weight and heaviness for use as a treatment product.
Clay	Clay powder can be mixed with a number of different ingredients to make foot masks. Gel seaweed, aloe gel, massage oil, water, lotion and ground herbs, yogurt, fruit juices, and essential oils can all be mixed with clay powders.
Moor mud	Moor mud is a thick, rich peat that is well known for its anti-inflammatory properties. It is a good choice for sore feet or arthritis.
Dead Sea mud	Dead sea mud is high in sulfur and is used for foot pain, inflammation, and arthritis.
Cryogenic products	Cryogenic or "ice" masks are cooling and pain relieving. They are revitalizing for sore, tired feet.
Paraffin and Parafango	Paraffin and Parafango masks are warming and soothing. They are often used for arthritis or to soften and smooth the skin.
Essential oils	Essential oils can be mixed into a clay base to provide a wide range of different therapeutic effects in the feet. For example, 6 drops of juniper berry essential oil can be mixed up with clay for a detoxifying mask. Two to 4 drops of peppermint make a revitalizing mask. Eight to 10 drops of German chamomile mixed with kaolin clay and hemp seed massage oil make a good mask for foot puffiness.
Other	A variety of other professional masking products with different properties are available through spa suppliers.

wipe off the toenails (that are covered in petroleum jelly) and to make sure that the foot is clean of the treatment product. If heated booties are used to warm the treatment product, they should be removed within 20 minutes, and flushing strokes should be used to encourage fluid to move toward the heart. Otherwise, the limb may feel swollen and heavy.

FINISHING PRODUCTS

To end the service, a gel, light lotion, cooling aroma foot mist, or foot powder finishing product may be applied. These products are usually chosen based on the concept of the service. For example, a treatment for athletes with foot pain might finish with a medicated foot powder, and a soothing treatment aimed at relaxation may use a lavender lotion. The therapist should wipe down the feet after they have been moisturized to remove any excess product, especially if the spa has tiled floors. Excess product can cause a client to slip and fall when getting off the massage table.

A Sample Spa Foot Treatment Procedure

The treatment described below shows just one way that the different elements of a foot treatment might be organized together. The different elements and the order of the steps can be changed to suit the individual therapist. For example, the massage step could come before the application of the treatment product, as it does in this sample, or it could come after the application of the treatment product. For an overview of the sample treatment, view the foot treatment snapshot and Figure 8-10.

SESSION START

The client begins the session dressed in a robe and seated in a comfortable chair with his or her feet in a decorative container that is filled with warm water and a soaking additive. A side table holds a cup of warm herbal tea. A hand towel, nailbrush, cleansing product, disposable or washable slip-

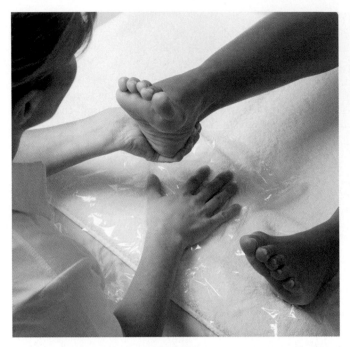

Figure 8-9   Placing a piece of cellophane under the foot before application of the treatment product.

pers, and an exfoliation product are placed to the side of the chair within easy reach of the therapist. A pedicure seat and foot rest is placed in front of the foot soak basin.

Snapshot: A Sample Spa Foot Treatment

Indications
Relaxation; foot pain; sore, tired feet; low energy; stress

Contraindications
Pitted edema, broken bones or fractures, infections, ingrown toenails, painful corns, gout, warts, athlete's foot, neuropathy, circulatory conditions

Supplies for the Treatment Table Setup (from the bottom to the top layer)
1) Massage sheet
2) Bath towel set horizontally at the bottom of the massage table
3) Top massage sheet
4) Blanket or bath sheet for warmth
5) Pillow for the client's head
6) Bolster

Supplies for the Foot Soak Setup
1) Comfortable chair for the client
2) Side table with a beverage such as hot herbal tea or lemonade
3) Pedicure chair with foot rest for the therapist (optional)
4) Foot soak container placed on top of a hand towel and filled with warm water and a soaking additive
5) Cleanser
6) Robe and slippers
7) Dry hand towel

Supplies for the Work Table Setup
1) Exfoliation product
2) Massage cream
3) Diaper wipes
4) Petroleum jelly
5) Treatment product
6) Application brush or vinyl gloves
7) Soda cooler
8) Hot, moist towels
9) Cellophane wrap or plastic bags
10) Thermal booties plugged in
11) Finishing product
12) Aroma mist
13) Paraffin dip plugged in
14) Essential oils (optional)

Procedure
1) Soak and cleanse the feet.
2) Exfoliate the feet.
3) Move the client to the treatment table.
4) Provide a foot massage.
5) Provide reflexology techniques.
6) Apply treatment product.
7) Massage the hands and arms and dip in paraffin.
8) Remove the treatment product from the feet.
9) Apply a finishing product to the feet using flushing strokes.
10) Remove the paraffin from the hands and apply flushing strokes up the arms.
11) Provide an aura mist.

STEP 1: SOAK AND CLEANSE

While the client soaks his or her feet, it is nice to provide a neck and shoulder massage. After this, take one foot out of the soak and place it on the foot rest. Apply a cleanser and gently scrub the nails with a nailbrush. Put the first foot back in the foot soak container and repeat with the second foot.

STEP 2: EXFOLIATION

Take the first foot out of the soak and put it on the foot rest. Apply an exfoliation product and scrub the foot. Rub a callus file across rough areas to the tolerance of the client if the laws of the state allow it. Callus files can feel too ticklish for some clients. If so, simply skip this step. Put the first foot back in the foot soak container and repeat with the second foot. Alternatively, the foot soak and exfoliation can take place on the treatment table.

STEP 3: MOVE THE CLIENT TO THE TREATMENT TABLE

Remove the client's feet from the soaking basin and place them on a hand towel so they can be dried. Put disposable or washable slippers on the client's feet and escort the client to the massage table (some clinics use washable mats that

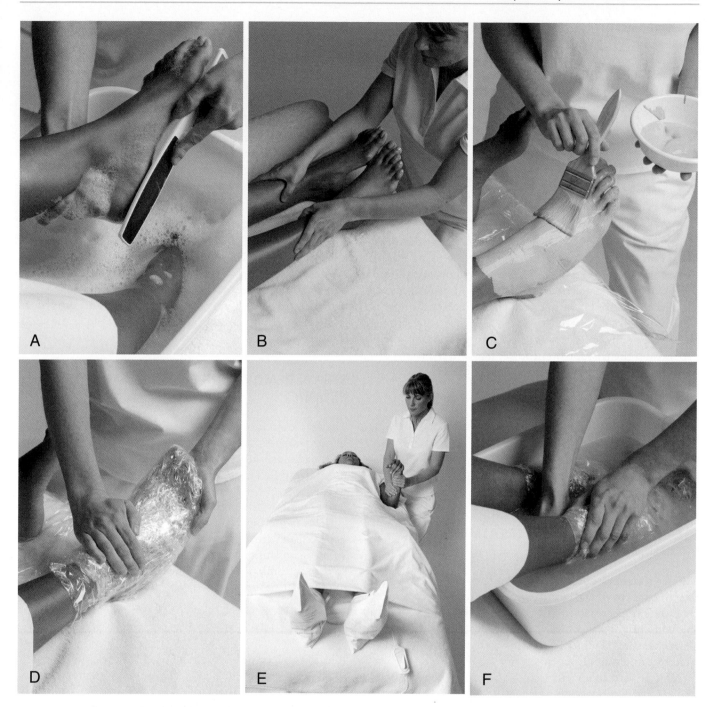

Figure 8-10   Reflexology foot spa treatment. (A) Soaking, cleansing, and exfoliating can be conducted with the client positioned on the treatment table, or the client can be soaked while seated in a chair and be moved to the treatment table after this step. This image shows the use of a callus file, which cannot be used by massage therapists in some states. **(B)** Foot massage and reflexology routine. **(C)** Application of treatment product. Cover the nail and the gap between the nail and the flesh with petroleum jelly and then apply the treatment product to the foot. **(D)** Wrap the foot in cellophane wrap (or a plastic bag) and insert the feet into heated booties or warm towels. **(E)** Process. Massage the face or treat the hands with an exfoliation, massage, and paraffin dip. **(F)** Removal of treatment product. Treatment product can be removed with hot towels or in a second foot bath, as shown here. Finish with a peppermint lotion, foot powder, or foot gel.

the client walks on to reach the treatment table). Turn away or leave the room so that the client can remove the robe and slip under the drape (the client can leave on the undergarments). Ask the client to position him- or herself with the feet at the very end of the massage table because this makes reflexology easier.

STEP 4: FOOT MASSAGE

Before the massage, a hot pack can be placed across the drape over the client's belly for warmth, and an eye pillow can be placed over the eyes to shut out light. Hot stones can also be placed on the client for warmth (see Chapter 12 for details on working with hot stones). Warm stones should not be placed on the face or over the client's eyes. If stones are placed on a client's face, the client has to hold the head still to keep the stones from sliding. This causes the client to tense his or her neck each time a technique is carried out.

The type of massage that is given during a foot treatment depends on the therapist. The lower legs and the upper anterior leg can also be massaged as part of the service.

STEP 5: REFLEXOLOGY

Remove the lubricant from the client's feet with a diaper wipe or hot, moist towels and apply the reflexology techniques to both feet. Specific reflexology points might also be dotted with an appropriate essential oil.

STEP 6: APPLICATION OF TREATMENT PRODUCT

The treatment product chosen depends on the goal and overall concept of the treatment. For example, a treatment that aims to increase circulation in the feet and stimulate the body might use seaweed or a kaolin clay with juniper berry essential oil added. A treatment that aims to revitalize tired feet might apply a peppermint mask.

A bit of petroleum jelly is applied to the cuticle and nail of each toe. The space between the nail and flesh at the tip of the toe is filled in with the jelly. This prevents treatment product from lodging in this space and making the toenails appear dirty at the end of the service.

A piece of cellophane is placed under each foot before the treatment product is applied. The therapist lifts the first foot by holding on to the ball of the foot with one hand. The product is applied underneath the heel with a brush using the other hand. After covering the heel, the foot is placed back down on the cellophane while the upper part of the foot is covered with the product. After the second foot has been covered in the same way, the cellophane is brought up and around each foot so that it completely covers the treatment product. The feet are slipped into thermal booties to process for up to 15 minutes.

STEP 7: PROCESS

Before moving on from the feet to any other body area, the therapist should always remember to decontaminate the hands. While the feet are processing in the treatment product, the arms and hands can be massaged and dipped in paraffin. Alternatively, the face can be massaged or the scalp can be treated.

STEP 8: REMOVAL OF THE TREATMENT PRODUCT

The feet are removed from the thermal booties and cellophane wrap. As the cellophane is pulled off the foot, the therapist uses it to remove as much of the treatment product as possible. The feet can either be rinsed off in a basin of warm water, or the treatment product can be removed with hot, moist towels. Special attention is paid to the nails and cuticles (which are covered in petroleum jelly). They are wiped clean with a tissue or rinsed with water until they are spotless. Flushing strokes are used to encourage circulation so that the limb does not feel heavy and swollen after wearing the thermal booties.

SESSION END

A lotion, gel, or powder can be used for the finishing step of the foot treatment depending on what is most appropriate for the treatment used. After this, the paraffin is removed from the hands and flushing strokes are applied up the client's arms. Finally, an aura mist can be spritzed in a high arch over the client to signal the end of the service.

SAMPLE TREATMENTS

Foot Loose Athlete Reprieve

Promotional Description

Whether you're a professional competitor, a weekend warrior, or you simply want a reprieve for your feet; the Foot Loose Treatment will bring relief. The session begins with a quick foot assessment aimed at identifying the "stressors" that make feet ache. Next the feet are soaked in a fizzy blend of menthol crystals and essential oils before being scrubbed with an antiseptic tea tree buff. The feet are soothed with penetrating massage strokes and reflexology point work. Next, Moor mud, long used in Europe for rheumatism, is applied in a generous layer before the feet are inserted into cozy heated booties. While the feet absorb the healing properties of the mud, the neck and shoulders are massaged.

Treatment Outline

1. Quick foot assessment
2. Soak and exfoliation
3. Massage
4. Reflexology (focus on reflexes of the muscular system)
5. Moor mud application
6. Neck massage while the Moor mud absorbs
7. Moor mud removal
8. Finish with the application of a medicated foot powder

Product Notes

Fizzy Menthol Soak

Purchase menthol crystals and citric acid from a soap making outlet. Use a pinch of each in a full basin of water.

Tea Tree Buff

Add 3 drops of tea tree essential oil to one Tbsp of exfoliation product just before applying it to the feet.

Massage Lotion

2 fl oz of massage cream with bay laurel (9 drops), sweet birch (4 drops), peppermint (2 drops), basil (2 drops), and lemon (11 drops)

Peppermint Beach Feet Tingle

Promotional Description

Tired? Run down? Do you need a day at the beach and just can't find the time? This treatment aimed at refreshing the feet is lighthearted and upbeat! The feet commune with the sea in an ocean soak with soothing seaweed. Next, sea salt is applied in a vigorous buff that removes hardened skin and stimulates circulation. A massage with aromatic lotions and reflexology techniques prepares the feet for the peppermint kelp mask that leaves feet refreshed and tingly. While the mask works its magic, your therapist will smooth your hands with a gentle buff and a massage. This treatment is almost as fun as a day at the beach!

Treatment Outline

Follow the directions for a basic foot treatment using the products described below. Peppermint products obtained from a spa supplier can also be used.

Product Notes

Ocean Soak

$\frac{1}{2}$ cup of sea salt, 1 tsp of seaweed powder, warm water. It's nice to include polished ocean stones and a clean, smooth-textured shell in the foot basin.

Sea Salt Scrub

Mix 2 Tbsp of foaming body wash with sea salt just before applying it to the feet.

Peppermint Kelp Mask

Mix $\frac{1}{2}$ cup of powdered kelp with $\frac{1}{2}$ cup of kaolin clay and add water until it reaches the consistency of a thick paste. Add $\frac{1}{2}$ cup aloe vera gel or a light lotion and mix the formula until it is smooth and creamy. Cover the mixture with plastic wrap and heat it until it is warm. Add 3 drops of peppermint essential oil directly to the mixture before applying it to the feet.

Ocean Body Mist

Add 10 drops of mandarin, 3 drops of basil, and 2 drops of sweet fennel to 2 oz of distilled water in a mist bottle.

The Garden Walk

Promotional Description

When your feet need gentle relief, the Garden Walk foot treatment is the answer. A rose petal soak is followed by a sweet sage buff and "sunshine" masque. A lavender lotion is used for a light reflexology session, and your hands receive a relaxing massage and paraffin dip. This treatment is soft and soothing like a walk along a shady garden path.

Treatment Outline

Follow the treatment steps for the basic foot treatment using the products described below.

Products

Rose Petal Soak

Add foaming body wash and 1 drop of rose essential oil to warm water and froth it into bubbles. Sprinkle rose petals on top of the bubbles.

Sweet Sage Buff

2 Tbsp of exfoliation cream, 1 drop clary sage, 1 drop Spanish sage, 2 drops lavender, and 3 drops mandarin essential oil

Sunshine Masque

$\frac{1}{2}$ cup milk powder, $\frac{1}{2}$ cup finely ground oatmeal, 1 Tbsp honey, 2 Tbsp aloe vera gel, and 4 drops of sweet orange essential oil. Add warm water until the mask achieves the consistency of a paste.

Lavender Foot Powder

1 Tbsp plain foot powder and 1 tsp of powdered lavender (powder the lavender in a coffee grinder)

Summary

Foot treatments are popular offerings on spa menus across the country. Although massage therapists cannot perform nail care as would be expected in a pedicure, they can mix and match treatment elements to design enjoyable foot care services.

When designing a foot treatment, the therapist often includes a foot assessment step, soaking and cleansing step, exfoliation, treatment mask, massage, and reflexology techniques. Other steps and techniques can be added based on the training and interests of the therapist.

Reflexology is a technique that is often used in foot treatments. It is a holistic therapy based on the belief that there are points on the hands, ears, and feet that correspond to every area of the body. Through stimulation of these points, the body is relaxed, allowing it to rest and recover. Reflexology routines can be designed to benefit every system in the body by focusing on the specific reflex points for the organs or glands that play a role in the particular system.

REFERENCES

1. The General Causes of Foot Pain. University of Maryland Medical Center. Available at http://www.umm.edu
2. Heart JA. Foot Pain and Shoe Size. Available at http://www.nlm.nih.gov
3. Runquist B: *Anatomy and Foot Loosening for Reflexology Seminar Materials.* Seattle School of Reflexology, 1996.
4. *Getting Nailed.* An ABC News 20/20 presentation. Available at http://www.spatrade.com
5. Ingham ED: *Stories the Feet Can Tell Thru Reflexology.* Revised by Byers DC. Ingham Publications, 1992.
6. International Institute of Reflexology. Available at http://www.reflexology-use.net

REVIEW QUESTIONS

Multiple Choice

1. A _____ is a foot treatment in which the cuticle is pushed back and trimmed, the nail is trimmed, and the nail is filed.
   a. Reflexology treatment
   b. Foot massage
   c. Pedicure
   d. Manicure

2. The border of the nail is partly covered by a fold of skin commonly called the _____.
   a. Cuticle
   b. Callus
   c. Plantar surface
   d. Dorsal surface

3. A small area of thickened skin that is caused by continued friction or pressure is called a _____.
   a. Cuticle
   b. Callus
   c. Plantar surface
   d. Dorsal surface

4. An individual who is certified or licensed to provide care of the nails or to apply, repair, or decorate gel nails or acrylic nails is called a _____.
   a. Massage therapist
   b. Esthetician
   c. Hand and foot specialist
   d. Nail technician

5. The arch of the foot refers to _____.
   a. Actually three strong arches (the medial longitudinal arch, lateral longitudinal arch, and transverse arch) that give the foot the strength to support the weight of the body
   b. Actually two strong arches (the longitudinal arch and the transverse arch) that give the foot the strength to support the weight of the body
   c. There is no true arch in the foot. Instead, the foot is flat.
   d. The ankle is sometimes referred to as the arch of the foot.

Matching

Please place an X by the techniques that are out of the scope of practice of a massage therapist. Place an A by techniques that the massage therapist can perform in a foot treatment.

_____ Polish is removed and the nail is trimmed and shaped with an emery board.

_____ Reflexology techniques are performed.

_____ The cuticle is pushed back and the excess is trimmed.

_____ A treatment product such as seaweed, mud, or paraffin is applied to the feet.

_____ The feet are soaked in a basin of warm water.

Fangotherapy

Key Terms

Clay: A variable group of fine-grained natural materials that is usually "plastic" when moist and are mainly mineral in composition.

Emulsion: A mixture of two or more liquids in which one is present as microscopic droplets distributed throughout the other.

Fango: The Italian word for mud; the term is used loosely to describe products that include mud, peat, and clay.

Moor mud: A low-moor peat from the Neydharting Moor in Austria that is well known for its anti-inflammatory effects. It is regularly mined and shipped to the United States for spa treatments.

Mud: Soft, wet earth that is mainly mineral in composition (derived from rock) with some percentage of organic matter (matter derived from plant breakdown).

Peat: Partially carbonized organic tissue formed by decomposition in water of various plants but mainly mosses of the genus *Sphagnum*.

Sphagnum: A genus of mosses that grows only in wet acid areas where their remains are compacted over time (sometimes with other plants) to form peat.

Sulfur: A chemical element that is an important constituent of many proteins and is often found in thermal pools and in some therapeutic muds. Sulfur is believed to reduce oxidative stress on the body and is used to treat arthritis, sore muscles, skin diseases, and other conditions.

angotherapy is the use of **mud**, **peat**, and **clay** for healing purposes (Fig. 9-1). The word *fango* is the Italian word for mud, so, strictly speaking, peat and clay should not be labeled as fango treatments. However, most spas use the term *fango* loosely, so to avoid confusion, the more general meaning of the word is adopted here.

Each of these materials (mud, clay, and peat) has its own special properties, but in general, they hold heat and are useful as a thermal application for chronic conditions. They also stimulate circulation and lymph flow, support detoxification, and help the body to relax. Some types of fango have anti-inflammatory and pain-relieving properties that make them useful for soft tissue injury. The sensation of being covered in thick, warm mud is a unique experience for clients, so services featuring fango are a regular and popular item on spa menus. This chapter aims to briefly describe the classic use of fango, identify different type of fango products, and build on the skills learned in previous chapters. New treatments (scalp and neck treatment, back treatment) are described in step-by-step detail, but discussions of services such as the full-body fango cocoon assume that the reader has achieved proficiency with the treatments outlined in earlier chapters. This chapter also introduces the use of fango for the different stages of inflammation in the healing process. This information will be of use to the massage therapists who work at medical spas or who regularly treat soft tissue injury in their private practices.

The reader may want to review Chapter 3 ("Foundation Skills for Spa Treatment Delivery"), Chapter 6 ("Exfoliation Treatments"), and Chapter 7 ("Body Wraps") before providing the treatments in this chapter. The therapist may also want to read the section on Indian head massage in Chapter 11 ("Ayurveda") for ideas on strokes to use during scalp and neck treatments.

Fangotherapy in Europe

Many early European spas originated around thermal areas with mineral hot springs. The mud around a hot spring was used for its therapeutic mineral content. It was common for a spring to hold religious significance for the local people, so bathing in the springs or using the mud from the area

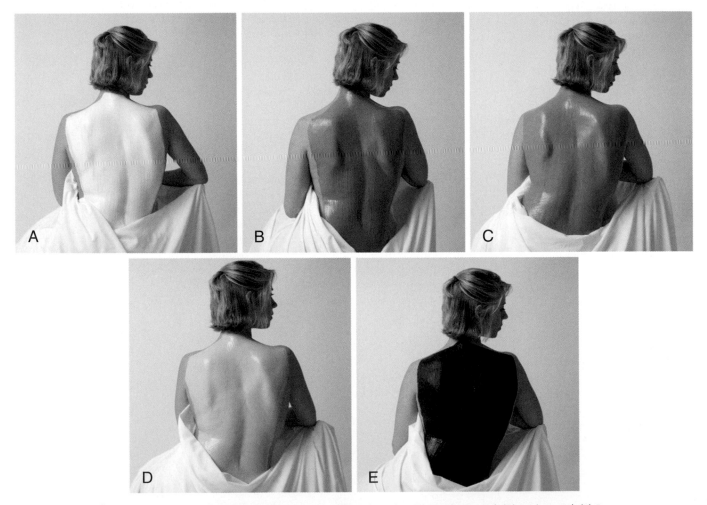

Figure 9-1   Clay, mud, and peat. (A) Kaolin clay. **(B)** Sedona clay. **(C)** Dead Sea mud. **(D)** Marine mud. **(E)** Peat.

was believed to give healing on both a spiritual and physical level.[1] Over time, research has shown that hot spring mud and the microorganisms that it contains have healing properties that are valuable for the treatment of a wide range of conditions.

As mentioned in Chapter 1, the Italian towns of Abano, Montegrotto, Galzignano, and Battaglia are famous for their thermal baths, which have a long history of use. Over the centuries, people have come to the area for the healing properties of the thermal fango (Euganaean Hills mud) that is found at the spas. Today, more than 170 hotels with spa facilities circle the 130 mineral springs. Traditionally, the mud was used in its natural state, but now it is "matured" in special tanks to improve its therapeutic properties. The maturation process, which was developed by the Pietro d'Abano Spa Research Centre, involves incubating the mud in Euganaean mineral water for 50 to 60 days, allowing the nonpathogenic microorganisms present to multiply. The mud is used to treat osteoarthritis, fibromyalgia, soft tissue injury, inflammation, and some skin conditions.

In Europe, fangotherapy usually takes place once or twice a year at health spas under a doctor's guidance. Although the regimen may vary from spa to spa, the patient will have fasted for at least 4 to 6 hours before the treatment. The treatment generally begins with mud applied to the body at a temperature of around 104° to 115°F (40° to 46°C). Full-body applications are left on for 20 minutes, and spot treatments are left in place for up to 30 minutes. The mud treatment is followed by hydrotherapy in the form of a mineral soak in the thermal waters of the region or a hot and cold contrast shower. Sometimes the patient is wrapped in blankets to increase perspiration after the hydrotherapy soak. The treatment ends with a massage and a long nap.

Fangotherapy in the United States

Evidence suggests that every major U.S. hot spring (and probably its associated mud) was used at some point by an Indian tribe.[1] The Native Americans considered a hot spring as sacred, neutral ground. Warriors could rest by a hot spring to heal a battle wound without worry of being attacked by another tribe. The early European settlers recognized the healing benefits of these hot springs and later developed them into commercial spas in the tradition of their homelands. Saratoga Springs in New York is an example of this type of early American spa.

In the face of modern medicine, spa therapy declined in the 1940s, and many of the European-inspired spa centers closed. With their closure, some of the specific knowledge about thermal waters and therapeutic mud at these locations was lost.[1]

The increasing focus on fitness and wellness has fueled the reemergence of the spa industry and, with it, the use of fango for healing. At the time of writing, fango treatments are mainly used for skin care in the United States. This may be because their therapeutic benefits have yet to be fully understood or appreciated. Another factor may be that most spa clients are familiar with the idea that fango improves the texture of the skin but may be less clear about its benefits for the musculoskeletal system and body. This is likely to change as information spreads about the use of fango treatments for decreasing pain from chronic conditions such as osteoarthritis or soft tissue injury, supporting detoxification, reducing stress, and relaxing the body.

Types of Products Used in Fangotherapy

All types of fango have heat-retention properties and can be warmed up and applied to relax the body or decrease muscular tension. Clay, mud, and peat have different therapeutic properties and uses. Clay is mainly mineral (derived from rock) and is the most "drawing" and stimulating of the fango substances. Mud is also predominantly mineral but has small amounts of organic components that give anti-inflammatory or analgesic properties. Peat is therapeutically the most active substance of the three because it is mainly organic and derived from the breakdown of plant material over thousands of years. A number of European studies had concluded that peat is anti-inflammatory, analgesic, a circulatory stimulant, antiviral, immune boosting, and endocrine balancing. Table 9-1 gives an overview of fangotherapy substances.

CLAY

Clay is a general term for a variable group of fine-grained natural materials that are usually "plastic" when moist. When viewed under an electron microscope, clay particles are about 100 times longer than they are wide. If water is added to dry clay, the moisture is held between the flat plates by surface tension so that the particles do not pull apart, but instead, slide easily over one another. This gives moist clay its smooth and creamy consistency.

Many different types of clay are commercially available from different soils and environments around the world. Clays from marine sediments or from areas around hot springs or geysers usually have a higher mineral content than other clays, but all commercially available clay have the same basic properties. First, clay holds heat, so it can be warmed and used to decrease muscle tension and relax the body. Second, clay is highly absorbent and is used to draw impurities and moisture from the surface of the skin. This "drawing" action stimulates circulation and lymphatic flow and purifies the skin. Finally, clays readily suspend to form an **emulsion** in water and other liquid substances. This property is useful in cosmetics because clay helps to hold other substances together and prevent separation. Clay is regularly used as an emollient and colorant in powders,

| Table 9-1 | Fangotherapy at a Glance |

COMPOSITION	CATEGORIES	MAIN TYPES	COMMERCIAL NAME	PROPERTIES	USES
Mainly mineral	Clay	Kaolinite Illite	Kaolin, China white, French green	Thermal, relaxing, circulatory stimulant, absorbs excess oil and draws out impurities, suspends to form an emulsion to hold cosmetic substances together, acts as a carrier for other therapeutic products	As a thermal agent to warm and relax the body, as a base for treatment products, for esthetics Cosmetic emulsions
		Semectite	Bentonite, Fuller's earth, MAS		
	Mud	Sulfur containing and "matured"	Dead Sea, Euganaean, Piestany, many others	Anti-inflammatory, circulatory stimulant, analgesic, antiseptic, immune boosting, thermal, detoxifying, relaxing, others	Arthritis, muscle pain or soreness, joint pain, inflammation, relaxation, revitalization, esthetics, others
Mainly organic	Low-moor peat High-moor peat	Mosses and other plants Mainly mosses	Moor mud, many others Many European types	Anti-inflammatory, circulatory stimulant, antiviral, antiseptic, immune boosting, endocrine balancing, thermal, detoxifying, relaxing, others	Arthritis, muscle pain or soreness, joint pain, inflammation, relaxation, revitalization, esthetics, others

liquid foundations, lotions, and skin masks. This characteristic also makes it useful as a carrier product for other therapeutic substances. Items such as seaweed, herbal infusions, essential oils, and natural food products (e.g., yogurt, honey, milk, fruit juices, mashed fruits) can be mixed into clay to make interesting treatment products. The use of clay is often associated with the areas in which it was mined. For example, Sedona clay is no more healing than other clays, but its link to the majestic red rocks of Arizona and to Native American healing traditions make it a popular choice with clients. Table 9-2 gives an overview of some popular and commercially available clay, and Table 9-3 offers some easy clay recipes for in-house treatment products.

MUD

Like clay, mud is mainly mineral in origin, but it contains 2% to 4% organic substances, which play an important role in its therapeutic use. Therapeutic mud is "matured" or "ripened" in natural mineral water. The maturing process for each mud may be slightly different, but it generally involves the oxidation and reduction of the mud over a period of up to 12 months. The process of maturing the mud is characterized by changes in the chemical composition of the mud and changes in its appearance.[2]

A good example is the maturing process used at the Piestany spa in Slovakia. The brown Piestany mud is matured to increase its **sulfur** content by "curing" the mud in outdoor storage units and exposing it to bacteria, which reduce the sulfates present in the mud to sulfides. This changes the mud's color from brown to black.[2] Up to 40,000 patients visit the spa each year to receive its famous fango treatment for arthritis.[3]

Sulfur is perhaps the most important component in the different kinds of therapeutic mud and occurs naturally in the vicinity of volcanoes and hot springs. Sulfur baths have been researched as a viable means of reducing oxidative stress on the body and decreasing inflammation in muscles and joints.[4] Sulfur-rich mineral and mud baths are useful in the treatment of osteoarthritis, rheumatoid arthritis, and other inflammatory conditions. Individuals report that they experience increased strength, decreased morning stiffness, better walking ability, and decreased pain after a course of sulfur mud treatment. Therapeutic mud is also used successfully for bursitis, tendonitis, sprains, strains, and other musculoskeletal injuries and disorders.

One of the most popular types of sulfur-containing therapeutic mud is that obtained from the Dead Sea region in Israel. The extremely saline water (27% salt) is 10 times saltier than the Mediterranean Sea and has a high concentration of calcium, magnesium, sodium, potassium, and bromine. Research on Dead Sea mud supports its use in the treatment of arthritis,[5] rheumatoid arthritis,[6] skin problems, and respiratory diseases.[7]

Table 9-2 | Overview of Popular Clays

CLAY TYPE	COMMERCIAL NAME	ORIGINS	APPEARANCE OR TEXTURE	COMMENTS
Kaolinite: From the Chinese word *kauling* meaning "high ridge," referring to the hill in the Jiangxi Province of southeastern China from which the clay was first obtained	Kaolin, China white, China clay	Southeastern China; Malaysia; Cornwall; England; and Georgia, United States	Fine-grained consistency, pure white color, smooth and creamy when wet	A good choice for in-house treatment products or as a carrier for essential oils
Illite: These clays are mica-like in structure and often originate from recently deposited deep-sea sediments; the most common clay found in nature	French green (French green clay classically refers to an illite clay that has been mined in France and sun dried)	Illite clays are found all over the world; the title "French green clay" does not always mean the product originated in France	Extremely fine-grained, pale in color, smooth and creamy when wet	A good choice for in-house treatment products but often more expensive than kaolin
Semectite: Expanding lattice clays that usually swell in water	Sedona clay	Sedona, Arizona: Formed from ancient ocean sediment and volcanic activity	Fine to medium textured, red in color, smooth to slightly abrasive	A good choice for treatments aimed at detoxification or that contain a Native American spiritual element
	Wyoming bentonite	Often from Mississippi and Alabama; associated with freshwater sediments	Consistency can be lumpy, gray or brownish in color	Because the consistency can be lumpy, this is a good clay to avoid unless it has been processed commercially
	Sodium bentonite	Associated with marine sediments and mined in many areas of the world	Gel-like in consistency and gray or brownish in color (may also be yellowish, pinkish, or greenish)	Used to regulate the viscosity in homemade skin care products; kaolin and French green clay are easier to use as treatment products
	Fuller's earth	England and other areas; the clay gets its name from "fulling," the process of removing grease from woolen cloth	When mixed with water, it crumbles into mud and has little natural plasticity; therefore, it has a lumpy, crumbly consistency	Kaolin and French green clay are a better alternative for in-house treatment products

| Table 9-3 | Creative Clay Mix-Ups* | | |

NAME	RECIPE	PROPERTIES	USES
Juniper clay	**Spot treatment:** 4 drops of juniper berry essential oil and water to the desired consistency. **Full-body treatment:** 8 drops of juniper berry, 10 drops of grapefruit, and 2 drops of lemon oil with water to the desired consistency	Stimulating, warming, detoxifying, circulatory and lymphatic stimulant, revitalizing	Foot mask for sore feet, full-body fango cocoon for detoxification, spot treatment for sore muscles
Coffee clay	**Spot treatment:** 1 shot of espresso and warm water or strong coffee to the desired consistency **Full-body treatment:** 3 shots of espresso and warm water or strong coffee to the desired consistency	Stimulating, firming, circulatory stimulant	Spot treatment for body contouring or cellulite
Peppermint clay	**Spot treatment:** 3 to 6 drops of peppermint essential oil and warm water to the desired consistency	Stimulating, cooling, revitalizing, analgesic, circulatory and lymphatic stimulant	Foot mask for tired feet, spot treatment for sore muscles, spot treatment for cellulite
Rose petal clay Lavender clay	**Spot treatment:** 1 tsp of dried and powdered rose petals or lavender, 1 drop of rose or 4 drops of lavender essential oil, and warm water to the desired consistency. **Full-body treatment:** 2 Tbsp of dried and powdered rose petals or lavender, 2 drops of rose or 8 drops of lavender essential oil, and warm water to the desired consistency	Relaxing, soothing, calming, softening	Foot or hand mask for a gentle treatment, full-body mask for a relaxation treatment
Pain-away clay	**Spot treatment:** 2 drops sweet birch oil, 2 drops eucalyptus oil, 1 drop German chamomile, hemp seed oil to desired consistency (do not use water). **Full-body treatment:** 6 drops sweet birch oil, 4 drops eucalyptus oil, 2 drops German chamomile oil, hemp seed oil to desired consistency (do not use water)	Analgesic, circulatory stimulant, antispasmodic, anti-inflammatory	Application to a specific joint, application to an area of pain (e.g., back, hamstring), spot treatment for sore feet
Egyptian clay	**Spot treatment:** 2 drops frankincense, 2 drops myrrh, 1 drop rose, and water to the desired consistency	Relaxing, softening, soothing, calming	For a treatment inspired by Egypt, for a full-body fango cocoon aimed at relaxation

Table 9-3   *(continued)*

NAME	RECIPE	PROPERTIES	USES
	Full-body treatment: 8 drops frankincense, 4 drops myrrh, 1 drop of rose, 1 drop of geranium, and water to the desired consistency		
Botanical clay	A variety of powdered herbs can be used and mixed with clay powder. Add 2 Tbsp of powdered herbs to every cup of clay. Use an herbal infusion or tea to mix up the clay powder. For example, a green tea and lemongrass make a nice botanical combination.	The properties will be based on the botanicals that are used in the mix	Foot or hand mask, full-body detoxification treatment, slimming treatment
Sunny clay	1/2 cup of powdered oatmeal is added to every 1/2 cup of clay powder and mixed with warm juice (apple, cranberry, pineapple, or orange work well) to the desired consistency.	Refreshing, softening, revitalizing	Foot or hand masks, full-body cocoons aimed at relaxation and revitalization
Natural food items clay	Natural food items can be blended with clay and water to form treatment products. For example, fresh pumpkin, fresh avocado, fresh mango, or fresh papaya might be mixed with clay and water in a blender to the desired consistency. Note: Blend the clay as little as possible because it can lose some of its permeability with overmixing.	Refreshing, relaxing, softening, stimulating	Foot or hand treatment, back treatment, hair treatment, full-body cocoon

* Each of these products can be mixed into any type of clay base. The reader will notice that the exact amount of clay or liquid is not indicated. This is because different clays hold water and mix up differently. The reader is advised to start with 1/2 cup of clay for a spot treatments and 1 cup of clay for a full-body treatment. More clay may be needed depending on the size of the client. The different liquids should be added until the desired consistency is reached. Aim for a creamy texture that is not too runny. To powder a botanical ingredient, dry it and place it in a coffee grinder.

PEAT

Sphagnum is the main genus of mosses that form a bog. As the *Sphagnum* moss decays, the bog becomes filled with a deeper and deeper layer of dead *Sphagnum*, which is known as peat. The lack of oxygen in the bog and the acidic conditions created by *Sphagnum* slow the growth of microbes. This is why human bodies unearthed from peat bogs thousands of years after burial are perfectly preserved. Because the rate of decomposition is very slow, the minerals usually recycled by living things remain in the peat.[8] This is why peat is therapeutically active and why gardeners use peat to build up the fertility of soil.

Peat is usually broken down into two main commercial categories: high-moor peat and low-moor peat. The basis for this is unclear, and the two types are often so similar that they are difficult to separate without information on their geographical origin.[9] Spas generally prefer to use low-moor peat (a well-known lowland peat is **Moor mud** from the Neydharting Moor in Austria) because it is thought to have a broader range of therapeutic properties than high-moor peat. This idea reflects the belief that compared with high-moor peat, low-moor peat is composed of a wider range of plant species, so it is likely to have a wider range of therapeutic properties. However, research gives no clear evidence of a significant difference in the therapeutic benefits of the two types of peat.

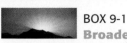

BOX 9-1
Broaden Your Understanding

Fango Benefits for the Skin
Estheticians value fango applications for the reason that clay, mud, and peat benefit the skin and improve the skin's texture. Because of its absorbent nature, clay is the most popular choice for oily skin types. Clay draws impurities out of the skin, stimulates circulation which aids in nutrient exchange, and retextures the skin by supporting natural exfoliation. Clay can also be softening, even for dry skin so long as it is kept moist while it is on the skin and not allowed to dry out.

Mud and peat soften the skin's texture, and some minerals may be absorbed from the mud into the skin, although the evidence for this is unclear. Some studies suggest that fango treatments help to normalize the pH of the skin, strengthen the barrier function of the stratum corneum, decrease transdermal water loss, and normalize sebum flow, making fango useful for both dry and oily skin.[18,19] After a full-body fango application, clients often notice the improved texture of their skin and its softness.

General Treatment Considerations

Before providing a fango treatment, assess the contraindications for the treatment and pay attention to the special storing, mixing, warming, and processing requirements for fango.

CONTRAINDICATED INDIVIDUALS

Clients with heart or circulatory conditions; who are pregnant; or have a fever, diabetic neuropathy, or a neurological disorder should not receive full-body hot fango treatments. Spot applications on such individuals may be appropriate for use depending on the medical condition, the temperature of the fango (98° to 102°F is recommended), the length of the treatment, and the other products that are being used.

BROKEN OR INFLAMED SKIN

The use of peat and mud is not advised on broken or inflamed skin. Although peat and mud are regularly used in Europe and by estheticians for skin care, broken skin is prone to infection. Peat and mud are not necessarily

checked for harmful pathogens or held to any standardized quality requirements. Clay can be used with oily skin that has minor blemishing, but severe acne, which might be located on a client's back, should not be treated except by an esthetician or dermatologist.

FANGO TEMPERATURE

Fango can be applied from room temperature up to 115°F. It is interesting to note that in Europe the fango is applied at a temperature of 104° to 115°F even in situations where acute inflammation is present. Despite the excellent results they achieve in Europe, it is better to err on the side of caution and not use hot temperatures for inflammation. Apply fango at room temperature or chilled to the area of injury, and apply heated fango to the rest of the body. Areas distal to the injury site should not be treated with fango to prevent stagnation in the distal tissue. An overview of the use of fango for soft tissue injury and inflammation with specific temperature recommendations is given below. A metal probe–type thermometer or a latte thermometer can be used to check the temperature of the fango.

MIXING AND STORING FANGO PRODUCTS

When using mud, clay, or peat, they should not be mixed or stored in metal containers because they may react chemically with the metal. Clays can lose some of their permeability if they are overprocessed or overmixed. It is recommended that fango products are heated only once in a double boiler, used shortly afterward, and the leftovers discarded.

PREVENTING DRY OUT

Mud and peat are not commonly allowed to dry out on the body. They are covered in plastic or with a hot, damp towel during the treatment to keep them moist. This is because the therapeutic properties of the mud are affected if the fango dries out and the microorganisms living in the fango are killed. For certain purposes (e.g., to draw blood to an area or oily skin on the back), clay can be allowed to dry out slightly but not completely. Clay that is too dry is not good for the skin because it can become irritated and dehydrated as the clay pulls out its moisture and oils. Use a moisturizing lotion after using a clay product on any area of the body.

The Full-Body Fango Cocoon

A full-body fango cocoon is indicated for a wide range of conditions, including low energy, low immunity, stress, muscle tension and soreness, chronic soft tissue conditions such as fibromyalgia, cellulite, contouring treatments, and for detoxification. Full-body applications of mud, clay, or peat are difficult to carry out in a dry room setting because product removal is time consuming and the client may get cold and impatient. Gel-based fango products are now available and are easy to remove in a dry room, but the fango in these products is significantly diluted. If a shower is not available, a gel-based product or spot treatment is recommended.

In the Full-Body Fango Cocoon Snapshot, after the fango has been removed, a foaming body wash is used to help clean off any remaining traces of fango if a gel-based product was not used and no shower is available. Although step-by-step directions for a cocoon wrap are described in Chapter 7, the reader will notice that this outline does not follow the directions exactly. As with any service, treatment steps can be mixed and matched depending on the facility, products, and the preferences of the individual therapist.

Snapshot: The Full-Body Fango Cocoon

Indications
Stress, muscle tension and soreness, chronic soft tissue condition, relaxation, detoxification, body contouring, revitalization

Contraindications
Heart or circulatory conditions, pregnancy, fever, diabetic neuropathy or neurological disorders, recent soft tissue injury, any condition contraindicated for massage

Supplies for the Treatment Table Setup (from the bottom to the top layer)
1) Blanket (wool or cotton) placed across the table (horizontally) so that the long edges are at 90 degrees to the table edges
2) Thermal space blanket placed horizontally (optional)
3) A plain flat sheet placed in a standard orientation with its long edges parallel to the edge of the table (if the fango needs to be removed in a dry room)
4) A plastic sheet placed horizontally
5) One bath towel placed horizontally at the top of the table
6) One bath towel placed horizontally at the bottom of the table
7) Drape
8) Bolster
A Fomentek might be used under the massage sheet if additional warmth is needed.

Supplies for the Work Table Setup
1) Dry brushes
2) Fango warming in a double boiler
3) Application brush or vinyl gloves
4) Bowl of warm water
5) Foaming body wash product
6) Massage cream
7) Aura mist
8) Soda cooler
9) Hot, moist towels
10) Dry hand towels
11) Disposable undergarments

Dry Room Procedure
1) Dry brush the posterior body areas.
2) Apply fango to the posterior body areas.
3) Turn the client supine using the flip-over method.
4) Dry brush the anterior body areas.
4) Apply fango to the anterior body areas.
5) Cocoon for 20 to 30 minutes. Massage the feet, face, or both while the fango is processing.
6) Unwrap.
7) Remove the fango from the client's body and remove the plastic sheeting under the client.
8) Cleanse and then massage each anterior body area.
9) Aura mist.
10) Turn the client prone.
11) Cleanse and then massage each posterior body area.

Procedure if a Shower is Available
1) Exfoliate or dry brush the posterior body areas.
2) Turn the client supine.
3) Exfoliate or dry brush the anterior body areas.
4) Apply fango using the sit-up method.
5) Cocoon for 20 to 30 minutes. Massage the feet, face, or both while the fango is processing.
6) Unwrap the client and remove some of the fango by hand (wear vinyl gloves for quick cleanup).
7) Move the client to the shower wrapped in the body plastic.
8) Change the table to massage sheets while the client showers.
9) Client returns to a clean massage table.
10) Full-body massage.
11) Aura mist.

The Fango Back Treatment Procedure

Fango back treatments can be given by massage therapists to decrease lower back or upper back pain, to release tense muscles, for general relaxation, or for revitalization. The therapist is encouraged to include a fair amount of massage in this treatment. Any other treatment product could be used in place of the fango in this outline depending on the treatment goals. An overview of this service is given in the Fango Back Treatment Snapshot and in Figure 9-2.

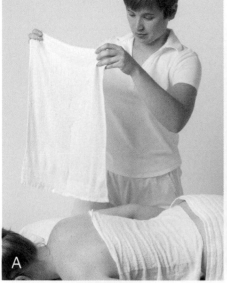
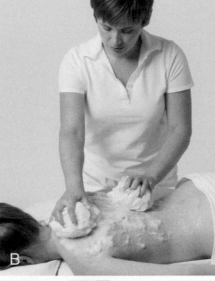
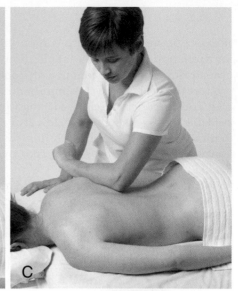
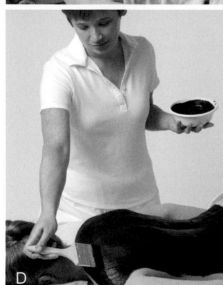
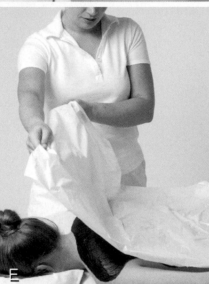
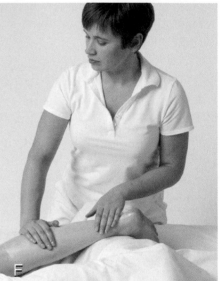
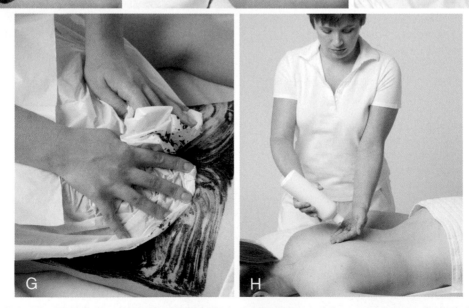

Figure 9-2   The fango back treatment. (A) Steam the back. **(B)** Exfoliate and cleanse. **(C)** Massage the back. **(D)** Apply the fango to the back. The product used in this picture is moor mud (a peat). **(E)** Cover the fango with plastic. **(F)** Process. Massage the posterior legs. **(G)** Remove the fango. Remove as much fango as possible with the plastic body cover. Remove the remaining fango with hot towels. **(H)** Apply a finishing product to the back.

Snapshot: The Fango Back Treatment

Indications

Late subacute to chronic back pain, stiff muscles from a workout or overexertion, stress, chronic muscular holding patterns, or for general relaxation

Contraindications

This particular outline is contraindicated for acute inflammation. Fango is also contraindicated for broken skin, severe back pain, and posterior leg pain from an undiagnosed cause or any condition contraindicated for massage.

Supplies for the Treatment Table Setup (from the bottom to the top layer)

1) Bottom massage sheet
2) Bath towel
3) Top massage sheet
4) Blanket or bath sheet for warmth
5) Bolster

Supplies for the Work Table Setup

1) Cleanser
2) Exfoliation product
3) Bowl of warm water
4) Massage oil or cream
5) Fango warming in a double boiler
6) Application brush or vinyl gloves
7) Plastic body wrap cut so that it will cover the back
8) Warm pack
9) Thermometer
10) Hot, moist towels
11) Soda cooler
12) Finishing product
13) Skin toner and cosmetic sponges
14) Aura mist

Procedure Option 1

1) Apply steamy towels to the back.
2) Cleanse the back.
3) Exfoliate the back.
4) Apply a skin toner to the back.
5) Massage the back.
6) Remove excess massage cream or oil.
7) Apply fango to the back and cover with plastic.
8) Drape the back and place a warm pack on top of the drape so that it keeps the fango warm.
9) Massage the posterior legs while the fango is in process.
10) Remove the fango.
11) Apply a finishing product.
12) Turn the client supine.
13) Massage the neck and shoulders.
14) Aura mist.

Procedure Option 2

1) Massage the posterior legs.
2) Massage the back.
3) Cleanse the back.
4) Exfoliate the back and skin tone.
5) Turn the client to the supine position.
6) Sit up the client and apply fango to the back.

7) Lay the piece of plastic body wrap across the top of the massage table.
8) The client lies back onto the body wrap plastic.
9) Massage the neck, face, and feet while the fango is in process.
10) Sit the client up and remove the fango with hot, moist towels.
11) Apply a finishing product to the back.
12) Lie the client down and aura mist to close the session.

SESSION START

In option 1, the client begins the treatment in the prone position. This requires the client to lie face down for approximately 40 minutes, which can be too long for some clients, especially those who are prone to respiratory congestion when in a face cradle. If this is a concern, use option number two described in the Snapshot.

STEP 1: STEAM THE BACK WITH HOT, MOIST TOWELS

Place two hot, moist towels on the back to steam the area and warm the tissue. A professional steaming unit (the type that is frequently used by estheticians in facials) can be used if it is available. If a professional unit is used, steaming can continue during the cleansing and exfoliation step because it warms the tissue and improves circulation.

STEP 2: CLEANSE THE BACK

Apply warm water to the back with the hands and then work a foaming cleanser into the skin with relaxing massage strokes.

STEP 3: EXFOLIATE THE BACK

Complete the cleansing step by using a small amount of exfoliation product on the skin. Work it in circular motions over the top of the back with two handheld loofahs or the bare hands. This feels stimulating and invigorating and improves circulation and lymphatic flow. Remove both the exfoliation and cleansing products with one hot, moist towel and apply a skin toner with cosmetic sponges.

STEP 4: MASSAGE THE BACK

Massage the back with Swedish, deep tissue, or other massage techniques for 10 to 20 minutes depending on the time available for the individual treatment. Remove the massage oil or cream with a hot towel and apply a toner to the skin with cosmetic sponges.

STEP 5: APPLY WARM FANGO

Check the temperature of the fango with a metal probe thermometer or a latte thermometer. It should be warmed to between 100° to 110°F. Apply a thick layer of warm fango to the back with a brush or massage it into the body with the hands while wearing vinyl gloves. Cover the fango with a precut piece of plastic wrap sheet and place an insulating blanket and warm pack (hydroculator pack, rice or flax seed microwavable pack) on top.

STEP 6: PROCESS: MASSAGE THE LEGS AND FEET

Massage the posterior legs and feet while the back processes in the fango. The treatment can be further tailored to the needs of the client by offering a sports-oriented massage with essential oils for sore muscles such as bay laurel or sweet birch or a firming massage with essential oils of grapefruit and thyme.

STEP 7: REMOVE THE FANGO

After 15 to 20 minutes, remove the fango with hot towels and apply a skin toner with flushing massage strokes. Most alcohol-free toners contain glycerine, which gives enough lubrication for massage.

STEP 8: APPLY A FINISHING PRODUCT

Apply a finishing product that is appropriate for the treatment goals. For example, a sore muscle treatment might end with a tingly fitness gel that contains pain-relieving camphor or peppermint. A general revitalization treatment might finish with a cream rich in citrus oils, which boost immunity and firm the tissues.

SESSION END

Turn the client into the supine position for a neck, shoulders, and face massage. Finish the service with an aura mist to fill the treatment room with a refreshing scent.

Sanitation

Some exfoliation mitts, textured cloths, and gloves are meant to be washed in a washing machine with hot water and dried in the dryer. If they cannot stand up to being washed, they should be disposed of after use on the client or wrapped up in plastic and sent home with the client.

The Fango Scalp and Neck Treatment Procedure

The scalp consists of five layers that include the skin, subcutaneous tissue, epicranius (including its aponeurosis the galea aponeurotica), loose connective tissue, and the pericranium. The skin, subcutaneous tissue, and galea aponeurotica are firmly attached to each other. The thin, sheet-like muscles of the scalp move the scalp, ears, and eyebrows. The thin, small muscles of the face create the movements that lead to facial expression. Every day, these muscles get a workout, and tension in facial and scalp muscles can play a significant role in tension headache pain or pathologies such as temporomandibular joint syndrome (TMJ). The fango scalp and neck treatment is indicated for neck tension, tension headache, face tension, relaxation, stress reduction, and revitalization. This service allows massage therapists to focus in on an area that is often touched on only briefly in a full-body massage. Although fango is used in this treatment outline, seaweed or melted shea butter can also be used with good results.

In this service, oil and fango are massaged through the hair to the scalp. Obviously, this will mess up the client's hair, and shampooing the hair is out of the scope of practice for massage therapists in most states. To avoid scope of practice conflicts, the therapist has three main options: 1) The client can be passed on to a cosmetologist who will finish the service by washing, cutting, or styling the client's hair; 2) The client can wash and condition his or her own hair (provide high-quality professional products) in a shower or tub; or 3) Most of the fango can be removed with hot, moist towels so that the client can go home and wash his or her own hair. In this case, the type of treatment product used is important. Most fango (or shea butter) will not damage the hair or irritate the scalp if it is left on for an extended period. Seaweed, on the other hand, may irritate the scalp, so it should be avoided in this instance. The scalp and neck treatment snapshot and Figure 9-3 provide an overview of this service.

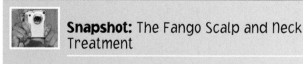

Snapshot: The Fango Scalp and Neck Treatment

Indications
Neck tension, face tension, stress reduction, relaxation, revitalization

Contraindications
Broken skin on the scalp, scalp condition, recent soft tissue injury such as whiplash, severe headache pain or migraine, illness, fever, any condition contraindicated for massage

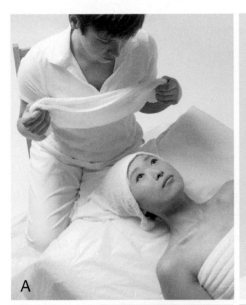

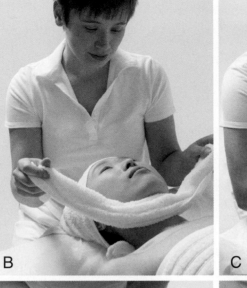

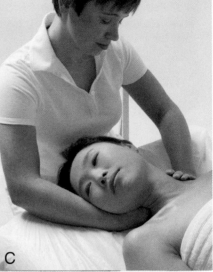

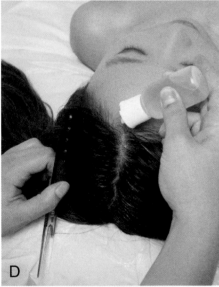

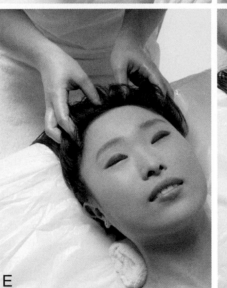

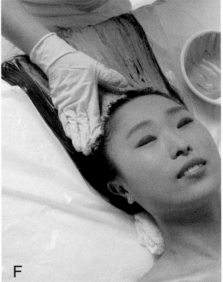

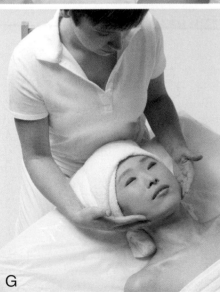

Figure 9-3   The scalp, hair, and neck treatment. (A) Place a hot, moist towel over the hair.
(B) Steam the face. **(C)** Massage the neck. **(D)** Oil the hair. **(E)** Massage the scalp. **(F)** Apply the
fango. The product used in this picture is a marine fango. **(G)** Face massage. The face massage
can take place while the fango is processing on the scalp, or it can be used as the final step of the
treatment.

Supplies for the Treatment Table Setup
(from the bottom to the top layer)

1) Bottom massage sheet
2) Plastic body wrap placed horizontally at the top end of the massage table
3) Top massage sheet
4) Blanket or bath sheet for warmth
5) Bolster
6) Hand towel rolled into a "sausage" to be placed under the client's neck
7) Warm pack for the belly
8) Eye pillow for the eyes
9) Warm pack or microwave booties for the feet.

Figure 9-4 shows the orientation of the plastic on the massage table and how it is used to protect the floor from fango accidents.

Supplies for the Work Table Setup

1) Soda cooler
2) Hot, moist towels
3) Scalp oil in a bottle with a flip-top lid warming in a hot water bath
4) Massage cream
5) Fango warming in a double boiler
6) Comb
7) Hair clip
8) Plastic hair cover or shower cap
9) Aura mist
10) Essential oils (optional)

Procedure

1) Comb out the hair if needed.
2) Steam the head and face.
3) Massage the neck.
4) Massage the scalp.
5) Apply fango to the scalp.
6) Massage the feet, hands, or both while the fango is processing.
7) Remove the fango from the hair.
8) Massage the face.
9) Clip the hair up and cover it with a plastic shower cap (optional).
10) Aura mist.

SESSION START

The client will need to remove his or her shirt and their socks (for foot massage) for this service. Clients often feel more comfortable if they leave on their underclothing but remove their clothes. This prevents their clothing from getting wrinkled or from bunching and restricting the client's movement. The client is bolstered as for massage and covered with a top sheet and blanket for warmth. A hand towel is rolled up and placed under the neck to give support. Warm packs placed on the belly or under the feet are soothing and comforting. If the client's hair is tangled, it is helpful to comb it out gently before the treatment starts.

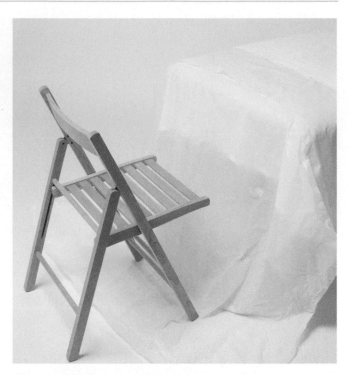

Figure 9-4   Orientation of the plastic for the scalp, hair, and neck treatment. Notice that the plastic is run under the chair to prevent fango from dropping onto the floor of the treatment room.

To begin the service, place 1 drop of an essential oil in the palm of the hands, rub them together briefly, and place them in an arch over the client's nose with the hands about 1 inch above the highest point of the nose. Ask the client to take a slow, relaxing breath. Essential oils that work well for this type of inhalation include lemon, Spanish sage, peppermint, rosemary, common sage, and *Eucalyptus*, although any oil could be used.

STEP 1: STEAM THE HEAD AND FACE

Remove a steamy towel from the soda cooler and place it around the top of the head. Place a second towel over the face. Allow the towels to steam the head and face for approximately 1 minute. Remove the towels and repeat this procedure with a second set of towels if desired. It is nice to scent these towels with essential oils or herbs. If they are scented, the therapist should use an oil that contrasts with the aroma used in the hand inhalation described above.

STEP 2: MASSAGE THE NECK

Remove the rolled hand towel that is supporting the client's neck and give a 10- to 15-minute neck massage using a full range of strokes and techniques. Include the upper chest area and arms if desired. Massage oil or a massage cream can be used for this massage.

STEP 3: MASSAGE THE SCALP

Test the temperature of the scalp oil in the bottle with the flip-top lid to ensure that it is not too hot. Part the hair down the middle and pour warm oil down the part from the hairline to the whorl of hair at the crown of the head. The whorl is the place where the hair changes the direction of its growth at the back of the head. Using soft pressure, zigzag the oil into the scalp, working out from the part toward the sides of the head. Direct pressure and gentle circular friction applied down the path of the parted hair stimulate the scalp and help to relax tight muscles. From the centerline created by the part, jump down 1 inch on one side of the head and create a new parting, flipping the excess hair over the other side of the head. Repeat the oil and massage sequence. Jump down another inch and create a new parting; then repeat the oil and massage sequence. Jump down another inch and create a third parting and repeat the oil and massage sequence. The final parting of the side of the head should start just above the ear. When one side has been oiled and massaged, the entire process is repeated on the other side of the head. This ensures that the entire scalp has been covered in oil. The therapist can now massage the scalp with a variety of techniques for an additional 5 to 10 minutes. Be sure to include the ears in the massage because this is an area that can hold a great deal of tension. A number of head massage techniques are shown in Chapter 11 in the Indian Head Massage section. At the end of the massage, the hair is combed straight back from the forehead in preparation for the application of fango.

STEP 4: APPLY WARM FANGO TO THE HEAD

Wearing vinyl gloves, apply warm fango from the hairline to the back of the head. The hair is then twisted up and a hot, moist towel is used to cover the fango and wrap around the head. A second dry towel is placed over the top of the hot, moist towel to insulate it.

STEP 5: PROCESS: MASSAGE THE FEET, HANDS, OR BOTH

The feet, hands, or both can be massaged while the fango is processing on the scalp. These areas can also be exfoliated or treated with an application of fango or a paraffin dip. For shorter treatments, the face is massaged while the fango is processing on the scalp and the service ends (as far as the massage therapist is concerned) with the removal of the fango from the hair.

STEP 6: REMOVE THE FANGO FROM THE HAIR

Remove the insulating towel and pull the hot, moist towel from the hair, taking as much fango as possible with it. A second and then a third hot, moist towel is placed over the hair and used to gently remove fango from the head. It is not possible to remove all of the fango or scalp oil from the hair in this manner, so the hair is now twisted and clipped up out of the way in anticipation of the final step of the service, the face massage.

STEP 7: FACE MASSAGE

Massage the face using either a heavy face cream or a light massage cream and then move onto the neck because both the head and neck will have been immobile for some time while the fango was processing. The face massage typically takes from 5 to 15 minutes depending on the time available. Face massage techniques are described in Chapter 3.

SESSION END

Spritz an aura mist in a high arch over the client to end the service and fill the treatment room with a refreshing scent. The session can end in three different ways: 1) Pass the client on to a cosmetologist for a shampoo, cut, and style; 2) Escort the client to a shower or soaking tub where he or she can relax and shampoo the hair; or 3) The client goes home to wash his or her hair.

Fango Applications for Musculoskeletal Injuries and Disorders

Massage and fango treatments are a powerful combination for the treatment of musculoskeletal injuries or conditions. Although some believe that mud therapy is a purely thermal process and therefore similar to any topical application of hot or cold, research in Europe suggests otherwise. In a study conducted in Italy, the level of hormone peptides from proopiomelanocortin, plasma beta-endorphin, and some hormones of the pituitary-adrenal glands were all decreased when mud pack treatments were used. The decrease in the levels of these peptides and hormones led to a reduction in the stress experienced by the patient, which, in turn, supported the healing process. These effects began after the first of 12 mud sessions and lasted for 30 days after the treatments had finished.[10]

In osteoarthritis, proinflammatory cytokines and nitric oxide play a role in progressive cartilage degradation and in the secondary inflammation of the synovial membrane of the affected joint. Mud pack treatment can positively affect the chemical mediators of inflammation and decrease damage to cartilage and the synovial membrane.[11-13] In Germany, a study conducted at the Department of Natural Cure, Blankenstein Hospital, in Hattingen, showed that peat components had positive effects on both the endocrine and immune systems.[14] A study in France showed that vascular changes induced by mud pack therapy are not fully explained by vasodilation in response to local temperature elevation. Although the other mechanisms involved could not be determined, it was concluded that mud packs could be successfully used to address vascular insufficiency in the lower limbs.[15]

The goal of this section is to encourage therapists to explore the use of fango in treatments to reduce inflammation, decrease stress, increase range of motion, increase circulation, and decrease adhesion formation and for conditions including soft tissue injury, fibromyalgia, osteoarthritis, and rheumatoid arthritis. It is assumed that a therapist using fango for such conditions understands the principles of hydrotherapy, has a solid understanding of pathology, and has prior knowledge and experience working with these conditions. For further information on these topics, therapists are referred to *A Massage Therapist's Guide to Pathology* by Ruth Werner[16] and *Massage for Orthopedic Conditions* by Thomas Hendrickson.[17]

ACUTE CONDITIONS

In *Massage for Orthopedic Conditions*,[17] Hendrickson summarizes the causes of pain as mechanical, chemical, and thermal. When abnormal tension is placed on soft tissue, especially over a period of time, it leads to tissue damage and inflammation, resulting in mechanical injury. Chemicals that are released as mediators of inflammation irritate nerve endings, leading to increased pain and muscle guarding. This, in turn, causes hypertonic muscles and ischemia (low oxygen), which increases the chemical toxicity of the tissue.

In an acute situation, in which pain, loss of function, redness, heat, and swelling are present, the therapist is unable to manipulate the soft tissue structures involved in the injury. The general treatment goal is to reduce inflammation, reduce pain, reduce sympathetic nervous system firing, and maintain any available range of motion unless passive movement is contraindicated, as with bursitis. Often, the therapist will apply an ice pack and gently massage the other areas of the body if the client can tolerate it. In some situations, the client is only able to tolerate the lightest touch, so only energy-work techniques are appropriate.

Mud or peat applications are ideal in this situation because they are more relaxing for the client than ice, and because the mud may affect the chemical mediators involved in the inflammatory process.[16,17] The application method is the same in most cases of inflammation, including rheumatoid arthritis, bursitis, osteoarthritis flareups, sprains, strains, tendonitis, tenosynovitis, and whiplash. Fango is applied to the area at the beginning of the treatment at a temperature of 50° to 75° F (10° to 24°C). A thermometer is used to monitor the temperature of the

product. Anti-inflammatory essential oils such as German chamomile and *Helichrysum* can be applied to the skin at a 10% concentration (60 drops of essential oil to every ounce of carrier product) before applying the mud. Although this may seem too high to American aromatherapists, this is the concentration used in Europe for topical applications and is very effective as long as the oils are not skin irritants. Essential oils for acute, subacute, and chronic inflammation are described in Table 9-4, and sample blends for the stages of inflammation are given in Table 9-5.

The soft tissue structures in an acute injury are already under extreme pressure because of the buildup of fluid in the tissue. The fango cannot be slathered on the body area as it would be in a normal treatment because the area is sensitive. Instead, the fango is moistened with mineral water until it has the consistency of a smooth paste. This paste is spread on a cotton cloth or pillowcase in a half-inch to 1-inch layer (Fig. 9-5). The cloth is placed gently over the affected body area with the mud facing toward the skin. It is left in place for up to 30 minutes while associated areas are massaged (as long as the client can tolerate touch). Warm fango (98°F or 36°C) can be applied to areas proximal to the injury site for its relaxing and soothing effect and to dissipate muscle spasms. Note that warm mud should not be applied to areas distal to the injury site because of the restricted blood flow in these tissues caused by the injury. Gently remove the mud with warm water and sponges at the end of the treatment.

> ### Sanitation
>
> To clean the cotton cloth or pillowcase used for the fango compress, rinse them in a bucket of hot, soapy water until most of the fango is removed. They can then be washed in the washing machine and dried with heat. Fango must be cleaned up in such a way to prevent damage to plumbing and equipment.

SUBACUTE CONDITIONS

As the body progresses into the late phase of subacute inflammation, fango can be applied directly to the body area at warmer temperatures (98° to 104° F) for 20 to 30 minutes, either before or after the massage (Fig.9-6). After it is applied, it is covered with a moistened cloth and an insulating blanket. It is important to use rhythmic joint mobilizations at the end of the session to encourage collagen to reorient itself along the lines of muscular stress. When an area is immobilized because of an injury, there can be a significant increase in adhesion formation. Carrot seed essential oil is particularly useful with cross-fiber friction techniques for decreasing adhesions and scar tissue.

Table 9-4	**Sample Essential Oils for Stages of Inflammation**	
ACUTE TO EARLY SUBACUTE	**LATE SUBACUTE**	**CHRONIC**
Sweet birch	Bay laurel	Bay laurel
White camphor*	Sweet birch	Sweet birch
German chamomile	White camphor*	White camphor
Cypress	Carrot seed	Clove
Fennel seed	Roman chamomile	Eucalyptus
Geranium	Eucalyptus	Fir needle
Grapefruit	Fir needle	Ginger
Helichrysum	Juniper berry	Juniper berry
Lavender	Lavender	Lavender
Lemon	Lemon	Sweet marjoram
Peppermint	Sweet marjoram	Peppermint
Myrrh	Peppermint	Scotch pine
Tea tree	Scotch pine	Rosemary
Wintergreen	Rosemary	Turmeric
Yarrow	Wintergreen	Wintergreen

* Brown and yellow camphor contain high concentrations (up to 80%) of safrol, which is toxic and carcinogenic. White camphor contains no safrol and is considered nontoxic and non-irritant.

Table 9-5	**Sample Essential Oil Blends for Stages of Inflammation**	
ACUTE TO EARLY SUBACUTE	**LATE SUBACUTE**	**CHRONIC**
Blends are at a 10% concentration	Blends are at a 3% concentration	Blends are at a 2.5% concentration
Blend 1: 2 oz of hemp seed oil, German chamomile (60 drops), *Helichrysum* (60 drops) Note: this blend will smell strong and be very expensive to create but it is highly effective.	**Blend 1:** 2 oz of hemp seed oil, bay laurel (10 drops), white camphor (6 drops), sweet birch (6 drops), rosemary (5 drops), lavender (9 drops)	**Blend 1:** 2 oz of hemp seed oil, atlas cedarwood (10 drops), ginger (5 drops), lemongrass (2 drops), lavender (10 drops), thyme (3 drops)
Blend 2: 2 oz of hemp seed oil, lavender (32 drops), German chamomile (9 drops), *Helichrysum* (9 drops), grapefruit (60 drops), sweet birch (9 drops)	**Blend 2:** 2 oz of hemp seed oil, sweet marjoram (9 drops), turmeric (7 drops), eucalyptus (6 drops), Roman chamomile (3 drops), spike lavender (11 drops)	**Blend 2:** 2 oz of hemp seed oil, bay laurel (10 drops), clove (2 drops), lemon (12 drops), fir needle (6 drops)

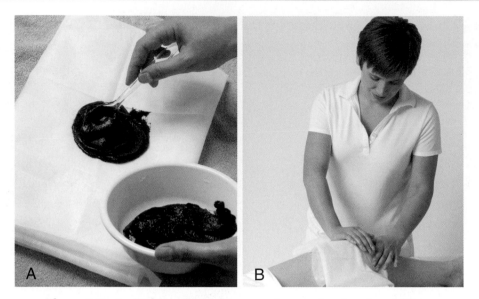

Figure 9-5   Application of fango for an acute or early subacute condition.

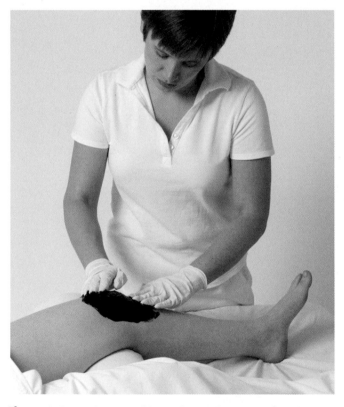

Figure 9-6   Application of fango for a subacute or chronic condition.

CHRONIC CONDITIONS

In the chronic stages of inflammation, the treatment goal is to lengthen and strengthen the tissue to prevent further microtearing and irritation. Hot fango can also be used for osteoarthritis that is not in a flareup, chronic plantar fasciitis, thoracic outlet syndrome caused by middle scalene or pectralis minor tension, and torticollis. A variety of massage techniques, including deep tissue, myofacial release, muscle energy technique, post-isometric relaxation (PIR), active isolated stretching (AIS), and many others can be used in combination with fango applications depending on the type of condition. For chronic conditions, the ability of fango to hold heat is particularly effective. It can be applied directly to the area in a half-inch to one-inch thick layer and left on for up to 30 minutes.

A full-body fango application is indicated for clients with fibromyalgia and chronic fatigue syndrome but should only be given with a doctor's release or an advanced understanding of these conditions. It is important to remember that a full-body application may be contraindicated for weakened individuals. Follow the steps outlined in the cocoon procedure in Chapter 7. If caution is required, the fango should be applied at a temperature closer to body temperature (98° to 104°F rather than 104° to 115°F) and should not be left so long (15 rather than 20 minutes).

SAMPLE TREATMENTS

Mindful Mud Cranium Care

Promotional Description

When was the last time you took care of your head? That's right—your head! Every day, the muscles of the scalp and face get a workout while we mull over the challenges in our day-to-day life. Over time, tension builds up, and the face and head feel tired and weary. Let your mind unwind while your neck, face, and scalp are massaged with soothing aromatic oils. Let tension melt while warm mud is slathered over your head to release everyday worries and relax your entire body. Leave with a smile, revitalized and invigorated by your well-cared-for cranium!

Treatment Outline

Follow the steps for the fango scalp and neck treatment

Scalp Oil Options

Brain Bliss

1 oz sunflower oil, rosemary oil (1 drop), lavender oil (4 drops), grapefruit oil (6 drops), nutmeg oil (1 drop)

Mindful Spirit

1 oz sunflower oil, frankincense (3 drops), sandalwood (4 drops), jasmine (1 drop), sweet orange (4 drops)

Psyche Connection

1 oz sunflower oil, neroli (2 drops), mandarin (6 drops), patchouli (1 drop), clary sage (3 drops)

Clarity

1 oz sunflower oil, rosemary (3 drops), geranium (1 drop), lemon (5 drops), lavender (3 drops)

Adobe Purification Ritual

Promotional Description

This specialized treatment inspired by Native American healing uses the rich red clay of Sedona. A stimulating exfoliation with blue corn and cactus cloth is followed by an application of the clay to the entire body. The clay draws impurities from the skin, soothes muscle tension, and relaxes the spirit. Warm juniper oil is massaged into the body to complete this healing experience.

Treatment Outline

Follow the directions for a cocoon described in Chapter 7 and use Sedona clay or mud for the treatment product. A nice way to enhance this treatment after the wrap is to send the client to continue the detoxification process in a steam room or sauna using pine or sage oil (sage sauna).

In-House Product for the Adobe Purification Ritual

Blue Corn Polish

$^{1}/_{2}$ cup ground blue corn, 1/4 cup plain moisture cream, 1 Tbsp plain body wash

Juniper Massage Oil

1 oz massage oil, juniper berry oil (6 drops), lavender oil (3 drops)

Sage Sauna or Sage Steam

2 cups of water, 2 drops of common sage (*Salvia officinalis*), 1 drop of rosemary. Throw the water on the heat source in the sauna or use this blend in the steam room. Do not place oils that have not been mixed in water on a heat source because they may burn or "pop."

Dead Sea Envelopment

Promotional Description

The Dead Sea region is a unique environment that yields a therapeutic mud famous throughout the world for its mineral-laden healing properties. The body is buffed with Dead Sea salts and enveloped in warm mud to absorb nutrients essential to the body. Muscle tension melts as the skin is rinsed clean of impurities and rich creams are applied to seal in moisture.

Treatment Outline

Follow the directions for a cocoon described in Chapter 7 and use Dead Sea mud as the treatment product. A variety of different support products can be used in this wrap. If the therapist wants to create a smell-scape or use plants indigenous to Israel, he or she can include products with olive, fig, citrus fruits, and avocado.

Moor Back Treatment

Promotional Description

Back pain can slow down your day and leave you feeling drained and irritable. This treatment using the healing peat from the Austrian Moors will bring relief from pain and revitalize the spirit. A 30-minute deep tissue massage and application of essential oils aimed at the muscular system complete this service.

Treatment Outline

Follow the steps for the fango back treatment.

Essential Oil Blends Ideas for the Moor Back Treatment

Body Balance Blend

2 fl oz massage oil, essential oils of rosemary (4 drops), lavender (7 drops), lemongrass (2 drops), clary sage (5 drops), mandarin (12 drops)

Overworked Muscles

2 oz massage oil (hemp seed oil is ideal), essential oils of bay laurel (8 drops), eucalyptus (2 drops), ginger CO_2 (1 drop), lemon (10 drops), white camphor (4 drops; it must be white camphor, not yellow or brown), myrrh (5 drops)

Burnout Relief

2 fl oz massage oil, essential oils of geranium (2 drops), grapefruit (15 drops), lavender (7 drops), cypress (5 drops), clove (1 drop).

Sulfur Mud Pack

Promotional Description

Do you experience achy joints and chronic muscular pain? If the answer is yes, then this healing treatment using sulfur muds from Europe may bring some relief. In Europe, mud is used to treat arthritis and muscle pain with remarkable results. The warm mud will be packed on areas of tension to warm the tissue and to bring its special healing properties to the body. Swedish and deep tissue massage techniques release tense muscles and calm the spirit.

Treatment Outline

The treatment outline should be based on the essential oils and fango temperatures that are most appropriate for the needs of the client. It is nice to have fango "processing" on one area while another is massaged.

Summary

Fangotherapy is the use of mud, peat, and clay for healing purposes. Although fango treatments are mainly used for skin care in the United States, massage therapists will find fango useful for spa treatments aimed at the reduction of soft tissue pain and dysfunction and to relax and revitalize the body.

The therapeutic substances used in fango spa treatments have different characteristics that affect their therapeutic properties and uses. Clay, which is mainly mineral (derived from rock), is the most absorbent of the fango substances. It is used to pull impurities from the skin and to stimulate circulation. Mud is also predominantly mineral but has small amounts of organic components that give it a wider range of properties. A mud may be anti-inflammatory, antiviral, and immune boosting. Peat is therapeutically the most active substance of the three because it is mainly organic and derived from the breakdown of plant material over thousands of years.

REFERENCES

1. Lund JW: *Balneological Use of Thermal Waters*. Klamath Falls, OR: Geo Heat Center, 2000.
2. Bergel RR: The biology and physics of peloids. *Demascope* 2000 (November), 2000.
3. Lund JW: Geothermal Spas in the Czech Republic and Slovakia. *GHC Bulletin*. 2000 (September);35–37.
4. Ekmekcioglu C, et al: Effect of Sulfur Baths on Antioxidative Defense Systems, Peroxide Concentrations and Lipid Levels in Patients with Degenerative Osteoarthritis. *Research in Complementary and Classical Natural Medicine* 2002;9:216–220.
5. Elkayam O, et al: Immediate and delayed effects of treatment at the Dead Sea in patients with psoriatic arthritis. *Rheumatol Int* 2000;19:77–82.
6. Sukenik S, et al: Mud pack therapy in rheumatoid arthritis. *Clin Rheumatol* 2000;11:243–247.
7. Carpio-Obeso MP, Shorr M, Valdez-Salas B: Desert ecosystems: Similarities, characteristics, and health benefits. *Rev Environ Health* 1999;14:257–267.
8. Kimmerer RW: *Gathering Moss, A Natural and Cultural History of Mosses.* OR: Oregon State University Press, 2003, p. 113.
9. Beer AM, Lukanov J, Sagorchev P: A new view on quality controlled application of peat in medical treatment. *Peatland International* 2003;1:25–28.
10. Pizzoferrato A, et al: Beta-endorphin and stress hormones in patients affected by osteoarthritis. *Minerva Med* 2000;91:239–245.
11. Grigor'eva VD, Orus-ool VK, Fedorova NE: Low-temperature peloids in rehabilitating osteoarthritis patients. *Vopr Kurortol Fizioter Lech Fiz Kult* 2001;5:8–11.
12. Bellometti S, et al: Both serum receptors of tumor necrosis factor are influenced by mudpack treatment in osteoarthritic patients. *Int J Tissue React* 2002;24:57–64.
13. Bellometti S, et al: Mud bath therapy influences nitric oxide, myeloperoxidase and glutathione peroxidase serum levels in arthritic patients. *Int J Clin Pharmacol Res* 2000;20:69–80.
14. Beer AM, et al: The effect of peat components on endocrine and immunological parameters and on trace elements. *Clin Lab* 2001;47:161–167.
15. Poensin D, et al. Effects of mud pack treatment on skin microcirculation. *Joint Bone Spine* 2003;70:367–370.
16. Werner R: *A Massage Therapist's Guide to Pathology*, 2nd ed. Baltimore: Lippincott Williams & Wilkins, 2002.
17. Hendrickson T: *Massage for Orthopedic Conditions*. Baltimore: Lippincott Williams & Wilkins, 2003.
18. Comacchi C, Hercogova J: A single mud treatment induces normalization of stratum corneum hydration, transepidermal water loss, skin surface pH and sebum content in patients with seborrhoeic dermatitis. *J Eur Acad Dermatol* 2004;18:372–374.
19. Carabelli A, et al: Effect of thermal mud baths on normal, dry and seborrheic skin. Clinical trial at the Universita di Pavia, Italy.

REVIEW QUESTIONS

Multiple Choice

1. _____ is a component of therapeutic mud, especially those that are obtained in the vicinity of volcanoes and hot springs.
   a. Mucilage
   b. Fango
   c. Sea salt
   d. Sulfur

2. *Fango* is the Italian word for _____:
   a. Seaweed
   b. A body wrap
   c. Relaxation by a mineral spring
   d. Mud

3. When a mud is "matured" it is:
   a. Processed to develop nonpathogenic microorganisms that make the mud more therapeutic
   b. Aged to make the mud smell more pleasing
   c. Dried or dehydrated to kill any pathogenic microorganisms
   d. Mixed with fresh plants to increase the range of chemicals

4. In Europe, fangotherapy is regularly used in the treatment of:
   a. Cancer
   b. Aids
   c. Arthritis
   d. Meningitis

5. Therapeutic peat falls into two main commercial categories. These are:
   a. Mainly black and mainly brown
   b. Mainly mineral and mainly organic
   c. High moor or dead sea
   d. High moor or low moor

6. In Europe, fango is applied to the body at this temperature, even in cases of acute inflammation.
   a. 56° to 66°F
   b. 24° to 32°F
   c. 78° to 89°F
   d. 104° to 115°F

Fill in the Blank

7. Full-body fango applications can last between _____ and _____ minutes.

8. When viewed under the electron microscope, clay particles are about _____ times longer then they are _____.

9. Kaolinite clay is generally _____ in color and was first mined in China.

10. At the Piestany spa in Slovakia the mud turns from brown to black when it is _____.

CHAPTER 10

Thalassotherapy

Chapter Outline

Key Terms

Algae: Algae occur in all marine and terrestrial ecosystems of the world wherever there is water. The terms *algae* and *seaweed* are often used interchangeably, which causes some confusion. Seaweeds are algae that have a particular growth form, but the term *algae* also includes a wide range of other terrestrial and aquatic organisms with different evolutionary histories.

Alginate: A substance found in seaweed that has therapeutic properties for skin and body and is often used as a thickening agent in cosmetic preparations.

Galvanic current machine: A machine used by estheticians in facial treatments. It has two different uses depending on the polarity of the current that is used. When the working electrode is the negative pole, it is used with a disincrustation solution to soften blocked sebum in pores. When it is set on the opposite polarity (positive pole is the working electrode), it is used to soothe the skin and encourage the absorption of a water-soluble treatment product.

High-frequency machine: Machine that generates a rapidly oscillating electrical current that is transmitted through glass electrodes. The current produces heat in the skin, which stimulates circulation. It also produces ozone, which acts as a germicide to kill bacteria.

Minerals: Naturally occurring substances that play a crucial role in the body's metabolic processes. They are required by the body to function properly.

Mucilage: A gelatinous substance found in plants and animals that is extracted for cosmetic purposes from plants such as seaweeds. It is composed of protein and polysaccharides and is used to give cosmetics a creamy substance and to moisturize and protect the skin.

Polysaccharides: A class of long-chain sugars composed of monosaccharides that are often used in skin care as antioxidants and water-binding agents.

Seaweed: Multicellular marine-based algae that fall into one of three main groups: green algae (*Chlorophycota* spp.), brown algae (*Phaeophycota* spp.), and red algae (*Rhodophyta* spp.).

Silicone: One of the elements present in seaweed that binds water to the skin and gives a silky feel when added to cosmetics.

Thalassotherapy: The use of marine environments and sea products, including seawater, sea mud, seaweed, and seafood, for healing and wellness.

Thalassotherapy is the use of marine environments and sea products, particularly seaweed, for healing and wellness. Joseph Conrad once said: "The true peace of God begins a thousand miles from the nearest land." In that single line, Conrad captured the magical, indescribable quality of the sea. The mystique of the sea may be one reason that treatments featuring seaweed are held in such high regard by spa clients. It is probable that the reliable results achieved by the use of seaweed in slimming treatments, revitalization treatments, esthetics, and relaxation treatments is the other reason for its popularity.

Seaweeds are multicellular marine-based **algae** that may fall into one of three groups: green seaweed (*Chlorophycota*), brown seaweed (*Phaeophycota*), and red seaweed (*Rhodophyta*).

Brown and red seaweeds are the most common types of seaweed used in cosmetic products or for spa treatments, although all seaweeds have some therapeutic value because of their high mineral content. Many seaweeds also have interesting forms of antimicrobial and other biological activity.

This chapter aims to give a brief history of thalassotherapy, review the relevant research on the benefits of seaweed for the body, and describe the use of seaweed in combination with other products such as cellulite creams. A slimming seaweed cocoon is described in step-by-step detail, and a seaweed breast treatment is outlined with a treatment snapshot. Therapists are encouraged to use seaweed as the treatment product in other services outlined in this book. For an overview of the types of seaweed that are used in thalassotherapy, see Table 10-1.

Table 10-1	Algae at a Glance				
TYPES	**BOTANICAL**	**COMMON**	**PROPERTIES**	**INDICATIONS**	**CAUTIONS**
Green (*Chlorophycota* spp.): 7000 species; 800 of these are "seaweeds"	*Ulva lactuca*	Sea lettuce	Antiviral, high vitamin C content, anti-inflammatory, demulcent	Inflammation, muscle soreness or pain, fibromyalgia, stress, low energy, low immunity, others	Skin irritation possible but unlikely, iodine or shellfish allergies
	Evernia prunastri (lichen)	Oak moss	Antiseptic, demulcent	Most often used as an absolute for base note in fragrances	6 to 12 drops maximum for a full-body treatment
Blue-green (*Cyanophycota* or *Cyanobacteria* spp.): Not seaweeds	*Spirulina maxima*, *Spirulina platensis*	Spirulina	Anti-inflammatory, stimulating, skin firming, moisturizing	Detoxification treatments, slimming treatments, low energy, stress, others	None
Brown (*Phaeophycota* spp.): 3000 species; most are seaweeds	*Laminaria* spp., *Sargassum* spp., *Fucus* spp., *Ascophylum* spp.	Kelps, wracks	Wound healing, hair growth, stimulates metabolism, detoxifying, aids cellular exchanges, revitalizing, stimulates circulation and lymphatic flow, heats the body	Detoxification treatments; slimming treatments; muscle pain or tension; low energy; stress; burnout; dry, rough, dull, saggy, dehydrated, or congested skin	There is some concern that full-body treatments using brown algae overstimulate the thyroid or affect thyroid medications; iodine allergies
Red (*Rhodophyta* spp.): 8000 species; most are seaweeds	*Chondrus crispus*, *Gelidium amansii*	Carrageen agar-agar (also known as Japanese isinglass)	Anti-inflammatory, circulatory stimulant, demulcent, stabilizer, used in cosmetic emulsions	Detoxification treatments; low energy; stress; slimming treatments; for dry, rough, dehydrated, or irritated skin	Skin irritation possible but unlikely; iodine or shellfish allergies

Spirulina

Spirulina spp. is a blue-green algae (Cyanophycota or Cyanobacteria) that is not a seaweed because it is unicellular and so not seaweed-like in appearance. Spirulina spp. is notable for its use as an agent to firm and moisturize the skin. It also has a wide range of biological activity with actions including anti-cancer,[16–18] immunostimulating,[17–19] antidiabetic,[17,20,21] anti-inflammatory,[12,17,22] antioxidant,[12] membrane stabilizing,[12] antiatherogenic,[23] anti-allergy,[17,22] blood vessel relaxing,[24] antiviral,[18] antiarthritic,[25] blood lipid lowering,[26] and antianemic[17] effects. It has been used to treat chronic hepatitis[12] and herpes simplex virus type 2.[27]

A Brief History of Thalassotherapy

The French recognized the therapeutic benefits of sea bathing in the early 1800s, and by 1824, they had set up facilities to warm seawater for treatments. In 1869, the term *thalassotherapy* (*thalassa* is the Greek word for sea), was coined by Dr. de la Bonnardiere. In 1960, the French Medical Academy officially defined thalassotherapy: "Thalassotherapie uses seawater, seaweed, sea mud or other sea resources and/or the marine climate for the purpose of medical treatment or treatment with a medicinal effect." In France, thalassotherapy is covered by medical insurance as a standard treatment for sore throats, digestive problems, arthritis, musculoskeletal injury, respiratory ailments, developmental disorders in children, endocrine imbalances, and skin conditions.

Therapeutic techniques in French thalassotherapy include: hydrotherapy using seawater; argotherapy, which uses seaweed packs on the body; fango therapy, which uses sea mud packs on the body; eliotherapy, the inhalation of aerosol-sized particles of seawater; kinesitherapy, which consists of floating in a relaxation pool filled with seawater; aquagym therapy, which is exercise in seawater; and sea diets, diets rich in seaweeds and seafood.

In the United States, thalassotherapy is most often used to firm, moisturize, and condition the skin. The American spa-going public may be familiar with the general benefits of seaweed for the skin but may not yet be exposed to the benefits of seaweed for full-body wellness, revitalization, and detoxification and as an energy booster. As with fango, this is likely to change as spa menus continue to expand and substances once valued primarily in esthetics are accepted for their full range of therapeutic properties.

The Therapeutic Benefits of Seaweed for the Body

The different forms of thalassotherapy may be effective because seaweed and seawater contain significant concentrations of **minerals**, and seaweeds contain many useful bioactive compounds that are absorbed by the skin. It is helpful for therapists to have a general understanding of the physiological actions of the main species of seaweed before designing thalassotherapy treatments. Empirical evidence, clinical studies, and research suggest that seaweed treatments can be used to support endocrine balance, support detoxification, support the elimination of excess fluid in body tissue, decrease the symptoms of fibromyalgia, decrease muscular pain, stimulate circulation and lymph flow, boost general immunity, give an energy boost, and facilitate relaxation and the decrease of stress.

The studies on seaweed show that it contains large amounts of polysaccharides, which have a wide range of biological activities, including antithrombotic, anticoagulant, anti-cancer, and antiviral effects.[1] The minerals that seaweeds accumulate from seawater account for up to 36% of their dry weight. Seaweeds have high concentrations of vitamins A, B1, B2, B3, B5, B12, C, D, E, and K. They also contain polyphenols and carotenoids, which play a role in protecting the body from oxidative stress.

A polysaccharide compound, isolated in 1994 from *Ulva* spp., a green marine algae, has significant antiviral activity, reducing replication rates of some strains of human and avian influenza viruses.[2] In Scottish folk medicine, the thin, mucilaginous nature of *Ulva* fronds made it useful as a cold compress for nosebleeds, migraines, burns, sores, and cuts. Research showing that *Ulva* spp. produces a biologically active steroid (3-O-beta-D glucopyranosyl-stigmasta-5, 25-diene) that reduces edema when applied topically supports this traditional use.[3]

Brown seaweed such as *Laminaria, Sargassum, Fucus,* and *Ascophylum* spp., stimulate metabolism, raise body temperature, and affect cell membrane transport, facilitating detoxification and contain iodine, which influences thyroid activity.[4] Brown seaweeds also contain alginate, a jelly-like carbohydrate used for its water-holding, gelling, emulsifying, and stabilizing properties. Alginate dressings are used on epidermal and dermal wounds to give a moist environment that leads to rapid granulation and healing.[5] Alginate has also been used as a medium for transdermal drug delivery systems[6] and to regulate abnormal collagen metabolism.[7]

Species of another seaweed genus, *Sargassum* spp. (known as *hai zao* in Chinese), have been used in traditional Chinese medicine since the eighth century AD. In Chinese medicine, *Sargassum* spp. is mainly used for the treatment of goiter because of its action on the thyroid, which helps to regulate metabolism. Other uses include the treatment of edema, other thyroid disorders, and pain from inflammation. Herbalists use *Sargassum* spp. to promote weight loss, but long-term use is avoided because of its action on the thyroid. The literature suggests that *Sargassum* spp. has a mild diuretic effect, is effective against herpes simplex type 1 and 2,[8] can be used as a topical antifungal agent,[9] has liver-protecting capabilities,[10] and contains antioxidants that protect the body from damage caused by free radicals, so it can slow the aging process.[11]

 BOX 10-2
Broaden Your Understanding

The Benefits of Seaweed for the Skin

France is the largest market for seaweed used in cosmetics with an estimated 5000 tons of wet seaweed being harvested and processed annually to meet the demand.[28] The vitamins, minerals, amino acids, sugars, lipids, and other components of seaweeds (e.g., alginic acid, silicone, alginates, agar-agar proteins, cellulose, mucilage, and fucosterol) make them useful for a variety of cosmetic products. For example, seaweed extracts react with skin proteins to form a protective gel on the skin's surface that reduces moisture loss.[29] Seaweed also appears to promote local vasodilatation and increased circulation of blood and lymph flow. This may be the basis for the widespread use of seaweeds to treat cellulite. Seaweed cleanses, purifies, tones, firms, softens, and hydrates the skin. It is recommended for most types of skin because of its balancing and soothing effects. It is used in acne treatments for its antibiotic and anti-inflammatory properties. It can also be used on clients with dry skin to retain moisture, stimulate circulation, and promote nutrient exchange. When used on mature skin, its firming and toning action has a positive effect on the appearance of fine lines and wrinkles. Zinc, a mineral found in most seaweed, acts as a biocatalyst. It is useful for stabilizing the skin by balancing glandular secretions. Commercially, zinc creams are used to treat acne, give protection against exposure to the sun, and regulate the sebaceous glands.

There is a large amount of research on the uses of seaweed for skin treatment. For example, citrinol, an acyclic diterpene alcohol found in Sargassum tortile, *a brown marine algae, is effective against gram-positive bacteria, including* Propionibacterium acnes, *the bacterium associated with inflammatory acne.[30] Interestingly, the activity of crinitol was shown to increase in the presence of antioxidants.*

In a study conducted in Japan and published in the Journal of Cosmetic Science,[31] Fucus vesiculosus extract (1% in a gel) applied topically to one cheek twice daily for 5 weeks decreased skin thickness and increased skin elasticity. With age, cheek skin usually increases in thickness and its elasticity decreases, leading to wrinkles and sagging skin. Extracts of Fucus vesiculosus *also aid the wound contraction and the granulation process[32] and show in vitro antibiotic activity against* Staphylococcus aureus, Pseudomonas aeruginosa, *and* Escherichia coli.[33] *An absolute (alcoholic extract) of* Fucus vesiculosus, *a brown marine algae, can be obtained commercially from some aromatherapy suppliers and mixed into creams and lotions by the therapist.*

Ascophylum nodosum, *another species of brown seaweed, contains large amounts of fuciodan, a sugar (alpha-L-fucose)-based polysaccharide that retains moisture and has immunostimulating, anticoagulating, and antiaging activity.[34–37] Two separate French studies published in Biomedical Pharmacotherapy show that fucose and fucose-rich polysaccharides penetrate the skin, decrease free radical scavenging, and increase the cell proliferation to slow down the aging of skin cells.[36,37] Frenchwomen traditionally used* Ascophylum nodosum *extracts to increase hair growth and soften rough and damaged skin.[38]*

Red seaweed such as carrageen extracted from Irish moss (Chondrus crispus) and agar-agar (Gelidium amansii; note: agar-agar is derived from the Malaysian word for seaweed) are good emulsifiers, balancers, and lubricants.[39] A study conducted by the Estée Lauder company showed that sulfated polysaccharides from red micro-algae have anti-inflammatory properties when applied topically to the skin.[40] The anti-inflammatory effects of red seaweed are recorded folk remedies from Ireland to Malaysia. For example, the Celts used Irish moss for sore throats and to soothe chapped skin, and the Malaysians used agar-agar for burns and skin irritation.

General Treatment Considerations

Before offering thalassotherapy treatments, it is important to understand the contraindications to seaweed, the different forms of seaweed products, how to dilute seaweed products for clients with sensitive skin, and how the odor of seaweed may affect the business. Because a slimming treatment is described in this chapter, some notes on cellulite and cellulite products are also included here.

CONTRAINDICATED INDIVIDUALS

Individuals with vascular problems, high or low blood pressure, who are pregnant, or who have a fever should only be given this treatment if first approved by their physician. Seaweed tends to increase blood flow and accelerate detoxification, which increases the load on the cardiovascular system and may cause complications in weakened individuals.

Brown seaweeds have high concentrations of iodine and may overstimulate the thyroid gland. In a healthy person, this usually results in a feeling of increased energy and well being at the end of the treatment. But for individuals with thyroid disorders or who are taking thyroid medications, a full-body treatment may throw the body out of balance. Until more research is available, it is best to err on the side of caution and avoid giving full-body brown seaweed treatments to clients with thyroid disorders. Choose green or red seaweed treatments instead, or only apply the seaweed to one area of the body, as in the seaweed back treatment.

When taking the client's health history, it is important to check for shellfish or iodine allergies. If a client is allergic to either shellfish or iodine, he or she should not receive a seaweed treatment.

SENSITIVE SKIN

In a seaweed cocoon, the trapped heat from the body causes perspiration and may make sensitive skin more susceptible to irritation. If the skin type of the client is fair or prone to sensitivity, choose a green or red seaweed product and avoid using brown seaweed. Alternatively, use a gentler aloe gel-based product because these are milder in action than powdered seaweed (Fig. 10-1). Seaweed products can also be diluted by adding kaolin clay or a fixed oil such as sunflower or sweet almond to the mix. Many premixed products cause irritation because poor-quality essential oils have been added to "improve" the smell of the seaweed product. To avoid this problem, buy unscented products that are as pure as possible and add therapeutic-grade essential oils to scent them if desired. If skin irritation occurs during a seaweed treatment, remove the seaweed product with cool towels and apply a fixed oil such as sunflower to the body in a heavy layer. Do not massage in the oil; instead, remove the excess oil with more cool towels. If a shower is available, the client should rinse in cool water until the irritation subsides.

The therapist should protect his or her hands from strong seaweeds, cellulite creams, and firming creams by wearing vinyl gloves while applying these products. The therapist's hands often become overexposed to such products during the course of a day at the spa and so are prone to sensitivity and even contact dermatitis.

PRODUCT FORM AND APPLICATION CONSIDERATIONS

Cosmetic products that contain seaweed take many forms. The seaweed may have been dried and powdered, blended as an extract into a lotion or gel base, dried and mixed with sea

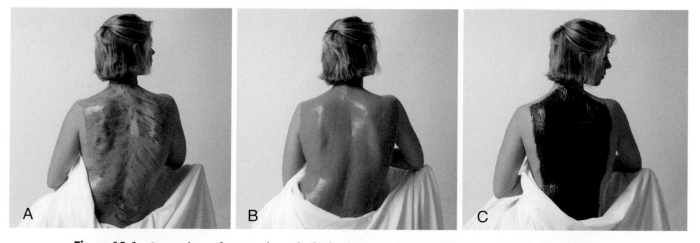

Figure 10-1   Comparison of seaweeds on the body. This figure shows the different consistencies of seaweed products that have been applied to the body. It is easy to see that a gel-based product would be easier to remove than a powdered product. **(A)** Gel seaweed. **(B)** Powdered seaweed mixed with kaolin clay, water, and lotion. **(C)** Powdered seaweed mixed with oil.

salts for hydro soaks, extracted for use in body mists and facial toners, or mixed with paraffin for easy removal. Absolutes (solvent extracts) of *Sargassum*, *Fucus*, and *Laminaria* spp. can be purchased from some aromatherapy suppliers and added to creams, oils, gels, cleansers, and other products for easy use.

The type of product chosen usually depends on the equipment available and the removal method used. For example, a clinic without a shower may choose a gel-based seaweed for easy cleanup and quick hot towel removal. A spa with a Vichy or Swiss shower may choose powdered seaweed for the treatment. Powdered products are thicker when mixed and stick to the body during hot towel removal. They are time consuming and difficult to remove without a shower. That said, there are ways to mix up powdered seaweed to make it easier to remove. Table 10-2 gives some ideas for mixing up powdered and gel seaweed for hybrid treatment products.

Several new seaweed gels on the market are designed to be applied with a brush in a generous layer and then left to

Table 10-2	Seaweed Mix-Ups*			
NAME	**RECIPE**	**PROPERTIES**	**USES**	
Sea Milk	Add ½ cup of milk powder to every ½ cup of seaweed powder. Use a small amount of hot water to dissolve the mixed powders. Add ½ cup of plain body lotion to the mix. Now add warm milk, cream, or buttermilk to the mixture until the desired consistency is reached.	Relaxing, soothing, calming, softening	Full-body application for sensitive skin, breast treatment, scalp and neck treatment	
Ocean Oil	16 oz of a cold pressed vegetable or nut oil is warmed on the stove. 2 Tbsp of seaweed powder is dissolved into this oil and heated on a low temperature for 20 minutes while stirring constantly. The mix is placed in a glass bottle and shaken each day for 1 week. The oil is strained through a coffee filter. Essential oils can be added to scent this product.	Stimulating, firming, circulatory stimulant, energizing, revitalizing, immune boosting	Full-body massage or as the massage oil in a larger seaweed treatment; as a product that can be applied to the skin before a therapeutic shower (Vichy, Swiss) or soaking treatment	
Peppermint Sea Twist	6 drops of peppermint essential oil is added to gel seaweed for a spot treatment or full-body application.	Stimulating, refreshing, cooling, revitalizing, analgesic, circulatory and lymphatic stimulant	Foot mask for tired feet, spot treatment for sore muscles, spot treatment for cellulite, full-body cocoon for refreshment	
Sea Shea	Melt shea butter in a double boiler until it is liquid. Mix powdered seaweed with warm oil until it dissolves and then add it to the shea. Allow the shea to cool while it is whipped with a wire whisk or in a blender. Use 1 Tbsp of powdered seaweed to every cup of shea butter.	Relaxing, revitalizing, softening, calming, gentle lymph and circulatory stimulant	Useful as a thick, after-treatment body butter, as a massage product, or as the treatment product in a full-body cocoon, neck and scalp treatment, or hand and foot treatment	
Marine Minerals	Gel seaweed is mixed with kaolin clay until a creamy, rich treatment product is produced. Essential oils can be added to the mix if desired.	Stimulating, slimming, detoxifying, softening, revitalizing, relaxing	Full-body cocoon, back treatment, foot treatment, breast treatment	

* Seaweed powder is usually mixed up with warm water, but a number of useful treatment products can be made by mixing seaweed powders with different liquids or oils. Each of these recipes can be used with any type of seaweed powder. The reader will notice that the exact amount of seaweed or liquid is not indicated. This is because different seaweed powders have been processed differently and so mix up differently. The reader is advised to start with 3 Tbsp of seaweed powder for a spot treatment and 1 cup of seaweed for a full-body treatment. More seaweed may be needed depending on the size of the client. The different liquids should be added until the desired consistency is reached.

absorb during a cocoon. At the end of the wrap phase, the gel is simply massaged into the skin with a finishing product rather than being removed. These products are simple to use and give satisfying results. Try out a number of different products for the ease of delivery and results before finalizing the treatment outline.

If a soaking tub or hydrotherapy tub is available, bathing in seaweed solutions is a relaxing way to experience thalassotherapy. Seaweed soaks remineralize the body, stimulate both circulation and metabolism, soften and cleanse the skin, and leave the body feeling energetic and revitalized.

Seaweed is usually heated before being applied. As with fango products, seaweed products should not be mixed, heated, or stored in metal containers because they may react chemically with the metal.

SEAWEED ODOR

Seaweed has a strong smell that some people like ("Oh, it smells like the ocean in here!"), and some people dislike ("That smell is giving me a headache and making my stomach upset!"). The smell is potent and may spread beyond the treatment room. This can be a problem in a small, busy clinic, and it should be considered by the owner before investing in the equipment needed to deliver the treatment. Some therapists add essential oils to seaweed products to "improve" the smell and to add to the therapeutic properties of the treatment. However, adding essential oils just to mask the smell is not usually very practical because a high concentration of essential oil is needed.

CELLULITE AND CELLULITE PRODUCTS

Before offering a slimming body service, it is useful to understand something about cellulite and why it occurs. *Cellulite* is a cosmetic term that refers to uneven, dimply areas of skin found on the thighs, hips, and buttocks of women. Although the formation of cellulite is usually found in mature women, it can begin as early as puberty. This condition is not restricted to overweight women but can occur in very slim women, too.

Three fat layers lie directly below the epidermis and dermis of the skin. The most superficial of these layers, known as the subcutaneous fat layer, has specialized fat storage chambers. These chambers are created by connective tissue that anchors the skin to muscle tissue. The characteristic dimpling of cellulite is caused by weakened connective tissue, which may be linked to increased levels of estrogen. When the fat cells swell against the weakened connective tissue, a bulge occurs, creating the dimpled appearance of cellulite. Men rarely develop cellulite because they store fat differently than women. In women, the fat storage chambers are organized into broad, vertical chambers. Men store fat in smaller chambers that are diagonally orientated and less likely to bulge.

It is also likely that poor lymph and blood flow contribute to the problem. As the fat cells swell, they place surrounding structures under pressure. This causes increased permeability of capillary walls, leading to localized fluid accumulation. If lymphatic flow is sluggish, this excess fluid is never removed and causes connective tissue strands to stiffen, pulling down on their anchor points and further increasing the bulging appearance of the skin.

There has been a great deal of research carried out on methods to reduce cellulite by nonsurgical means. Treatments include intensive massage techniques, often with electrical suction devices; topical creams; compression wraps; and intramuscular injections. However, there is little evidence for the effectiveness of these treatments, making it ethically difficult to sell them to clients.

Although it is difficult to reduce cellulite, its appearance can at least be improved. Cellulite creams are a popular and accepted means of improving the appearance of cellulite. These products are often used with tension wraps (described in Chapter 7), which compress the tissue so that it appears slimmer for a period of time after the wrap is removed. Sometimes cellulite or firming products are activated with heat and so applied underneath very warm treatment products such as Parafango or paraffin.

Cellulite and firming creams contain ingredients that stimulate circulation and lymph flow and heat the tissue. The most widespread ingredient in cellulite and firming creams is aminophylline (its chemical cousin, theophylline, is also used). In vitro, aminophylline causes fat cells to shrink, which has led to its popularity.[12]

Another trendy ingredient is Yohimbine from the bark of *Pausinystalia johimbe*, a tree that is grown in West Africa along the coast of Nigeria and Gabon. Yohimbine is well known as a male sex stimulant and is often added to bodybuilding formulas because compounds in its bark are precursors of testosterone. The compounds in yohimbine increase local circulation, which may help to break down fatty deposits. Products containing yohimbine often alarm therapists because some cause the skin to turn fire-engine red. This is not skin irritation, but the skin feels very warm for about 20 minutes after the application. Cellulite and firming creams that increase local circulation make very effective sore muscle creams, so they can be used as a treatment product in services for athletes.

The Slimming Seaweed Cocoon Procedure

A full-body seaweed treatment is indicated for a wide range of conditions, including low energy, low immunity, stress, muscle soreness, fibromyalgia, detoxification, relaxation, body slimming, and cellulite reduction. Both the hot sheet wrap procedure and the cocoon procedure described in

Chapter 7 can be used with seaweed as the treatment product to meet the general treatment goals described above. The procedure explained in this chapter aims to help define the contours of the body, so it includes a cellulite product and skin-firming product.

Slimming treatments are popular with clients who are preparing for a big event and want to look their best in tight-fitting clothing or a special outfit such as a prom dress. This treatment can also be marketed to men who want to sculpt their physique, especially bodybuilders in the last stages of preparation before a competition. In any case, this service also supports full-body relaxation and revitalization. The slimming seaweed cocoon snapshot and Figure 10-2 give an overview of this service.

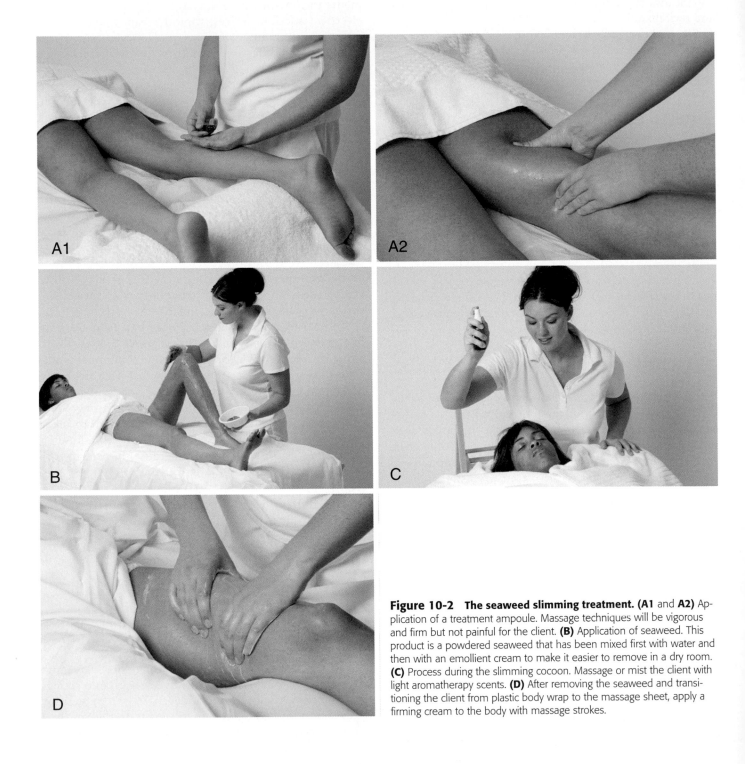

Figure 10-2   The seaweed slimming treatment. (A1 and **A2)** Application of a treatment ampoule. Massage techniques will be vigorous and firm but not painful for the client. **(B)** Application of seaweed. This product is a powdered seaweed that has been mixed first with water and then with an emollient cream to make it easier to remove in a dry room. **(C)** Process during the slimming cocoon. Massage or mist the client with light aromatherapy scents. **(D)** After removing the seaweed and transitioning the client from plastic body wrap to the massage sheet, apply a firming cream to the body with massage strokes.

Snapshot: The Slimming Seaweed Cocoon

Indications

To slim the contours of the body, detoxification, stress, to promote revitalization and boost energy

Contraindications

High or low blood pressure, varicose veins, poor circulation, thyroid disorders or thyroid medications, shellfish or iodine allergies, sensitive skin, pregnancy, heart conditions, thrombosis or deep vein thrombosis

Supplies for the Treatment Table Setup (from the bottom to the top layer)

1) Blanket (wool or cotton) placed horizontally across the table so that the long edges are at 90 degrees to the sides of the table
2) Thermal space blanket placed horizontally across the table (optional)
3) A plain flat sheet placed with the long edges parallel to the long edges of the table (if the product needs to be removed in a dry room)
4) A plastic sheet placed horizontally across the table
5) One bath towel placed horizontally at the top of the table
6) One bath towel placed horizontally at the bottom of the table
7) Disposable undergarments or dry hand towels to act as a drape
8) Bolster

A Fomentek might be used under the massage sheet if additional warmth is needed.

Supplies for the Work Table Setup

1) Exfoliation product or dry brushes
2) Cellulite cream
3) Seaweed warming in a double boiler
4) Application brush or vinyl gloves
4) Firming product
5) Skin toner
6) Soda cooler
7) Hot, moist towels
8) Aura mist

Procedure

1) Exfoliate the posterior body areas.
2) Apply a skin toner to the posterior body.
3) Massage cellulite cream into target areas of the posterior body.
4) Turn the client supine.
5) Exfoliate the anterior body areas.
6) Apply a skin toner to anterior body areas.
7) Massage cellulite cream into target areas of the anterior body.
8) Apply seaweed to the body using the sit-up method.
9) Cocoon and massage the face, feet, or hands while the seaweed is processing.
10) Remove the seaweed with hot, moist towels.
11) Apply firming cream to the body.
12) Aura mist.

SESSION START

The client begins the treatment in the prone position and bolstered as for massage. A warm pack (e.g., hydroculator, flax seed pack) can be placed on the lower back to warm the area and give comfort for the client.

STEP 1: EXFOLIATION OF THE POSTERIOR BODY

Any type of exfoliation treatment can be used, but because the treatment goals include detoxification, dry skin brushing is appropriate. An exfoliation with sea salts is also stimulating and maintains an ocean theme. Chapter 6 describes exfoliation techniques in step-by-step detail. As each body area is exfoliated, a skin toner is applied to balance the pH of the skin. This is especially important with seaweed treatments because it helps to prevent skin irritation.

STEP 2: APPLY A CELLULITE CREAM TO TARGET AREAS OF THE POSTERIOR BODY

After exfoliating the posterior body, a cellulite cream is massaged into target areas such as the posterior thighs, gluteals, and waistline. Some therapists advocate the use of intensive massage in these areas based on the idea that they break down fat deposits and move them out of the tissue. How exactly the fat deposits are moved out of their connective tissue chambers is not clear unless the connective tissue is damaged. Some spas or therapists buy expensive machines that use a suction massage to lift and manipulate the tissue. Local circulation is visibly increased, but whether this results in a decrease of cellulite is unproven. Intensive or painful massage techniques are not recommended because they could bruise the client, lead to varicose veins, or cause undue discomfort. Good results are achieved with standard massage strokes and the application of seaweed over top of the cellulite cream.

STEP 3: EXFOLIATE AND APPLY CELLULITE CREAM ON THE ANTERIOR BODY

The client is turned into the supine position so that the anterior body areas can be treated. Each area is exfoliated, and a skin toner is applied before a cellulite cream is applied with regular massage strokes to target areas such as the anterior thighs, belly, hips, and upper arms.

STEP 4: APPLICATION OF SEAWEED

The sit-up method is used to apply seaweed to both the anterior and posterior body. First, the knees are bent and the seaweed is applied to both the anterior and posterior sides of the legs. The legs are flattened against the plastic body wrap, and the client is asked to sit up (first remove the bolster). The seaweed is applied to the back and gluteals, and the client is asked to lie back down. Finally, the belly and upper chest, followed by the arms, are treated, and the client is wrapped in the plastic.

STEP 5: COCOON

The plastic wrap is pulled around the client and tucked in loosely. Next the outer wrapping materials are pulled up and around the client. The bath towel at the top of the massage table can be used around the client's head in a turban drape or tucked into the top of the cocoon. The feet are wrapped with the towel at the bottom of the massage table. Hot water bottles, heat lamps, or flax seed packs can be used for additional warmth if needed.

STEP 6: PROCESS: MASSAGE THE FACE, FEET, OR BOTH

While the client is processing in the cocoon, a relaxing face massage can be given using a face cream. Offer the client a sip of water or herbal iced tea through a flexible straw and mist the client with an aroma mist or spring water. After the face massage has been completed, the feet can be massaged. During any type of cocoon, enhancers such as a face massage, hot stone foot massage, reflexology, scalp treatment, or other special extra can be used to fill out the treatment and make it exceptional for the client.

STEP 7: UNWRAP

To remove the wrap, first take off the blankets. The therapist now has two options for removing the plastic based on the equipment available at the practice.

Option 1: Leave the client loosely wrapped in the plastic and take him or her to a shower. If the shower is outside the treatment room, drape the client with a bathrobe or sheet. Take the plastic from the client as he or she steps into the shower and throw it away. Put massage sheets on the massage table while the client is showering.

Option 2: If there is no shower, the plastic sheeting needs to be removed completely from underneath the client as the client is cleaned off with hot towels. To remove a plastic sheet, a clean sheet will need to have been placed under the plastic when the table was made up.

Unwrap the plastic, leaving the client covered by the breast drape and anterior pelvic drape that were put on before the client was wrapped up. Remove the product from the client's arms, upper chest, and abdominal area and ask him or her to hold onto the breast drape and sit up. Remove the product from the back and the posterior arms. Roll up the plastic sheet until it sits as close to the gluteals as possible. Wipe the feet with a hot towel and ask the client to bend the knees and hold up the feet. Roll up the dirty side of the plastic that is

underneath the client's feet. Place the client's clean feet on the massage sheet, which was underneath the plastic (the knees are still bent). Remove the spa product from both legs with hot towels and roll the plastic up as high as possible under the gluteals. Place the clean legs flat on the massage sheet and cover them with a sheet or towel for warmth. The client then lies back down on the massage sheet and slightly lifts the hips so that the plastic can be removed. The client is now draped with a massage sheet for the rest of the treatment.

STEP 8: APPLY FIRMING PRODUCTS

Some firming products are so strong that they are only applied to target areas of the body, but others are meant to be applied to the entire body. Sometimes the products are combined in a treatment. The strong product is applied to target areas and then the rest of the body is treated with a gentler product. Read the directions and cautions on all firming products carefully to ensure that they are used correctly.

SESSION END

After the application of a firming product, use an aura mist to signal the end of the treatment and to fill the room with a refreshing scent.

Sanitation

During the cleanup for a cocoon, it is important to spray the thermal space blanket with alcohol and allow it to air dry before putting it in a closed cabinet. Reusable mixing bowls, application brushes, and the soda cooler should be washed with hot, soapy water and sprayed with alcohol. Product bottles that were handled during the treatment should also be wiped down with alcohol before they are put away.

The Seaweed Breast Treatment

The breast, which has no muscle tissue, is composed of glandular tissue surrounded by fat. It is sensitive to estrogen, progesterone, and prolactin levels during the menstrual cycle and pregnancy. As elsewhere in the body, an intricate system of blood and lymphatic vessels bring nutrient-rich blood to breast tissues and carry metabolic wastes away for elimination. When breast tissue is compressed or restricted, usually by bras, metabolic wastes may build up in the tissue.[13] There is some evidence that this may cause a woman to experience greater tenderness during menstruation or increase a woman's chances of developing breast cancer.[14]

In the United States, breast massage and spa treatments for improving breast health generate a somewhat wary reception from therapists and clients alike. This may be because massage was once linked to prostitution and therapists worry that their professionalism will be called into question if they give a treatment for breast health. Breast massage is often avoided in massage schools because of state laws or discouragement from school accreditation bodies. Some states allow therapeutic breast massage with informed client consent, and others have legislation that requires therapists to take an advanced training and certification. Many men are rightly concerned about providing breast massage in cross-gender spa treatments. Even with informed client consent, male therapists are at risk in such a setting.

The American public is uncertain of the benefits of breast massage and breast treatments for disease prevention. Services aimed at improving the appearance of breast tissue are often more readily accepted. Therapists are rarely given training in breast massage at massage schools, so they have to seek out specialized instruction if they want to learn. Specialized training is important because it covers a wide range of topics from the psychology of touch and good ethical practice, to proper lymphatic drainage and the anatomy of the structures involved. *Breast Massage*, written by Debra Curties, is a particularly helpful guide for massage therapists interested in learning more.[15]

Although many spas do not offer treatments that involve working with breast tissue, some spas do, so it is important for therapists to know how to approach this type of service professionally. When working with breast tissue in a spa setting, avoid the nipples and areola and use firm, steady pressure at all times. Therapists should make sure that they check the laws in their state and obtain the client's *written* consent before offering a breast treatment.

The Seaweed Breast Treatment Snapshot given here presents an outline for novice therapists to help them understand the treatment steps that might be used in such a service. This service should be considered as an "advanced treatment," so specialized training in breast massage is recommended for novice therapists to build a solid foundation of knowledge. Experienced therapists might use this snapshot as a starting point when designing an original breast service. The goals of this treatment are to tone breast tissue and improve breast health by increasing circulation and lymph flow. An esthetician would add treatment steps for smoothing and moisturizing the skin to improve the appearance of the breasts. This outline is meant to be used as a "wellness" treatment rather than an active therapy for a diagnosed disease. Therapists with an advanced understanding of breast cancer or other serious breast conditions may include seaweed or therapeutic mud in their treatments to stimulate lymphatic drainage and the elimination of metabolic wastes from breast tissue. It is important to recognize that breast treatments may be against the law, so it is the therapist's responsibility to be aware of the relevant laws, regulations, and restrictions that apply in their state.

Snapshot: The Seaweed Breast Treatment

Indications
Sluggish lymphatic flow, poor circulation, to encourage breast health, stress, to firm and tone the breast tissue

Contraindications
Iodine allergies, broken or inflamed skin, high blood pressure, pregnancy or nursing, fever or illness, current breast cancer (unless the therapist has an advanced understanding), lymphatic insufficiency (unless the therapist has an advanced understanding)

Supplies for the Treatment Table Setup (from the bottom to the top layer)
1) Massage sheet
2) Top massage sheet
3) Blanket or bath sheet for warmth
4) Bolster
5) Pillow for the client's head

Supplies for the Work Table Setup
1) Plastic body wrap cut to fit over the upper chest
2) Cream cleanser
3) Gentle exfoliation product
4) Skin toner
5) Cosmetic sponges
6) Essential oil support lotion
7) Seaweed warming in a double boiler
8) Soda cooler
9) Hot, moist towels
10) Vinyl gloves
11) Aura mist

Procedure
1) Steam the breasts and upper chest with a professional steamer or with hot, moist towels.
2) Cleanse the area with a cream cleanser; remove the cleanser with hot, moist towels.
3) Exfoliate the area; remove the exfoliation product with hot, moist towels.
4) Apply a skin toner to the area.
5) Apply seaweed to the area.
6) Cover the area with plastic and a blanket.
7) Massage the hands, feet, or face.
8) Remove the seaweed with hot, moist towels.
9) Provide a breast massage (optional—with written consent only).
10) Apply a skin toner to the area.
11) Apply an essential oil support lotion to the area.
12) Aura mist.

Essential Oil Support Lotion
1 oz plain lotion, lavender (3 drops), grapefruit (5 drops), juniper berry (2 drops), frankincense (4 drops), lemon (4 drops)

Other Seaweed Treatments

The therapist is encouraged to try out seaweed products in a number of the other treatment outlines offered in this book. For seaweed back treatments or neck and scalp treatments, follow the appropriate outlines in Chapter 9 and substitute seaweed for fango. For a seaweed foot service, follow the outline for a basic foot treatment in Chapter 8 and use seaweed as the treatment product. Consider using a seaweed gel with a hot stone massage to bring clients the rejuvenating qualities of both of these treatments. In this case, the gel is used instead of massage oil. Seaweed powders can be blended with sea salts to offer in the gift store as an energizing soaking product for home use.

BOX 10-3
Broaden Your Understanding

What is a Facial?
Currently, the most popular treatment offered at spas is massage. The second most popular treatment is a facial. In most states, facials are outside the scope of practice of massage therapists and can only be given by a licensed or certified esthetician. Although massage therapists do not usually give facials, they may help to inform clients of the benefits of facials, which helps to sell additional services for the spa.

Each facial should be tailored to meet the skin type and specific needs of the client. The overall goals of a facial are to deep clean the pores, remove impurities from the skin, nourish and condition the skin, and improve or normalize skin function for better skin health. The session begins with a consultation and an analysis of the client's skin (**A**). This may be done with a Woods lamp, a fluorescent light that is used to identify the skin type. Next the skin is cleansed and exfoliated (**B**), massaged (**C**), and steamed (**D**) before ripe pimples or other blemishes such as comedones (blackheads) and milia (whiteheads) are extracted manually (**E**). This step may include the use of a disincrustation solution and a galvanic machine. The disincrustation solution is an alkaline product that helps to soften hardened sebum in the pores. A **galvanic current machine** may be used to help the solution penetrate the skin. The facial mask is applied to further draw impurities from the skin or to nourish and recondition the skin after it has been deep cleansed (**F**). Seaweed is perhaps the most beneficial natural product that might be used in a facial mask because of its ability to improve the moisture content of the skin, tone and firm tissue, and stimulate nutrient exchange in the skin. Sometimes a galvanic current machine is used to encourage the absorption of a nutrient-rich, water-soluble treatment product. A **high-frequency machine** may also be used (**G**). The ozone generated by this type of current has germicidal properties and helps to kill bacteria on the skin. The facial usually ends with the application of a moisture-rich finishing cream.

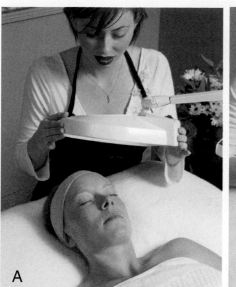

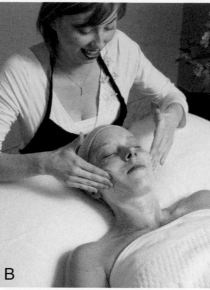

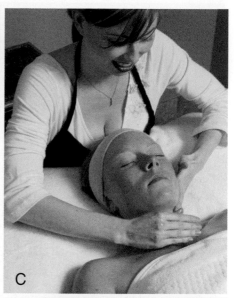

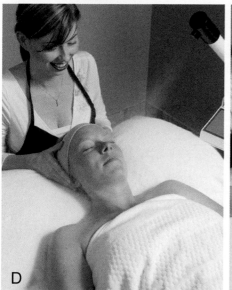

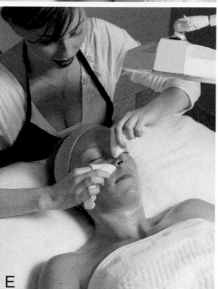

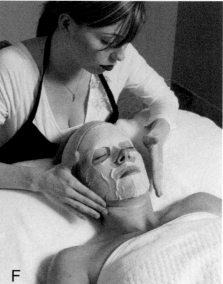

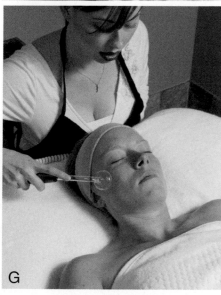

SAMPLE TREATMENTS

French Thalassotherapy

Promotional Description

The finest seaweeds from the coast of Brittany are used in traditional methods to relax and revitalize the body. A sea salt exfoliation is followed by a purifying kelp mask that detoxifies and smoothes. Vitamin rich creams are massaged into the skin to finish this elegant and graceful treatment.

Treatment Outline

Follow the treatment steps for a cocoon in Chapter 7 using seaweed as the treatment product. A sea salt exfoliation is covered in Chapter 6.

Sea Sculpt

Promotional Description

Slim the silhouette with revitalizing elements from the sea. This service targets problem areas such as the hips, thighs, belly, and upper arms, with powerful seaweeds and essential oils. First, a vigorous dry brush stimulates lymphatic flow and circulation. A cellulite cream rich in essential oils and natural botanicals helps to flush the tissue in stagnation-prone areas before the body is covered in rich, detoxifying seaweeds. An application of firming gel finishes this service and leaves the body feeling radiant and toned.

Treatment Outline

Follow the steps for the slimming seaweed cocoon. All natural products can be made in house if preferred by the therapist.

In-House Products for the Sea Sculpt Treatment

Slimming Massage Oil

Warm 16 fl oz of sunflower oil slowly on the stovetop and add 2 Tbsp of seaweed powder. Mix the powder into the oil over the heat for about 20 minutes. Store the mixture in a glass bottle for 1 week and shake the bottle daily. Filter the excess seaweed through a coffee filter and place the filtered oil in 2 fl oz bottles. Add the following essential oils to each of the two ounce bottles: grapefruit (25 drops), thyme (2 drops), juniper berry (5 drops), and white camphor (3 drops). Essential oil safety note: It is important to use white camphor rather than brown or yellow camphor because brown and yellow camphor contain high concentrations (up to 80%) of safrol, which is toxic and carcinogenic. White camphor contains no safrol and is considered nontoxic and non-irritant. All three camphors are fractions obtained during the distillation of *Cinnamomum camphora*. White camphor is the lightest fraction (lowest boiling point) and should be colorless to very pale yellow.

Cellulite-Activating Cream

Mix 2 oz of plain massage cream with grapefruit (20 drops), clove (2 drops), sweet fennel (4 drops), and spike lavender (10 drops).

Seaweed Firming Gel

2 oz of plain seaweed gel (the kind that is meant to be left on the body) and juniper berry (5 drops), sweet fennel (5 drops), and grapefruit oil (26 drops).

Mermaid Shimmer

Promotional Description

Feeling scaly and water logged? This combination of treatments filled with the benefits of sea products is more relaxing than a day at the beach! The body is descaled with an invigorating Dead Sea mineral scrub. Next, target areas are massaged with a firming cream to increase local circulation and reduce water retention. The body is cocooned in a thick kelp mask while the feet are massaged with essential oils and reflexology techniques. To finish the service, rich creams are massaged into the body to relieve muscle tension and deeply hydrate the skin.

Treatment Outline

Follow the directions for the slimming seaweed cocoon and modify the end of the service to use a full-body massage instead of an application of firming creams.

Summary

Thalassotherapy is a broad term for many different types of treatment that are based on sea products or seawater. It includes seawater hydrotherapy, the application of seaweed or seamud packs, exercise in seawater, relaxation by floating in seawater, diets rich in seaweed or seafood, and even the inhalation of aerosol-sized particles of seawater. Therapists will find that seaweed has many benefits for both body and skin, providing a number of treatment options that are possible to deliver in a dry room setting.

REFERENCES

1. Burtin P: Nutritional value of seaweeds. *Electronic Journal of Environment, Agriculture and Food Chemistry* [serial online]. 2003;2.
2. Ivanova V, et al: Isolation of a polysaccharide with antiviral effects from Ulva lactuca. *Prep Biochem* 1994;24:83–97.
3. Awad NE: Biologically active steroid from the green alga Ulva lactuca. *Phytother Res* 2000;14:641–643.
4. Kuznetsova TA, et al: Immunostimulating and anticoagulating activity of fucoidan from brown algae. *Antibiot Khimioter* 2003; 48:11–13.
5. Limova M, Campbell K: Evaluation of two calcium alginate dressings in the management of venous ulcers. *Ostomy Wound Management* 2003; 49:26–33.
6. Elliott WJ, Prisant LM: Drug delivery systems for antihypertensive agents. *Blood Press Monit* 1997;2:53–60.
7. Tajima S, et al: Alginate oligosaccharides modulate cell morphology, cell proliferation and collagen expression in human skin fibroblasts in vitro. *Arch Dermatol Res* 1999;291:432–436.
8. Zhu W, et al: Isolation and characterization of a sulfated polysaccharide from the brown alga Sargassum patens and determination of its anti-herpes activity. Biochem Cell Biol 2003;81:25–33.
9. Mohapatra BR, Bapuji M, Sree A: Antifungal efficacy of bacteria isolated from marine sedentary organisms. *Folia Microbiol* 2002;47:51–55.
10. Wong CK, Ooi VE, Ang PO: Protective effects of seaweeds against liver injury caused by carbon tetrachloride in rats. *Chemosphere* 2000;41: 173–176.
11. Yan X, Nagata T, Fan X: Antioxidative activities in some common seaweeds. *Plant Foods Hum Nutr* 1998;52:253–262.
12. Gorban EM, et al: Clinical and experimental study of spirulina efficacy in chronic diffuse liver diseases. *Lik Sprava* 2000;6:89–93.
13. Singer RS, Grismaijer S: *Dressed to Kill: The Link Between Breast Cancer and Bras.* New York: Avery Publishing Group, 1995.
14. Heieh CC, Trichopoulos D: Breast size, handedness and breast cancer risk. *Eur J Cancer* 1991;27:131–135.
15. Curties D: *Breast Massage.* New Brunswick, Canada: Curies-Overzet Publications, 1999.
16. Dasgupta T, et al: Chemomodulation of carcinogen metabolizing enzymes, antioxidant profiles and skin and forstomach papillomagenesis by Spirulina platensis. *Mol Cell Biochem* 2001;226:27–38.
17. Chamorro G, et al: Update on the pharmacology of Spirulina (Arthrospira), an unconventional food. *Arch Latinoam Nutr* 2002;52: 232–240.
18. Hirahashi T, et al: Activation of the human innate immune system by Spirulina: Augmentation of interferon production and NK cytotoxicity by oral administration of hot water extract of Spirulina platensis. *Int J Immunopharmacol* 2002;2:423–434.
19. Blinkova LP, Gorobets OB, Baturo AP: Biological activity of Spirulina. *Mikrobiol Epidemiol Immunobiol* 2001;2:114–118.
20. Rodriguez-Hernandez A, et al: Spirulina maxima prevents fatty liver formation in CD-1 male and female mice with experimental diabetes. *Life Sci* 2001;69:1029–1037.
21. Rarikh P, Mani U, Iyer U: Role of Spirulina in the control of glycemia and lipidemia in type 2 diabetes mellitus. *J Med Food* 2001;4:193–199.
22. Remirez D, Ledon N, Gonzalez R: Role of histamine in the inhibitory effects of phycocyanin in experimental models of allergic inflammatory response. *Mediators Inflamm* 2002;11:81–85.
23. Kaji T, et al: Repair of wounded monolayers of cultured bovine aortic endothelial cells is inhibited by calcium spirulan, a novel sulfated polysaccharide isolated from Spirulina platensis. *Life Sci* 2002;70: 1841–1848.

24. Paredes-Carbajal MC, et al: Effects of dietary Spirulina maxima on endothelium dependent vasomotor responses of rat aortic rings. *Life Sci* 1997;53:57–61.
25. Remirez D, et al: Inhibitory effects of Spirulina in zymosan-induced arthritis in mice. *Mediators Inflamm* 2002;11:75–79.
26. Iwata K, Inayama T, Kato T: Effects of Spirulina platensis on plasma lipoprotein lipase activity in fructose-induced hyperlipidemic rats. *J Nat Sci Vitaminol* 1990;36:165–171.
27. Hernandez-Corona A, et al: Antiviral activity of Spirulina maxima against herpes simplex virus type 2. *Antiviral Res* 2002;56:279–285.
28. Economic Appraisal of Seaweed. Available at http://www.w-isles.gov.uk/minch/seaweed/seaweed-04.htm
29. Michalum N, Michalum MV: *Skin Care and Cosmetic Ingredients Dictionary*, 2nd ed. Albany, NY: Milady, Thomson Learning, 2001, p. 73.
30. Kubo I, et al: Antibacterial activity of crinitol and its potentiation. *Nat Products* 1992;55:780–785.
31. Fujimura T, et al: Treatment of human skin with an extract of Fucus vesiculosus changes its thickness and mechanical properties. *J Cosmet Sci* 2002;53:1–9.
32. Fujimura T, et al: Effects of natural product extracts on contraction and mechanical properties of fibroblast populated collagen gel. *Biol Pharm Bull* 2000;23:291–297.
33. Mearns-Spragg A, et al: Cross-species induction and enhancement of antimicrobial activity produced by epibiotic bacterial from marine algae and invertebrates, after exposure to terrestrial bacteria. *Lett Appl Microbiol* 1998;27:142–146.
34. Kuznetsova TA, et al: Immunostimulating and anticoagulating activity of fucoidan from brown algae. *Antibiot Khimioter* 2003;48:11–13.
35. Berteau O, et al: Characterization of a new alph-L-fucosidase isolated from the marine mollusk Pecten maximus that catalyzes the hydrolysis of alpha-L-fucose from algal fucoidan (Ascophyllum nodosum). *Glycobiology* 2002;12:273–282.
36. Fodil-Bourahla I, et al: Effect of L-fucose and fucose-rich oligo- and polysaccharides (FROP-s) on skin aging: penetration, skin tissue production and fibrillogenesis. *Biomed Pharmacother* 2003;57:209–215.
37. Peterszegi G, et al: Studies on skin aging. Preparation and properties of fucose-rich oligo- and polysaccharides. Effect on fibroblast proliferation and survival. *Biomed Pharmacother* 2003;57:187–194.
38. IMPAG: Active Algae Ingredients: Out of the Biosphere Reserve into Cosmetics. *IMPAG News* 2002;12. Available at http://www.impag.de
39. Miller ET: *Salon Ovations: Day Spa Techniques*. Albany, NY: Milady Publishing, 1996.
40. Matsui MS, et al: Sulfated polysaccharides from red microalgae have anti-inflammatory properties in vitro and in vivo. *Appl Biochem Biotechnol* 2003;104:13–22.

REVIEW QUESTIONS

Multiple Choice

1. The different forms of thalassotherapy may be effective because seawater contains a concentration of:
   a. Mica crystals
   b. Essential oils
   c. Analgesic components
   d. Minerals

2. This nation embraced sea bathing in the early 1800s and developed facilities to warm seawater by 1824:
   a. England
   b. France
   c. Germany
   d. Italy

3. *Thalassa* is the Greek word for:
   a. Water
   b. Rain
   c. Sea
   d. Seaweed

4. Thalassotherapy does not include:
   a. Inhalation of fine particles of seawater
   b. Seafood diets
   c. Desert clay
   d. Flotation in seawater

5. Seaweed is defined as a:
   a. Plant that needs large amounts of sunlight to thrive
   b. A marine-based algae
   c. A blue-green algae
   d. A green algae from the genus of *Spirulina* spp.

Matching

6. Red algae _____ A. *Chlorophycota* spp.

7. Green algae _____ B. *Rhodophyta* spp.

8. Brown algae _____ C. *Phaeophycota* spp.

9. Blue-green _____ D. *Spirulina* spp.

10. Not seaweed _____ E. *Cyanophycota* spp.

Introduction to Ayurveda for Spa

Chapter Outline

Key Terms

Abhyanga: Massage with oil provided by one, two, or more therapists.
Ayurveda: The traditional natural medicine system of India dating back more than 5000 years.
Doshas: One of three subtle energies (vata, pitta, kapha) that hold together two of the five elements.
Kapha: A dosha that is a combination of earth and water.
Pitta: A dosha that is a combination of fire and water.
Prakriti: The constitution or inherent characteristics of a person, including his or her physical type, mental type, and emotional type.
Shirodhara: The application of a thin stream of oil to the forehead to reduce vata disorders and bring calm to the mind and body.
Taila: Medicated massage oil that is made by cooking herbs into a fatty base such as sesame or coconut oil.
Ubtan: An herbal paste used to support detoxification and smooth the skin. It is applied externally to the body.
Vata: A dosha that is a combination of space and air.
Vikrti: An individual's diet, environment, work stress, mental or emotional trauma, relationships, or physical injury may cause their prakriti (dosha constitution) to become unbalanced. The unbalanced state is referred to as a vikrti state.

Ayurveda is both a traditional medical system and a philosophy that offers keys for creating harmony and balance in life. In Sanskrit, *ayur* means life, and *veda* means knowledge.[1] Traditional Ayurveda, which developed in Southern India and Sri Lanka, includes many elements of practice that require years of careful and dedicated study. The ayurvedic physician will have had at least 5 years of specific training and 1 year of supervision in a hospital. He or she will follow a rigorous patient examination process before arriving at a diagnosis and treatment plan. The eight branches of traditional ayurveda are integrated into a holis- tic practice. These include surgery; medicine; gynecology; pediatrics; toxicology; ear, nose, and throat; rejuvenation; and virilification therapy (treatments that improve fertility). In each of these branches, detoxification, diet, yoga, herbal medications, external treatments (e.g., massage), and meditation play a role in the healing or strengthening process.

Although there are some spas in the United States and the United Kingdom that are designed as ayurvedic medical centers where ayurvedic physicians work together with a highly trained support staff, most American spas do not focus on the treatment of disease. Instead, they adopt

Table 11-1   Traditional and Ayurveda-Inspired Body Treatments

NAME	BRIEF DESCRIPTION	MAIN INDICATIONS
Shirodhara	A thin, thread-like drizzle of refined sesame oil is poured across the forehead to bring calmness of mind, body, and spirit.	Aggravated vata, insomnia, and anxiety
Udvartana	An invigorating massage delivered with the application of an herbal paste.	Increased circulation; cleanses, exfoliates, and tones the skin; stimulates weight loss; supports detoxification; good for kaphas
Garshan[8]	Wearing raw silk gloves, one or two therapists briskly massage the client.	Increased circulation, toxin removal, weight loss, used to increase energy. Good for kaphas
Swedana	This is an herbal steam bath usually given after a massage.	Detoxification, balancing for vata and kapha types.
Vishesh[8]	This is a firm massage that uses deep strokes and squeezing movements.	Detoxification, muscle soreness; particularly indicated for kapha types
Pizzichilli	Large amounts of warm oil are poured over the body while two or more therapists perform massage.	To decrease muscle pain and to bring flexibility to joints; indicated for vatas but contraindicated for pitta types.
Pinda	The client is massaged by one or two therapists who hold muslin bags full of rice, milk, and herbs. This leaves the client very relaxed and the skin smooth.	Indicated for dry, rough skin; this is very relaxing and has a particular and unmistakable fragrance; cooling for pittas
Kati basti[8]	A massage using heat and specific medicated oils to address lower back pain.	Lower back pain, rigidity of the lower spine
Abhyanga	A massage performed by one, two, or more therapists working in synchronicity. The strokes are varied depending on the dominant dosha of the client.	To bring balance to the doshas, increase circulation, and aid detoxification
Bindi	*Bindi* means point or origin. Spas combine different elements to make their own unique bindi treatments. These elements might include a hydro soak, botanical mask, exfoliation, and herbal wrap.	To bring balance to the doshas, to increase circulation and detoxification, and to smooth the skin
Dosha wrap	Like the bindi treatment, spas mix and match elements for this wrap. It usually includes a custom blend of oils for the client's dosha, an exfoliation, massage, and wrap in warm towels or sheets.	To bring balance to the doshas, to increase circulation and detoxification, and to smooth the skin

Table 11-2 | The Five Elements (Panchamahabhutas)

ELEMENT	BODY PART	SENSES	QUALITY	TASTE	ACTION
Space (also called ether)	Relates to spaces in the body: Mouth, nostrils, abdomen, respiratory tract, cells, and so on	The ears: Sound	Smooth, soft, subtle, porous, non-slimy	No taste	Creates softness, lightness, and porosity
Air	Relates to movement: Muscles, pulse, respiration, peristalsis, movement in cells, and so on	The skin: Touch	Rough, light, dry, cold, soluble	Astringent and slightly bitter	Creates lightness, dryness, and emaciation
Fire	Relates to metabolism, digestive processes, and intelligence	The eyes: Sight	Rough, bright, heating	Pungent	Creates an increase in temperature, burning sensations, improved eyesight, improved digestion
Water	Relates to plasma, blood, saliva, digestive liquids, mucous membranes, and cytoplasm	The tongue: Taste	Cold, fluid, moist, heavy, slimy, emollient, purgative	Sweet with astringent, sour, saline	Creates moisture, glossiness; increases fluid content
Earth	Relates to bones, teeth, nails, muscles, tendons, skin, hair, cartilage	The nose: Smell	Heavy, dull, thick, firm, immobile, compact, strong, rough, emollient, purgative	Sweet	Creates firmness, strength, hardness

elements of ayurveda that focus on positive life choices, general detoxification, relaxation, enhanced spiritual awareness, and gentle exercise. This is a positive practical use of a complex traditional healing method that might otherwise be inaccessible and so readily dismissed by Westerners.

This chapter aims to introduce some of the core concepts of ayurveda that support the practice of ayurvedic body treatments that are commonly offered at spas. This chapter focuses on Indian head massage, abhyanga, shirodhara, and udvartana, which are well suited to dry room delivery. Other external treatments are also described. The resources section at the back of the book lists a number of reputable training centers and equipment sources for those interested in pursuing more information on ayurveda.

Core Concepts

The foundation of traditional ayurveda is based on the belief that everything in the universe is composed of five elements (*panchamahabhutas*). These elements (eternal sub-

stances) provide a means for understanding the nature of the universe and ourselves. They are space (sometimes referred to as ether), air, fire, water, and earth. Each of these elements has specific qualities that intermix in the body and when combined with the soul, form a unique individual. The five elements can be related to different parts of the body, to the senses that help us interpret the world, and to particular actions that produce change (Table 11-2).[2] Specific combinations of the five elements make up the three **doshas** (tridoshas).

THE THREE DOSHAS (TRIDOSHAS)

The doshas, known individually as **vata**, **pitta**, and **kapha**, can be viewed as vital body energies and as the energies that underlie all things in the world. In nature, the doshas govern different times of the day or night and different seasons or climates (Fig. 11-1). In the body, each dosha governs specific physiological functions. The way that the doshas combine in an individual governs the body type, mental and emotional characteristics, and personality. Although every individual has elements of all three doshas, one or more of

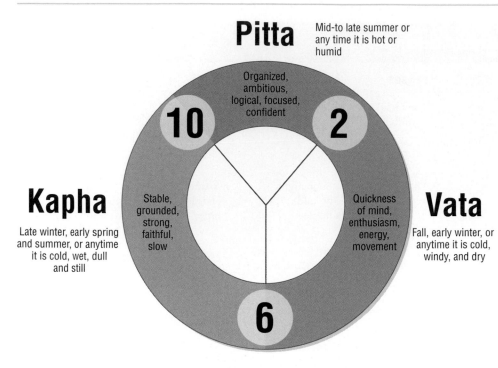

Pitta Mid-to late summer or any time it is hot or humid

Organized, ambitious, logical, focused, confident

Kapha
Late winter, early spring and summer, or anytime it is cold, wet, dull and still

Stable, grounded, strong, faithful, slow

Quickness of mind, enthusiasm, energy, movement

Vata
Fall, early winter, or anytime it is cold, windy, and dry

10   2   6

Attention and attunement to the natural world and its rhythms is one way to keep the doshas in balance. In Ayurveda, time, the seasons and the phases of life are governed by the doshas. Through mindfulness to the dosha clock and dosha season, greater harmony, balance, and health are achieved.[1]

Wake up: It is best to wake up during vata time (by 6:00 AM) to start the day with vata qualities (quick and energetic). Sleeping into kapha time (past 6:00 AM) gives the day kapha qualities (slow and heavy).

Exercise: Exercise is best during the early phases of kapha time (6 to 10 AM and 6 to 10 PM) because the body will be at its strongest and have the most stamina. Exercise during the middle of the day tends to aggravate pitta and can lead to feelings of irritability.

Work: Focus, organization, planning, and clear communication are at their best during pitta time from 10:00 AM to 2:00 PM. In the evening pitta cycle from 10:00 PM to 2:00 AM, pitta qualities enhance the dream state.

Main meal: Pitta governs metabolism and the absorption of nutrients from food. For this reason, it is important to eat the main meal during the middle of the day during pitta time, around 12:00 noon. Digestive processes slow during kapha time, so avoid eating anything heavy after 6:00 PM.

Sleep: To fall asleep quickly and to have a sound sleep throughout the night, ayurveda recommends bed before 10:00 PM (before kapha time ends). This allows a complete night's rest before the next kapha cycle begins.

Figure 11-1   A dosha-mindful day.

the doshas is dominant. This unique dosha combination is referred to as a person's doshic **prakriti** (constitution) and is believed to be determined by karma from the person's previous lives.[3]

In the simplest terms, an individual is healthy when the three doshas are in a state of balance. An unbalanced dosha state (**vikrti**) allows disease to take root. When an individual practices ayurveda, he or she is mindful of the activities and life choices that aggravate and pacify their particular prakriti. This allows the individual to make choices that promote balance and harmony and thereby decrease stress and disease.

Although an individual may have a dominant dosha, this does not mean that the doshas are static. Like everything in life, the doshas are in a constant state of transition. A certain situation may aggravate one dosha but pacify another dosha. Sometimes a client will exhibit physical, mental, and

emotional traits that indicate that he or she is decidedly a kapha (prakriti), but his or her current condition suggests that he or she has a pitta imbalance (vikrti). During the treatment session, the therapist will aim to pacify the pitta imbalance, and the long-term treatment goal might be to bring overall balance to the client's kapha-dominant prakriti.

Ayurvedic physicians use an in-depth 8- or 10-fold examination process to determine which dosha needs to be pacified in order to bring balance and healing to the body.[2] In a standard spa setting, a questionnaire is used to gather general data about a client's dosha state before the ayurvedic-inspired body treatment. The answers on the questionnaire help the therapist to make choices about the delivery of the treatment and the products that might be useful for the client. The questionnaire offered here is easy to use and is not too complicated (Fig. 11-2). The first

DOSHA QUESTIONNAIRE

Client's Name: _____ **Date:** _____

	Section One: Prakriti
	Directions: Choose the answer that describes you most accurately. No answer may fit perfectly, so simply make the best possible choice with the answers provided. Place a V, P, or K in the box to the left.

☐ ☐ ☐	My size at birth was small (V) My size at birth was average (P) My size at birth was large (K)
☐ ☐ ☐	I am thin and either short or very tall (V) I am medium in height and body (P) I am tall and sturdy or short and stocky (K)
☐ ☐ ☐	I have difficulty gaining weight (V) I gain or lose weight easily (P) I tend to gain weight easily (K)
☐ ☐ ☐	I have long, tapered fingers/toes (V) I have fingers/toes of medium length (P) I have square hands and shorter toes/fingers (K)
☐ ☐ ☐	I have knobbly, prominent joints (V) I have well-proportioned joints (P) I have large, well-formed joints (K)
☐ ☐ ☐	I have a delicate chin and a small forehead (V) I have a moderate chin and a medium forehead that have a tendency toward lines and folds (P) I have a large jaw and large forehead (K)
☐ ☐ ☐	I have uneven or buck teeth that are sensitive to either hot or cold (V) I have even teeth of medium or small size that tend to yellow (P) I have large, white, even teeth (K)
☐ ☐ ☐	My lips are thin and narrow (V) My mouth is of medium size (P) My lips are full (K)
☐ ☐ ☐	My skin is dry, rough, cold to touch (V) My skin is fair, soft, warm to touch (P) My skin is pale, cold, clammy, and tends to be oily (K)
☐ ☐ ☐	My hair is fine, coarse, brittle, and fine to medium in texture (V) My hair is fine, fair, or reddish (P) My hair is thick, oily, lustrous, and wavy (K)
☐ ☐ ☐	My neck is thin, very long, or very short (V) My neck is of regular proportion (P) My neck is solid and strong (K)
☐ ☐ ☐	My eyes are small, narrow, or shrunken, and my eye color is dull (V) My eyes are of average size and light colored (P) My eyes are large and lustrous (K)
☐ ☐ ☐	The shape of my face is long and angular (V) The shape of my face is heart-shaped, and I have a pointed chin (P) The shape of my face is rounded and full (K)
☐ ☐ ☐	My tongue tends to be dry with a thin, gray coating (V) My tongue tends to have a yellowish or orange coating (P) My tongue tends to be swollen with a thick, white coating (K)

Figure 11-2   Dosha questionnaire.

☐	I have a high tolerance to heat and enjoy hot weather (V)
☐	I have a low tolerance to heat and enjoy moderate to cool weather (P)
☐	I have a high tolerance to heat and prefer hot, dry, and windy weather (K)
☐	My normal body temperature is cool, and I tend to have cold hands and feet (V)
☐	My normal body temperature is warm, and I often feel too warm or hot (P)
☐	My normal body temperature is cold (K)
☐	My sleep is light and fitful (V)
☐	My sleep is sound but sometimes disturbed (P)
☐	I enjoy deep, prolonged sleep (K)
☐	I have short bursts of energy, but my endurance is low, and I run out of steam easily (V)
☐	I have moderate energy, moderate endurance, and good reserves (P)
☐	I have good endurance and large reserves of energy (K)
☐	In heat, I perspire minimally (V)
☐	In heat, I perspire profusely (P)
☐	In heat, I get clammy but I don't perspire freely (K)
☐	I am always doing different things: I have a tendency to fidget (V)
☐	My activity level is focused and moderate (P)
☐	I can be sluggish and even lazy (K)
☐	I have a lot of ideas that I have difficulty putting into action: I have a restless imagination (V)
☐	I am organized, efficient, intelligent, and tend toward perfectionism (P)
☐	I am steady, calm, and not easily disturbed but do not like to be rushed (K)
☐	I am good at remembering recent events but have poor long-term memory (V)
☐	I have a good memory (P)
☐	Information absorbs slowly, but once it does, I have excellent long-term memory (K)
☐	I am creative and expressive: I often change my beliefs (V)
☐	I am goal-oriented, ambitious, and have strong convictions that govern my behavior (P)
☐	I am contented and calm. I have steady, deeply held beliefs that I will not change easily (K)
☐	I have difficulty making decisions and change my mind often (V)
☐	I make rapid decisions and feel that they are good (P)
☐	I take a long time to make a decision but stick to the choices I make (K)
☐	I dislike routine and need a lot of change (V)
☐	I enjoy planning and organizing my life (P)
☐	I like routine and don't like it when things change (K)
☐	When stressed, I become fearful, anxious, and insecure (V)
☐	When stressed, I become confrontational, aggressive, judgmental, and hot tempered (P)
☐	When stressed, I have a tendency to withdraw. Sometimes I am greedy and possessive (K)
☐	I am a free spirit: I don't carefully plan my life but go with the flow (V)
☐	I am an achiever and I am ambitious. I carefully plan each step of my life (P)
☐	I feel safe, steady, and calm in my life. I would prefer it if things remain as they are (K)
☐	On a good day, I am secure, grounded, and settled (V)
☐	On a good day, I am confident, warm, brilliant, and witty (P)
☐	On a good day, I am warm-hearted, loving, and active (K)
☐	On a bad day, I am cold, distant, and insecure (V)
☐	On a bad day, I am jealous and controlling (P)
☐	On a bad day, I am possessive, lackadaisical, and clinging (K)
☐	I know a lot of people, but I have few close friends (V)
☐	I have a few good friendships. I seem to make enemies without meaning to (P)
☐	I have many loyal and close friendships (K)
☐	I spend the money I have impulsively and easily (V)
☐	I plan how I will spend money (P)
☐	I spend money reluctantly and I like to save (K)

Totals: Place the total number of V's under vata, the total number of P's under pitta, and the total number of K's under kapha in the spaces provided. _____ Vata _____ Pitta _____ Kapha

Figure 11-2 *(continued)*

DOSHA QUESTIONNAIRE

Section Two: Indications of Imbalance
Directions: Choose the answer that describes you most accurately and place a V, P, or K in the box at the left. If none of these descriptions fit, place an NA in the box to the left.

☐ Recently, my skin has been dry or I have dry patches (V)
☐ Recently, I have had heat rashes and spots (P)
☐ Recently, my skin has been oilier than usual (K)

☐ Recently, my hair has been dry, and brittle, and I have split ends (V)
☐ My hair seems to be thinning or graying more rapidly than usual (P)
☐ My hair has been excessively oily lately (K)

☐ I feel underweight and can't seem to gain weight even though I am trying (V)
☐ I keep gaining and losing the same 10 pounds (P)
☐ I'm overweight, and I am having difficultly losing weight (K)

☐ Lately, I feel cold a lot (V)
☐ These days, I often feel hot and irritated (P)
☐ Lately, I've been feeling cold and dull (K)

☐ I keep waking up and have difficulty getting back to sleep (V)
☐ I have difficulty getting to sleep but once asleep, I sleep soundly (P)
☐ I am sleeping excessively (9 to 10 hours), and I don't want to get up (K)

☐ I feel exhausted, restless, and nervous (V)
☐ I feel tense and tired but determined to get the job done (P)
☐ I feel lethargic and have low energy and I have difficulty taking on new tasks (K)

☐ Lately, I feel indecisive, chaotic, and forgetful, and I have difficulty focusing and concentrating (V)
☐ Lately, I feel judgmental of others, overly ambitious, and often negative (P)
☐ Lately, I feel uninspired and resistant to change, and I'm having difficulty retaining information (K)

☐ When stressed, I feel tearful and anxious (V)
☐ When stressed, I feel angry, aggressive, and confrontational (P)
☐ When stressed, I feel like I want to hide away from the world (K)

Totals: Place the total number of V's under vata, the total number of P's under pitta, and the total number of K's under kapha in the spaces provided. _____ Vata _____ Pitta _____ Kapha

Therapist's comments: _____

_____

_____

_____

_____

Figure 11-2 *(continued)*

set of questions (section one) helps to determine the clients dominant dosha (or doshas) and prakriti, and the second set of questions (section two) helps to determine any current dosha imbalance (vikrti). For example, if the client marks a high number of P boxes and some V or K boxes in the first section, he likely has a dominant pitta prakriti (remember that all three doshas will always be present in each person's constitution even although one or two will be dominant). If he marks a high number of V boxes in the second section, he likely has a vata imbalance. The therapist will want to pacify vata even though their client is a dominant pitta.

When the therapist and client have reviewed the questionnaire, they are ready to choose which type of treatment will suit the client's particular dosha or address the client's dosha imbalance. The dosha profiles below will help the therapist and client to understand the characteristics of each of the doshas and the types of treatments that support dosha balance. A ready-to-copy questionnaire appears in the appendix section at the back of the book.

The Dominant Vata Profile

Vata is the strongest of the three doshas and combines the elements of space and air. The word *vata* means to move or to enthuse. These words describe the vata tendency to move so quickly or to move so much that balance is lost. It is not surprising then that vata is the dosha most likely to become unbalanced. Table 11-3 provides an overview of the vata profile for quick reference.

General Vata Qualities. Vata governs both the physical and mental movements of the body, including the thought processes; circulation of blood; conduction of impulses in the nervous system; elimination of wastes; and muscular movements such as walking, lifting, and speaking. The vata season is autumn and early winter and any day that is cold, dry, and windy. Each dosha will have its own qualities. Vata qualities are described as dry, light, cold, subtle, unstable, rough, clear, and transparent.

Vata Body Type. People with vata as the dominant dosha tend to be thin or angular. They may be short or very tall. Their skin and hair are typically dry and rough, their teeth are large, their mouth small and thin, and their eyes are dull and dark. Vatas are highly active and have difficulty gaining weight despite being fond of sweet foods.

Vata Mental and Emotional Characteristics. The vata mind is restless, sensitive, and flexible. Although recent or minor events may be recalled with exacting precision, long-term memory is weak. A balanced vata is creative, filled with enthusiasm, artistic, and open minded. This sensitivity of mind, however, often leads the unbalanced vata to emotional insecurity, anxiety, and even to deep-seated or irrational fear. Vatas sleep little, and the sleep they do get is easily interrupted.

Factors that Aggravate or Pacify Vatas. Vatas are easily aggravated by situations that are overstimulating. These might include noisy parties, an overindulgence in TV or Internet surfing, confrontational situations, or conditions in which others are stressed or intense. Vatas need quiet sounds or calming music, gentle talk, soft touch, and a structured routine. Foods should be warming; uncooked or raw foods are kept to a minimum. When a vata is out of balance, he or she may experience joint pain, arthritis, constipation, high blood pressure, heart disease, and mental instability.

Spa Techniques that Pacify Vata or a Vata Imbalance. Vata qualities are described as dry, light, cold, subtle, unsta-

ble, rough, clear, and transparent. An individual who is a dominant vata or who has a vata imbalance will need to pacify these qualities with treatments that are oily, heavy, warm, obvious, stable, smooth, dark, and opaque. For the Western therapist, using these words to match a treatment to a client can feel a bit challenging. Instead of getting attached to these words, the therapist is encouraged to view them as metaphors and to use them to explore ayurvedic influences, promote creativity, and have fun. For example, a classic treatment for vata or a vata imbalance is the shirodhara treatment in which a thin stream of oil is played across the forehead. The oil is oily (balances dry), heavy (balances light), warm (balances cold), obvious (balances subtle: oil is being poured on the head, and this is observable and palpable), stable (balances unstable: the sensation of the oil running down the head pulls the mind's eye to one point, which helps to focus the mind, creating stability), smooth (balances rough: the oil feels smooth), dark and opaque (balances clear and transparent). The treatment happens with the client's eyes covered or closed in a darkened and quiet room. During this treatment, it is common for the client to explore internal mental and emotional spaces that are not as *clear* and *transparent* as everyday experience.

In another example, the vata client or client with a vata imbalance is not contraindicated for the udvartana treatment (a treatment in which an herbal paste is smoothed onto the body and then buffed off with towels), but the treatment needs to be modified. The **ubtan** (herbal paste) should be mixed up with extra oil (oily balances dry), and it should not be buffed off (buffing is rough, and the vata is already "rough"). Instead, the paste can be removed with hot, moist towels, making long, smooth sweeps (warm and smooth balances cold and rough) or in a soaking tub (warm and wet balance cold and dry).

The massage for a vata or client with a vata imbalance should be oily (balances dry), warm (balances cold), smooth (balances rough), and precise (balances subtle). Strokes should be long and flowing with a firm pressure and an even rhythm. Irregular movements, abrupt transitions, fussy and inefficient draping, tapotement, and pressure that is either too deep or too light will aggravate vata. The appropriate massage oils for vata include sesame, olive, almond, and ghee (clarified butter). Extra oil can even be applied to the body and allowed to soak in during a cocoon after the massage has ended. Warm packs (hydroculator, flax seed, corn, microwavable, other) can be used to provide extra warmth during the massage. Applying warm oil to the abdominal area and covering it with a heated towel and then a warm pack is particularly comforting for vatas. Grounding elements introduced during the massage also help to pacify vata. Hot stones might be placed on areas of particular tension (heavy balances light; warm balances cold), or the therapist may use guided meditation to help vatas focus the mind. In traditional spa treatments (i.e., treatments that are not inspired by ayurveda), the client might be treated with mud (heavy,

Table 11-3 Vata Dosha Profile

FACTORS THAT AGGRAVATE	AGGRAVATED VATA DISEASE	FACTORS THAT PACIFY
Rainy, cold, or windy weather The seasons of fall and early winter Vata-increasing foods (foods that are cold, dry, light, bitter, and astringent, including raw vegetables, dried fruits, red meat, stimulants such as coffee or soda, dried beans) Physical overexertion Irregular eating Snacking between meals Lack of sleep Mental overstimulation Emotional upset	Arthritis Rheumatoid arthritis Musculoskeletal disorders Paralysis Cardiovascular disorders Digestive disorders Constipation Diarrhea Foot diseases and disorders Mental instability	Quiet time Chanting or calming music Massage with warm sesame oil Warm, natural colors Sweet, gentle, and calming scents Vata-decreasing foods (foods that are rich, oily, and moderately spicy, including dairy products; grains; natural sweeteners such as honey; cooked vegetables; sweet, sour, and heavy fruits; chicken; seafood and turkey; herbs and spices) Regular sleep Structured routine Grounded and creative exercise such as gardening and dance
VATA MASSAGE AND FOOT BATH	**VATA HERBS**	**VATA ESSENTIAL OILS**
Vata Massage Long, smooth strokes and efficient draping; quiet music or silence; darkened room; extra oil; warm packs; grounding elements such as guided breathing exercises, guided meditation, or warm stones placed on areas of tension. Massage oils include sesame, olive, almond, and ghee (clarified butter). **Vata Foot Bath** (using herbs recognizable to Western therapists) Fill a muslin bag with ½ cup of mixed herbs that include ground ginger, sandalwood, eucalyptus leaf, calamus, and basil. Cover this bag with boiling water and allow it to steep for 20 minutes while it cools. Add cool or hot water as needed to adjust the temperature for the foot soak.	Traditional herbs that are used to pacify vata or to make vata taila are listed below. Ayurveda suppliers are listed in the back of the book. Suppliers have a variety of premade taila that are easy to use. Agnimantha (*Premna integrefolia*), ashwagandha (*Withania somnifera*), bala (*Sida cordifolia*), bhringaraj (*Eclipta alba*), bilva (*Aegle marmelos*), brihati (*Solanum indicum*), chandana or sandalwood (*Santalum album*), gokshura (*Tribulus terrestris*), jatamansi or spiknard (*Nardostachys* spp.), kantakari (*Solanum xanthocarpum*), neem (*Azadirechta indica*), patola (*Trichosanthes cucumeria*), prasarini (*Paederia foetida*), Punarnava (*Boerrhavia diffusa*), tulsi or sacred basil (*Ocimum sanctum*), vacha or calamus (*Acorus calamus*)	Angelica, anise, basil, bay laurel, birch (sweet), black pepper, cajeput, camphor (white), caraway, cardamom, cedarwood (atlas), cinnamon (caution), clove bud (caution), eucalyptus, sweet fennel, frankincense, geranium, ginger, jasmine, lavender, lemon, lemongrass, myrrh, nutmeg, orange (sweet), rose, spikenard, sage (clary), turmeric, valerian, wintergreen **Sample Vata Massage Blend** 2 oz sesame or almond oil, cardamom (12 drops), clary sage (8 drops), ginger (6 drops; buy the ginger CO_2), spikenard (3 drops), lemongrass (1 drop) **Sample Vata Aura Mist Blend** 2 oz purified water in a mist bottle, bay laurel (8 drops), eucalyptus (3 drops), jasmine (2 drops), sweet orange (10 drops), lavender (4 drops)

opaque, stable), seaweed (wet, smooth), or shea butter (oily, smooth, heavy) cocoons.

The Dominant Pitta Profile

In Sanskrit, *pitta* means to heat or to burn. Pitta is considered the dosha of transformation and is composed of the el-

ements of fire and water. Table 11-4 provides an overview of the pitta profile for quick reference.

General Pitta Qualities.   Pittas' functions include digestion, heat production, appetite, intellectual tasks, vision, the softness and suppleness of the body, and the imparting of color to the body. The pitta season is middle and late

Table 11-4	Pitta Dosha Profile	

FACTORS THAT AGGRAVATE	AGGRAVATED PITTA DISEASE	FACTORS THAT PACIFY
Hot or humid weather Mid to late summer Hot rooms or being overdressed in a warm environment Irregular meals Pitta-increasing foods (foods that are salty, sour, light, pungent, too oily, or acidic, including cheese, yogurt, hot peppers, tomatoes, garlic, onion, citrus fruits, tofu, peanuts, fish, red meat) Excessive mental activity Long periods indoors Alcohol consumption Uncommitted relationships	Burning sensations in the body Impaired vision Skin disorders and itching skin Indigestion and diarrhea Ulcers Blood disorders Jaundice Excessive perspiration and foul body odor	Soft music The sound of water Massage with coconut oil Cool colors with blue, green, or cream hues Pitta-decreasing foods (basmati rice, oats, wheat, unprocessed sugars such as maple syrup, vegetables that are not spicy, grapes, raisins, apples, nuts in moderation, chicken, turkey) Increased water intake Walks by water or in cool forests Stable relationships

PITTA MASSAGE AND FOOT BATH	PITTA HERBS	PITTA ESSENTIAL OILS
Pitta Massage Slow, calming strokes and efficient draping; darkened room; rhythmic and melodic music; and moderate oil and a grounded massage therapist. Massage oils include coconut, sunflower, safflower, and ghee (clarified butter). **Pitta Foot Bath** (using herbs recognizable to Western therapists) Fill a muslin bag with ½ cup of mixed herbs that include chamomile flowers, lavender flowers, peppermint, and lemongrass. Cover this bag with boiling water and allow it to steep for 20 minutes while it cools. Add cool or hot water as needed to adjust the temperature for the foot soak.	Some traditional herbs that are used to pacify pitta or to make pitta taila are listed below. Ayurveda suppliers are listed in the back of the book. Suppliers have a variety of premade taila that are easy to use. Agaru (*Aquilaria agalocha*), bala (*Sida cordifolia*), brahmi or gotu kola (*Centella asiatica*), ela or cardamom (*Eletteria cardamomum*), guduchi (*Tinospora cordifolia*), laksha (*Lacifera lacca*), manjishtha (*Rubia cordifolia*), musta (*Cyperus rotundus*), sariva (*Cryptolepis buchanani*), Shatavari (*Asperagus racemosus*), sveta chandan or white sandalwood (*Santalum alba*), ushira or vetiver (*Vetivera zizanoides*), yastimadhu or licorice	Camphor (white), cardamom, chamomile (German or Roman), champaca, coriander, fennel (sweet), gardenia, geranium, jasmine, lemongrass, lime, myrrh, peppermint, rose, sandalwood, spikenard, turmeric, valerian, wintergreen, yarrow **Sample Pitta Massage** Blend 2 oz olive or coconut oil, coriander (9 drops), geranium (2 drops), lavender (8 drops), vetiver (1 drop), peppermint (1 drop), sandalwood (9 drops) **Sample Pitta Aura Mist Blend** 2 oz purified water in a mist bottle, jasmine (4 drops), lime (20 drops), lemongrass (1 drop)

summer or any day that is hot and/or humid. Pitta qualities are described as hot, sharp, bright, liquid, slightly oily, sour, and pungent.

Pitta Body Type. People with pitta as their dominant dosha will tend to be of medium build and gain or lose weight easily. They often have light or red hair that is fine and soft in texture. Their hair may gray or fall out prematurely. They have hot, sweaty bodies and experience intense hunger pains. Pittas' eyes are light blue or gray in color and may easily turn red in the summer, after bathing, or after intense mental work. Pittas tend to have fair skin with promi-

nent freckles, birthmarks, or moles; the nose and chin are pointed. Pittas sleep soundly but lightly and may sleep for short periods of time. They like strong foods with sweet, bitter, or intense flavors.

Pitta Mental and Emotional Characteristics. The pitta mind is aggressively sharp with a clear memory and the ability to precisely articulate their thoughts and ideas. Pittas are ambitious, organized, and focused. They have a tendency to become emotionally intense and are prone to irritability and jealous behavior. They may become perfectionists and show little latitude to individuals around them that are vague or indecisive. When pittas are in balance, they are confident, bold, and brilliant. When they are out of balance, they are irritable, aggressive, impatient, and critical.

Factors that Aggravate or Pacify Pitta.
Pittas are aggravated by overheated rooms, overexposure to the sun, or too much clothing in overwarm environments. Although pittas are strong and determined in an argument, too much confrontation leads to imbalance. Pittas should have regular meals and drink adequate amounts of cool water. Excessive alcohol or spicy foods as well as eating while emotionally upset aggravate pitta. Pittas must balance mental activity with outdoor time. Walking in green forests or next to water is particularly calming.

Spa Treatments that Pacify Pitta or a Pitta Imbalance.
Pitta qualities are described as hot, sharp, bright, liquid, slightly oily, sour, and pungent. An individual who is a dominant pitta or has a pitta imbalance will need to pacify these qualities with treatments that are cool, soft, dark, solid, slightly dry, sweet, and mild. A classic treatment for the dominant pitta or a client with a pitta imbalance is pinda. Pinda is a treatment in which the body is massaged with muslin bags full of rice and herbs that have been cooked in milk. Pinda is cooling (balances hot), soft (balances sharp: the muslin bags create the sensation of being massaged with rice pudding), slightly dry (balances slightly oily: no oil is used, so the treatment is not as oily as a massage or shirodhara), sweet (balances sour: the milk, herbs, and rice smell sweet and yet exotic), and mild (balances pungent: this is a gentle treatment that is not too stimulating). Some ayurveda treatments are contraindicated for pittas. The pizzichilli treatment in which large amounts of warm oil are poured over the client while he or she is massaged is too hot and too oily for pittas. Similarly, swedana, a herbal steam bath, may also be too hot for a pitta. A pitta may enter the steam but need to come out sooner than a vata or kapha.

The pitta massage must be moderate in temperature or cooling, smooth, dark, calming, precise, and varied. Pittas may become critical and aggravated if they feel the therapist is not grounded and focused on the massage. The massage rhythm must be slow and calming because too many fast movements are irksome. Light or cooling oils are used in moderation. The appropriate massage oils for pitta include coconut, sunflower, safflower, and ghee (clarified butter). Warm packs and heavy blankets are only used if the day or treatment room is particularly cold. In traditional spa treatments (i.e., treatments that are not inspired by ayurveda), the client might be offered mint (cooling) cocoons, floral aromatherapy (sweet) cocoons, and mud treatments (soft, dark, and solid).

The Dominant Kapha Profile

Kapha means to keep together, to embrace, and also phlegm. A combination of earth and water, kapha expresses itself in nature as the solid structures of rocks and mountains. Table 11-5 provides an overview of the kapha profile for quick reference.

General Kapha Qualities
The kapha is the most stable of the doshas, and this stability functions as both physiological and psychological strength in the human body through anabolic or building processes, mucous membranes, phlegm, fat, and the lymphatic system. The kapha season is late winter and spring or any day that is cold, wet, dull, and still. Kapha is the dosha that is the least likely to go out of balance. Kapha qualities are described as heavy, cold, soft, viscous, sweet, stable, and slimy.

Kapha Body Type.
People with kapha as their dominant dosha are likely to be tall and solidly built or short and stocky with a large frame and a tendency to gain weight. Kapha hair is thick, soft, dark, and oily. They have round faces; large, expressive eyes; full mouths with small, white teeth; and pale, often oily, skin. Kaphas have a steady appetite and slow metabolism. They like bitter, pungent, and sharp tastes. They need the most sleep of all the doshas and sleep soundly when other dosha types would be disturbed.

Kapha Mental and Emotional Characteristics

The kapha mind absorbs information slowly but has a strong long-term memory. Kaphas speak slowly and precisely after carefully considering their position on a topic. They are the most loyal, patient, and compassionate of the dosha types, with a loving and emotionally secure nature. The stability and grounded nature that gives kaphas their reserves of strength and their steadiness of personality also makes them reluctant to change or release possessions. When in a balanced state, kaphas are content, supportive of others, loving, and affectionate. When they are out of balance, they sleep too much; overindulge in food; have a predisposition to laziness; and may exhibit greedy, possessive behavior.

Factors that Aggravate or Pacify Kapha.
Kaphas require plenty of vigorous exercise, bright colors, and upbeat music. Overeating, oversleeping, and eating very salty or very sugary foods aggravates kapha and leads to an unbalanced state in which the kapha feels bored, listless, and too dependent on loved ones. An out-of-balance kapha may be prone to obesity or its opposite, emaciation; to conditions of excess mucus; to loss of joint function (kapha governs body lubrication); to depression; and to mental confusion.

Spa Treatments that Pacify Kapha or a Kapha Imbalance.
Kapha qualities are described as heavy, cold, soft, viscous, sweet, stable, and slimy. An individual who is a dominant kapha or has a kapha imbalance will need to pacify these qualities with treatments that are light, warm, sharp, liquid, pungent, variable, and dry. For example, a

Table 11-5 | Kapha Dosha Profile

FACTORS THAT AGGRAVATE	AGGRAVATED PITTA DISEASE	FACTORS THAT PACIFY
Wet, cold, dull, or still weather The seasons of late winter and early spring Kapha-increasing foods (foods that are heavy, oily, cold, sweet, salty, or sour, including dairy products; sweets; sweet fruits such as avocados, bananas, coconut, and citrus fruits; nuts; red meat; dark meat; oily fish; salt; cold, carbonated drinks) Lack of exercise Overeating Too much sleep and taking naps Overdependence on loved ones Not allowing change	Weight gain or obesity Skin irritations Anorexia Disorders caused by excess mucus Goiter Indigestion Allergy and asthma (in traditional ayurveda, these two disorders as well as chronic eczema are believed to be inherited from life in the womb) Diabetes (starts as kapha and exacerbates pitta and vata in latter stages) Sinus problems	Regular exercise Regular mental stimulation Change of routine Kapha-decreasing foods (foods that are light, dry, warm, spicy, bitter, and astringent, including most grains; vegetables; light fruits such as apples, pears and berries; beans; and spices) Bright colors Upbeat music Stimulating and mucus-reducing scents such as eucalyptus, rosemary, and white camphor Relationships that encourage appropriate autonomy
KAPHA MASSAGE AND FOOT BATH	**KAPHA HERBS**	**KAPHA ESSENTIAL OILS**
Kapha Massage Stimulating, fast paced, firm, and non-oily. Powders (dry ubtan) may be used instead of oil. If oil is used, it should be lightweight and warming such as safflower, apricot kernel, sunflower, sesame, and mustard oil. **Kapha Foot Bath** (using herbs recognizable to Western therapists) Fill a muslin bag with ½ cup of mixed herbs that include basil, ground ginger, eucalyptus leaf, and common sage leaf. Cover this bag with boiling water and allow it to steep for 20 minutes while it cools. Add cool or hot water as needed to adjust the temperature for the foot soak.	Some traditional herbs that are used to pacify kapha or to make kapha taila are listed below. Ayurveda suppliers are listed in the back of the book. Suppliers have a variety of premade taila that are easy to use. Chitraka (*Plumbago zeylonica*), deodar or Himalayan cedar (*Cedrus deodar*), kavavira (*Nerium indicum*), manjishtha (*Rubia cordifolia*), neem (*Azadirechta indica*), nirgundi (*Vitex negundo*), punarnava (*Boerrhavia diffusa*), tulsi or sacred basil (*Ocimum sanctum*), vacha or calamus (*Acorus calamus*)	Anise, angelica, basil (sweet), bay laurel, birch (sweet), black pepper, cajeput, camphor (white), caraway, cardamom, cedar (atlas), clove bud (caution), cinnamon (caution), eucalyptus, frankincense, fir, ginger (buy the CO_2), myrrh, nutmeg, parsley, peppermint, pine needle, rosemary, sage (common), tea tree, thyme, turmeric, valerian, wintergreen **Sample Kapha Massage** Blend 2 oz sunflower oil, myrrh (12 drops), cinnamon (2 drops), sweet birch (4 drops), eucalyptus (4 drops), common sage (4 drops), rosemary (4 drops) **Sample Kapha Aura Mist Blend** 2 oz purified water in a mist bottle, bay laurel (4 drops), thyme (4 drops), fir (2 drop), anise (2 drops)

classic treatment for kapha or a kapha imbalance is udvartana, in which the body is massaged with an herbal paste (ubtan). In this case, the herbs are used dry (like a herbal powder) or they are blended with water or milk and no oil is used (dry balances slimy). Udvartana is stimulating (balances heavy), warming (balances cold), textured, and rough (balances soft: dry hand towels are used to buff off the herbal paste), spicy (balances sweet: ubtan contains mustard powder and various spices), and vigorous (balances stable). It invigorates and energizes the body, balancing the kapha tendency to remain at rest.

In another example, the kapha client or client with a kapha imbalance is not contraindicated for the shirodhara treatment, but the treatment needs to be modified. Instead of oil (the kapha is already "slimy and viscous"), warm milk or salt water is used (liquid, light, variable).

The massage for a kapha is the most stimulating and the least oily of the dosha massages. Their massage must be vigorous (e.g., a sports massage), fast paced, warming, firm, and non-oily. In a traditional ayurveda setting, massage for kaphas might be done with powders, alcohol, or silk gloves (a massage with silk gloves is called gershan) to avoid adding more oil to the kapha constitution. Lightweight or warming oils are used when a dry massage is not desired. Appropriate massage oil for kaphas include safflower, apricot kernel, sunflower, sesame, and mustard oil used in moderation. Similar to vatas, kaphas need warmth and can be heated with hot water bottles and warm packs.

General Treatment Considerations

Before offering ayurveda-inspired treatments, the therapist should consider skin sensitivity issues, the contraindications for each treatment, and how to represent and promote these treatments to clients.

ACCURATE REPRESENTATION OF AYURVEDA IN A SPA

There are many authentic ayurvedic physicians who feel disturbed and even angry about this nontraditional use of their ancient healing art.[2] First, there is a concern that spas are offering an oversimplified piece of a metaphorical and complicated system. Ayurveda is closely linked to Hinduism, which is not strictly a religion but rather the practice of Dharma, the code of life. The concept of a person having a dominant dosha, which is central to the practice of ayurveda, is interwoven with a belief in karma and previous lives. Many Westerners do not believe in karma and, in fact, hold quite opposite views. All clients can benefit from ayurveda no matter what their personal beliefs may be. However, the cultural context of ayurveda should not be ignored and is something that should be considered and accurately represented during the treatment.

As responsible therapists, it is important that we educate clients about the holistic practice of ayurveda and provide references to books or referrals to authentic ayurvedic physicians for clients wishing to learn more. It is also important to clearly define the treatment goals for any ayurveda services offered and to represent those services appropriately. For example, many spas use ayurvedic principles as a starting point for developing an otherwise original service. There is nothing wrong with this as long as it is reflected in the promotional literature. To say that a service is "inspired by" ayurveda is different than saying it *is* ayurveda.

TREATMENT NAMING

To avoid confusion, traditional treatment names should only be used for authentic and traditional treatments. For example, in one case, a spa brochure included a "panchakarma herbal wrap." Not knowing any better, the client would probably assume that this is an authentic ayurvedic treatment. Panchakarma (also spelt *pancha karma* and *pancakarman*) is, in fact, a detoxification treatment consisting of five different cleansing methods. These methods include emesis (therapeutic vomiting), purgation (use of a specific laxative), enema, nasya (administration of massage to the nasal cavity with a finger dipped into ghee), and detoxification of the blood (through a specific type of bloodletting).[1] Clearly, this is not a treatment that would ever be offered by a massage therapist.

SKIN SENSITIVITY

In India, where ayurveda originated, the climate is generally hot, and the local people have thick, strong hair and skin that are generally not prone to sensitivity. Some of the ingredients that are used in ayurveda can cause sensitivity in fair-skinned individuals. For this reason, the therapist should err on the side of caution and dilute products with aloe gel, milk, or a plain fixed oil (as opposed to the medicated taila, which will be described later) before their application to fair-skinned individuals.

HAIR ISSUES

Many ayurvedic services begin with an Indian head massage and foot soak. In an Indian head massage, oil is massaged through the hair to the scalp. The shirodhara treatment also coats the client's hair and scalp in oil. Obviously, this messes up the client's hair, and shampooing the hair is out of the massage scope of practice in most states. The therapist has three main options: 1) The client is passed to a cosmetologist who will finish the service by washing, cutting, or styling the client's hair; 2) The client is escorted to a shower or soaking tub where he or she washes and conditions the hair; 3) The therapist removes most of the oil with hot, moist towels so that the client can go home and wash the hair. In all cases, hair issues must be discussed with the client when making the appointment so that the client is prepared for the service.

Abhyanga

In India, massage is part of daily life, and it is common to see mothers, with a blanket spread across the ground, massaging their children in the open marketplace or to see women chatting and massaging each other's shoulders. Self-oiling and self-massage are also common practices.

Abhyanga is the Sanskrit word for oil massage. Abhyanga can be performed by the client or by one, two, or more therapists working together in a coordinated manner on a client. The strokes and massage oils are varied depending on the dosha of the client (review the dosha profiles for details).

India is a large country, so the techniques used vary in different regions. There are however, five general strokes that are used in traditional massage (Figure 11-3). These are the sweep, tapping, kneading, rubbing, and squeezing.[4]

The sweep (similar to effleurage) is applied from the navel out toward the distal areas of the body in brisk, straight strokes. On the legs, the sweep starts at the greater trochanter and ends at the feet. On the upper body, the sweep starts at the navel, sweeps up to the shoulder ("jump" the breast drape), and then sweeps down to the hands.

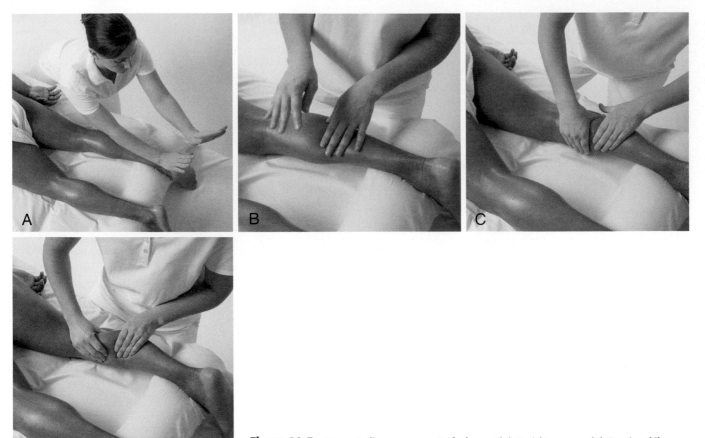

Figure 11-3   Some Indian massage techniques. (A) Straight sweeps. **(B)** Tapping. **(C)** Kneading. **(D)** Squeezing.

Sweeps are used to "open" and "close" a body area and are repeated up to 25 times on one area. Tapping (similar to tapotement) is used to awaken the body, alert the nerve endings, and increase circulation. It is done with open palms and relaxed fingers. After the area has received the tapping technique, it is kneaded (similar to petrissage) at a depth that is tolerable to the client. The area is kneaded thoroughly and completely before the therapist moves on to the fourth technique, which is rubbing. Rubbing (similar to friction) can be done on dry skin (except for vatas) or performed with oil. It can be deep (applied with the knuckles or thumbs) or light and superficial (applied with the fingertips). It can be performed quickly or slowly. Although some specific techniques rub in a counterclockwise direction, most often the rubbing is in clockwise circles. As the therapist reaches a marma point, the rubbing takes a particular form (see below under Marma Points). The fifth step in the massage sequence is squeezing. Using both hands, the therapist lifts an area of muscle with a squeezing and crossing torque-like motion. In bony areas such as the fingers and toes, a combination of squeezing and twisting is used to mobilize the area. To finish the fingers and toes, a drop of oil is placed on the finger so that it fills the gap between the nail and the flesh. The massage sequence ends for each body area just as it began with straight sweeps working out from the navel to the distal areas of the body.

MARMA POINTS

Marma points are energy centers in the body that are traditionally used with Indian massage and ayurvedic healing.[5] The name *marma* means secret, hidden, and vital. They connect the physical body with subtle energy bodies and often relate to specific organs or body areas. They are massaged in order to restore the body to normal function, balance the body's energies, and either energize or relax the body as necessary for improved health. Although specific marma points and gentle balancing methods are described in this text, it should be understood that this is a brief introduction to a complex system of healing. In fact, many traditional ayurveda physicians warn against the practice of marma therapy by anyone without specific training. This draws attention to the need for sensitivity and respect by the therapist when working with these dynamic points.

Marma points are located on the body by taking finger measurements from identifiable starting points. An individual's marma points are specific to his or her body. For this reason, the client's fingers are traditionally used to do the measuring. Marma points can be quite large (as much as 6 inches across), so in a modified treatment, it is best for the therapist to approximate and palpate for the point while allowing the client to relax.

These points are primarily massaged with the thumb (sometimes the fingertips, knuckles, fist, palm of the hand, or heel of the foot are used) after a drop of warm oil or a specific taila (medicated oil) has been applied to the point. Most often, the point is massaged in clockwise circles to strengthen and tone the tissue, but sometimes counterclockwise motions are used.[6] Direct pressure for 1 to 3 minutes can be used to stimulate a point.[3] Often, the therapist will begin at the center of the point and make ever larger circles until the entire point has been massaged for 3 to 5 minutes.[7] The pressure should be firm but not hard. If the client experiences any discomfort, the pressure on the point is too deep. Table 11-6 provides an overview of some marma points, and Figure 11-4 shows the general position of the points. In Table 11-6, specific essential oils are given for each point, but the therapist chooses the essential oil for each point based on the dosha and condition of the client and on the treatment goals. It should also be noted that many of the oils indicated by ayurvedic therapists are quite strong (e.g., cinnamon and basil) and should only be used in a diluted form (6 drops to 1 fl oz of carrier oil is recommended).

Abhyanga often uses medicated oils called tail or **taila** (*tila* means sesame oil). To make taila, a base oil such as sesame or coconut oil is cooked with herbs to infuse the oil with the properties of the plant. The herbs used in taila tend to be tonic or nervine, and the oil is often (but not always) named after the main herb in its recipe. For example, whereas masha taila is composed of masha (*Phaseolus* spp., a type of bean) and sesame oil, jyotishmati taila is composed of jyotishmati (*Celastrus paniculata*, or celastrus or oriental bittersweet) and apamarga (*Achyranthes aspera*, or prickly chaff flower). Sometimes a full-body massage is performed with taila and sometimes specific marma points are massaged with a particular taila to treat a symptom or condition. In one example, the respiratory system might be supported by massaging the two amsaphalaka marma points (one on each of the upper medical borders of the scapula) with strong clockwise circles using mahanarayan taila (mahanarayan taila is a combination of 14 herbs and sesame oil that is used for muscle pain, joint pain, and to support the respiratory system). Taila ingredients for the different doshas are outlined in each dosha profile overview, but it is easiest to purchase taila from specialist ayurveda stores, some of which are listed in the resources section at the back of the book.

Essential oils can also be used to make dosha-pacifying blends or to anoint a specific marma point. Heating oils are indicated for pacifying vata and kapha. These are commonly spicy oils such as ginger, nutmeg, pepper, thyme, and cinnamon. Sweet oils, such as the floral oils of rose, ylang ylang, jasmine, and neroli, or cooling oils, such as German chamomile, and yarrow, pacify pitta but aggravate kapha.

Root oils, which are energetically grounding, are good for vatas. These oils include ginger and angelica. Many oils are neutral and balancing for all of the doshas. This group includes lavender, clary sage, and frankincense. Each dosha profile overview provides a starter list of essential oils and blends for that particular dosha.

It should be noted that if the season or conditions of the day are decidedly of one dosha, any individual, regardless of his or her dominant dosha or dosha imbalance, might be given a massage with an oil blend that pacifies the qualities of the day. For example, if the day is cold, dry, and windy, a vata-pacifying blend and warm packs might be used on all individuals. This is because even the pitta will be cold on such a day and need vata qualities pacified to feel in balance.

THE ABHYANGA PROCEDURE

As mentioned previously, abhyanga can be performed by one, two, or more therapists. In the routine described here, two therapists work together in synchrony with a specific series of strokes. Therapists are encouraged to use this routine as a starting point and add or delete strokes as they deem appropriate. The process of developing a synchronized routine often leads both therapists to innovative ways to stretch or move the body.

The therapists must decide who will be the leader and who will be the follower. The leader sets the pace of the massage strokes and never leaves the client's body; the leader always maintains contact with the client in some way. The follower gets everything that is needed for the treatment (e.g., extra oil, hot herbal towels, eye pillow) and follows the leader's pace. The Abhyanga Snapshot and Figure 11-5 give therapists an overview of the treatment.

Snapshot: Abhyanga

Indications
To facilitate detoxification, balance or pacify a particular dosha, decrease muscle pain, decrease stress and mental exhaustion, bring balance to the body, maintain health

Contraindications
Broken or inflamed skin, high blood pressure, serious heart or circulatory conditions, illness or fever, any condition contraindicated for massage

Supplies for the Treatment Table Setup (from the bottom to the top layer)
1) Bottom massage sheet
2) Top massage sheet
3) Blanket or bath sheet for warmth
4) Two hand towels for draping
5) Bolster
6) Warm packs (optional)

(continues on page 228)

Table 11-6 Selected Marma Points

POINT NUMBER	NAME	MEANING	LOCATION	FUNCTION OR ASSOCIATION	ESSENTIAL OILS
1	Adhipati	Overlord	Top of the head	Seventh chakra, pineal gland, Prana (life-force), Self realization	Frankincense, myrrh
2	Simanta	Summit	Fissures of the skull (five)	Seventh chakra, nervous system, Prana	Frankincense, myrrh, camphor, mint oils
3	Sthapani	What gives support or fixes	Point between the eyes	Sixth chakra, Prana, the pituitary gland, inner vision	Sandalwood, camphor, basil, mint oils, lavender
4	Avarta	Calamity	Midpoint above the eyes (two)	Vata, Prana, sight, body posture	Camphor, mint oils, eucalyptus
5	Utkshepa	What is upwards	Above the ear (two)	Vata, the mind, large intestine, sense of smell, increasing awareness	Sandalwood, basil, spikenard, valerian
6	Shankha	A conch shell	Temple (two)	Vata, large intestine, sense of touch, clear hearing	Lavender, peppermint, eucalyptus, ginger
7	Apanga	Looking away	Outer corner of the eye (two)	Sense of sight, clarity of thought	Sandalwood, vetiver, rose
8	Shringataka	Where four roads meet	Soft palate of the mouth (four)	Vitality, taste, sight, hearing, smell, nourishment to Prana and the mind	Myrrh, frankincense, mint
9	Phana	A serpent's hood	Side of the nostrils (two)	Prana, sense of smell, balance of energy between the left and right side of the body	Camphor, eucalyptus, peppermint
10	Krikatika	Joint of the neck	Inferior to the external occipital protuberance on either side of the neck (two)	Body posture, subconscious mind, lubrication and contentment of the brain	Atlas cedarwood, mint, ginger, eucalyptus
11	Vidhura	Distress	Behind and below the ears (two)	Controls hearing, increases awareness of inner sounds	Sandalwood
12	Sira Matrika	Mother of the blood vessels	Base of the neck (eight): Four on each side of the neck on either side of the trachea	Blood flow to the head, nervous system	Angelica, spikenard, valerian, cypress, sandalwood, cajeput, rosemary, myrrh
13	Manya	Honor	Anterior neck inferior to the ear (two)	Speaking honorably, plasma, blood, circulatory system, throat, sense of taste, tongue	Cardamom, rosemary, tea tree, juniper, geranium, lavender
14	Nila	Dark blue	The main points are lateral to the trachea on both sides (two)	Upward-moving Prana, speech, thyroid, heat absorption, improvement of voice and power of speech	Sandalwood, chamomile, coriander, rose, peppermint
15	Amsa	Shoulder	Shoulder on the trapezius (two)	Fifth chakra, heat absorption, upward movement of Prana, brain, dream state	Jasmine, sandalwood, chamomile, mint, sage

Table 11-6 *(continued)*

POINT NUMBER	NAME	MEANING	LOCATION	FUNCTION OR ASSOCIATION	ESSENTIAL OILS
16	Amsaphalaka	Shoulder blade	Shoulder blade (two)	Respiratory system, joint lubrication, energy circulation, fourth chakra	Eucalyptus, mint, camphor
17	Brihati	Wide	Area of the upper back (two)	Courage, valor, heat absorption, third chakra, lymphatic system	Cardamom, camphor, eucalyptus
18	Parshvasandhi	The side of the waist	The lateral aspect of the lumbosacral joint (two)	Second chakra, adrenal glands, ovaries, reproductive system, immune system	Nutmeg
19	Nitamba	Buttocks	The upper gluteal region (two)	Plasma, lymphatic system, skeletal system, urinary system, kidneys, kapha	Cardamom, camphor, lemongrass, juniper, cypress, orange
20	Kukundara	What marks the loins	Top of the sacrum (two)	Blood formation, circulation, menstruation, second chakra, water element	Rosemary, turmeric, myrrh, angelica, cypress, juniper, birch
21	Katikataruna	What rises from the hip	Hip (two)	Bones, lubrication of the joints, skeletal system	Myrrh, camphor, wintergreen, eucalyptus, sage
22	Apalapa	Unguarded	Axilla (two)	Nervous system, nerve flow to the arms	Valerian, spikenard, basil
23	Stanarohita	Upper region of the breast	Above and to the center of the nipples (two)	Muscular system, nervous system, lungs, Prana	Sage, valerian, myrrh, juniper, sandalwood, eucalyptus, camphor
24	Hridaya	Heart	Heart	Circulatory system, blood, plasma, power of the mind, vitality, strength, immunity, fourth chakra, higher self, consciousness	Sandalwood, jasmine, rose, eucalyptus, ginger
25	Apastambha	What stands to the side	Upper area of the abdomen, lateral to the sternum (two)	Kapha digestion, bone, fat	Myrrh, ginger, cinnamon, eucalyptus
26	Nabhi	Navel	The navel	Third chakra, digestion, balancing energy, pitta dosha, element of fire in the body, power of action	Digestive oils, jasmine, rose, sandalwood
27	Basti	Bladder	Lower abdominal area	Muscular system, body fat, urinary system, reproductive system, second chakra	Nutmeg, valerian, sandalwood, clove, camphor
28	Guda	Anus	Anus	First chakra, reproductive system, excretion, earth element	
29	Kakshadhara	What upholds the flank	Top of the shoulder (two)	Muscular system, body posture	Eucalyptus, turmeric, myrrh
30	Lohitaksha (arm)	Red-jointed	Center of the deltopectoral triangle (two)	Lymphatic system, peripheral circulation to the legs	Eucalyptus, mint, cardamom, rose, myrrh

Table 11-6 *(continued)*

POINT NUMBER	NAME	MEANING	LOCATION	FUNCTION OR ASSOCIATION	ESSENTIAL OILS
31	Bahvi	Relates to arm	Inside of upper arm (two)	Plasma, healthy tissue growth, lymphatic system, circulation	Camphor, cardamom, mint, thyme, ginger
32	Ani (arm)	Point of a needle	Lower area of upper arm (two)	Pancreas, kidneys	Ginger, cardamom, parsley, juniper
33	Kurpara	Elbow joint	Medial and lateral side of the elbow (two)	Blood, circulation, balancing Prana, right elbow controls liver, associated with liver diseases, left elbow controls spleen, pancreas	Coriander, myrrh, turmeric (right elbow), ginger, cardamom, myrrh or turmeric (left elbow)
34	Indrabasti (arm)	Indra's arrow	Center of the forearm (two)	Digestive system, balancing Prana, small intestine	Anise, fennel, ginger, cardamom
35	Manibandha	Bracelet	Wrist (two)	Skeletal system, movement of the hands, lubrication of the joints, peripheral circulation, expression of the self in the world	Angelica, birch, myrrh, wintergreen, vetiver, spikenard, valerian
36	Kurchashira (hand)	The head of kurcha	Base of the thumb joint (two)	Digestive system, stomach, head, mind, nervous system, fire	Digestive oils, myrrh, camphor, sandalwood, valerian, spikenard
37	Kshipra (hand)	Quick to give results	Between the thumb and index finger (two)	Plasma, respiratory system, heart, lungs, Prana, passion, connection to will	Eucalyptus, sage, fennel, sandalwood, cardamom
38	Kurcha (hand)	A knot or bundle	Bottom of the thumb (two)	Seeing, sensory keenness, Prana, vata, nerve energy	Sandalwood, rose, chamomile, camphor, mint, clove
39	Talahridaya (hand)	Center of the surface	Center of the palm of the hand (two)	Energy flow, health, balance, respiratory system, heart, lungs, circulation, calling healing energy, releasing negative energy	Cardamom, rose, orange, ginger, eucalyptus, camphor
40	Lohitaksha (leg)	Red-jointed	In alignment with the inguinal ligament (two)	Lymphatic system, downward movement of energy	Camphor, eucalyptus, rose, myrrh, sage
41	Urvi	What is wide	The midregion of the upper thigh (two)	Plasma, water element, kapha	Atlas cedarwood, juniper, parsley, cardamom
42	Ani (leg)	Point of a needle	Lower area of upper leg (two)	Circulation of body fluids downward, balance	Yarrow, rose, sandalwood, Atlas cedarwood, ginger
43	Janu	Knee joint	Knee (two)	Lubrication of the joints, circulation to the legs, liver (right knee), spleen and pancreas (left knee)	Lime, myrrh, coriander (right knee), ginger, lemon, cardamom, turmeric (left knee)
44	Indrabasti (leg)	Indra's arrow	Center of the lower leg (two)	Digestive system, digestive fire, small intestine	Lavender, fennel, ginger, black pepper

Table 11-6 *(continued)*

POINT NUMBER	NAME	MEANING	LOCATION	FUNCTION OR ASSOCIATION	ESSENTIAL OILS
45	Gulpha	Ankle joint	Ankle joint (two)	Bone, fat, reproductive system, circulation of Prana, lubrication of the joints	Clary sage, vetiver, jasmine, rose
46	Kurchashira (foot)	The head of kurcha	Base of the big toe (two)	Muscular system, posture, digestion	Myrrh, camphor, ginger
47	Kurcha (foot)	A knot or bundle	Bottom of the big toe (two)	Seeing, sensory keenness, mental clearness	Sandalwood, rose, chamomile
48	Talahridaya (foot)	Center of the surface	Center of the sole of the foot (two)	Respiratory system, power of circulation, earth element, heart	Sandalwood, rose, cardamom, rosemary, ginger
49	Kshipra (foot)	Quick to give results	Between the big toe and the second toe (two)	Lymphatic system, respiratory system, heart, lungs, flow of Prana	Camphor, cardamom, eucalyptus

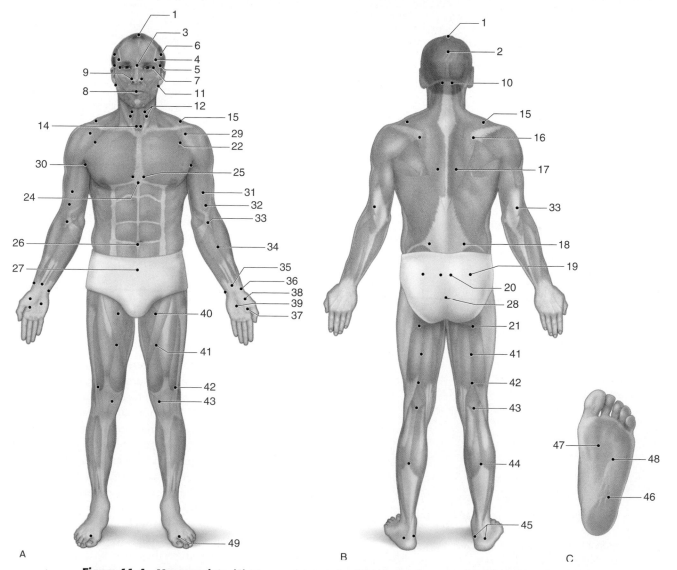

Figure 11-4   Marma points. (A) Marma points: anterior. **(B)** Marma points: posterior. **(C)** Marma points: foot.

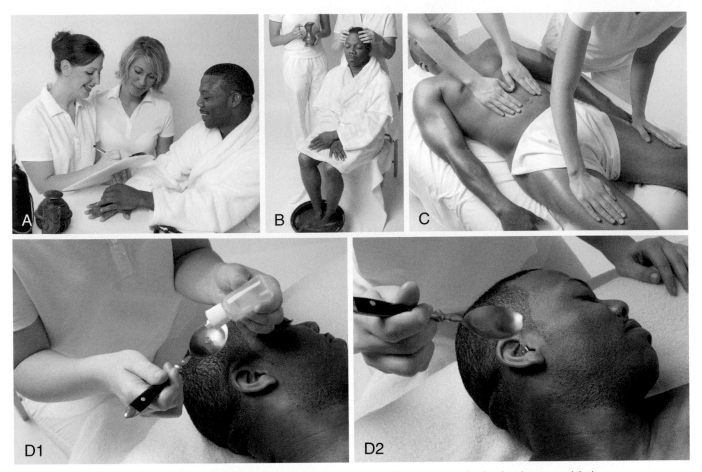

Figure 11-5   The Abhyanga treatment. (A) Dosha questionnaire. **(B)** Foot soak and Indian head massage. **(C)** Abhyanga tandem massage. **(D1** and **D2)** Session end: oil the ears.

Supplies for the Work Table Setup
1) Dosha questionnaire
2) Two bottles (one for each therapist) of a massage oil or taila appropriate for the dosha
3) Spoon (used for oiling the ears)
4) Dry hand towel
5) Aura mist

Supplies for the Foot Soak Setup
1) Foot soak container (copper is traditional; jasmine or other flowers floating on the surface are a nice touch)
2) Comfortable chair
3) Bath towel placed under the foot soak container
4) Pitcher of extra warm water
5) Exfoliation product for the feet
6) Robe or spa wrap
7) Dry hand towel
8) Slippers

Procedure
1) Client fills out dosha questionnaire.
2) Foot soak and Indian head massage are done.
3) The client is moved to the treatment table.
4) Posterior massage based on dosha.
5) Client turned to supine position.

6) Vata only: Application of heavy oil to the abdominal region. Cover this with a warm towel and a warm pack.
7) Anterior massage based on dosha.
8) Oil the ears.
9) Aura mist.

Session Start

The client is taken to the treatment room to change into a robe (or spa wrap) and slippers and fill out a dosha questionnaire. Juice, traditional fruits or food, or Indian tea can be served while the questionnaire is completed. This introduces the nourishing element of ayurveda. The therapists return to the treatment room after a suitable length of time (15 to 20 minutes) and reviews the questionnaire. The leader may ask the client additional questions as needed to help determine the client's dominant dosha and dosha imbalances. After this initial discussion has been completed, the leader gives directions to the follower to prepare the appropriate foot soak. While the foot soak is prepared, the leader describes the basic principles of ayurveda and some of the factors that might aggravate the client's particular dosha or dosha imbalance. Some spas or therapists hand out informative brochures that give directions for following home-based routines to support balance in the doshas.

Step 1: Foot Soak and Indian Head Massage

The treatment begins with a traditional foot soak and Indian head massage. The foot soak is the spiritual element of welcoming and purifying the client. Herbal blends for appropriate dosha foot soaks are listed in the dosha profile overviews. The leader steps behind the client and massages the shoulders and head with warm oil using the Indian head massage techniques described below at his or her discretion. The follower periodically fills the foot soak container with more warm water and washes, exfoliates, and massages the client's feet while they soak.

Indian head massage is an art form that is deeply relaxing and rejuvenating. In a typical session, the head, neck, and shoulders are massaged; marma points are stimulated; and the scalp and hair are oiled and invigorated. The following techniques provide an introduction to Indian head massage. Figure 11-6 shows the techniques used in this Indian head massage.

Oiling the Simanta and Krikatika Marmas. The
Simanta (summit) marma falls along the lines of the sutures of the skull, so it covers a large area.[7] The first point to oil in this area is found by measuring 8 finger widths up the head using the point between the eyebrows as a starting point. A generous amount of oil is poured on this spot and then the hairs are lifted and twisted to stimulate the point.[4] The second point to oil is found at the point where the client's hair forms a whorl. After the point is oiled, the hairs over this point are lifted and twisted to stimulate the marma. Between these two points is the Adhipati (overlord), which is located at the top point of the skull. This marma has a ruling action over the Simanta marma and controls the seventh charka, pineal gland, and nervous system. Oil and stimulate this point with hair twisting. To oil the Krikatika (joint of the neck) marmas, the client is asked to bring the head forward so that the chin sits on the chest. The points are directly beneath the occipital protuberance on each side of the neck. Oil and stimulate these points with hair twisting. Using zigzag finger movements, work the oil evenly through the hair and into the scalp. Go back to each of the points that were oiled and use gentle circular finger friction in clockwise circles to release the energy and tension in these areas.

Pounding. Place both hands together in a prayer position. While keeping the wrists loose and flexible, the edge of the joined hands is used in a tapotement-like action over the entire head.

Circular Finger Friction. Reaching up under the client's hair, the entire scalp is massaged with gentle circular finger friction. The forehead, above and behind the ears, and the base of the skull are also massaged in this manner. The point between the eyebrows, down the sides of the nose, under the eyes, under the cheekbones, and then down around the edges of the mouth and across the lower part of the cheek are massaged with circular fingers.

Skull Squeeze. Interlace the fingers over the top of the skull and press the hands together gently. Repeat this four to six times, working over the anterior and posterior sections of the skull. Place one hand on the forehead and the other at the back of the head and repeat the skull squeeze.

Massaging Specific Marma Points on the Face. There
are two marma points called Phana (a serpent's hood) on the side of each nostril. These points can be massaged with strong circular strokes to decrease headache pain, decrease sinus pressure, and decrease congestion. Usually, the whole side of the nasal bone is treated. The Apanga marma points are located on the outer corner of the eye and are massaged to relieve headaches caused by eye strain. These points also help to clear the upper sinuses. Shankha (conch) is the name of the point located on each temple. These points aid sleep and are associated with directing energy to the brain. The points named Utkshepa (what is cast upward) reside above the ear and are gently massaged to calm vata and the mind. Just above the center of each eyebrow is a point called Avarta, which is massaged to decrease vata and improve energy and adaptability. The Sthapani marma resides between the eyebrows and is often called the "third eye." This point is discussed further in the shirodhara section below.

Ear Massage. Rub oil into the external regions of the ear, pulling the ear backward as the oil is applied. Pull the earlobe in a downward and backward direction and then pull the earlobe across the opening of the ear to stretch it.

After the head massage, the therapist can massage the shoulders and upper arms of the client by pulling the robe off the shoulders (but leaving it to cover the rest of the body). If the client is wearing a spa wrap, the shoulders will already be exposed. When the massage of the head and shoulders is complete, the client's feet are removed from the foot soak and dried by the follower. The client is moved to the treatment table, and both therapists briefly leave the room or turn away while the client gets onto the table in the prone position.

Step 2: Massage

The speed of the strokes, the depth of the strokes, and the use of additional features such as a warm pack are all determined by the dosha or dosha imbalance of the client. Review the dominant dosha profiles for details. This routine is shown in Figure 11-7. Regardless of the series of strokes that are used, the two therapists must practice together to become proficient and achieve harmony.

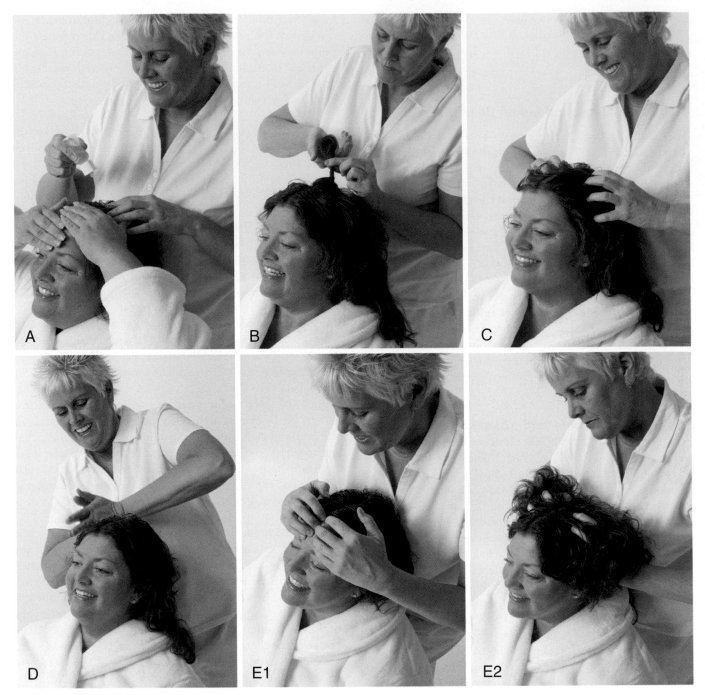

Figure 11-6   Indian head massage techniques. (A) Oiling the Simanta and Krikatika marmas. **(B)** Twisting and pulling the hair over marmas. **(C)** Using zigzag finger movements to work oil evenly through the hair and into the scalp. **(D)** "Pounding." **(E1** and **E2)** Circular finger friction.

Ground and Center.   The leader then adjusts the drape (use a gluteal drape) to allow access to the back and the posterior legs at the same time. The leader moves to one side of the table while the follower moves to the other side of the table. The therapists match their breathing to the client's breathing; they cross their hands and place one hand on a hip and one hand on a shoulder.

Application of Oil to the Posterior Body.   The leader applies oil from the lower back, up the back, down the arm

to the hand, back up the arm, and down the back to the hip on one side. At the same time, the follower applies oil from the hip, down the leg to the foot, and back up the leg to the hip on the same side. They repeat this process on the second side.

Spreading the Oil in Tandem.   The leader works the oil across the upper body while the follower works oil across the legs until it is even. The leader spreads the oil from the lower back, up the back, and down to the hands. At the same

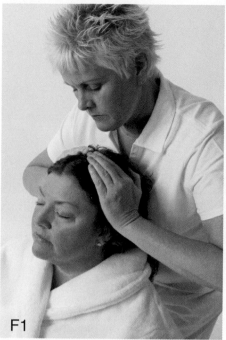

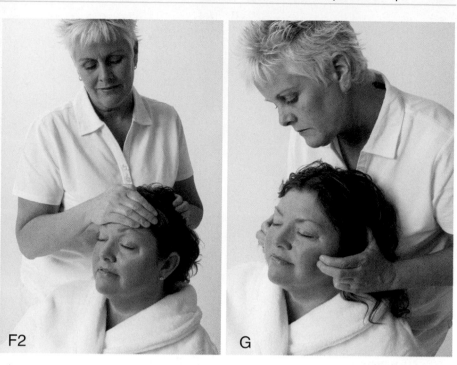

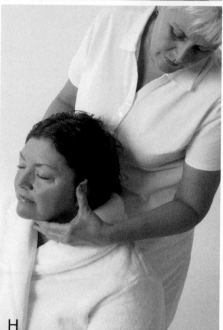

Figure 11-6 *(continued)* **(F1** and **F2)** Skull squeeze. **(G)** Massage marma points on the face. **(H)** Ear massage.

time and with the same rhythm, the follower spreads the oil from the hips to the feet. The leader's hand should be on the lower back (at the beginning of the stroke) at the same time that the follower's hands are at the hips (the beginning of the stroke).

Posterior Leg Massage. The leader joins the follower at the hips for the posterior leg massage. Each of the five traditional strokes (sweeps, tapping, kneading, rubbing, squeezing, end with a second set of sweeps) is performed on each leg simultaneously covering the entire area. The therapists watch each other carefully so that the strokes are

occurring in the same area at the same time. Each stroke begins at the greater trochanter and moves toward the feet. (The energy is "pushed" out from the core of the body, the navel, and toward the extremities; in this case, the feet.) Begin the sequence with 20 to 25 straight sweeps and hold the foot at the end of the last stroke. Progress from straight sweeps to the tapping technique, followed by kneading, rubbing, and finally squeezing. Marma points can be incorporated into the routine at the discretion of the leader or treatment designer. End the posterior leg sequence in the same way it began, with 20 to 25 straight sweeps, and hold at the foot on the last stroke.

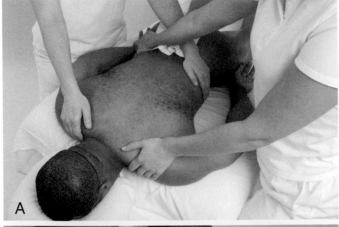

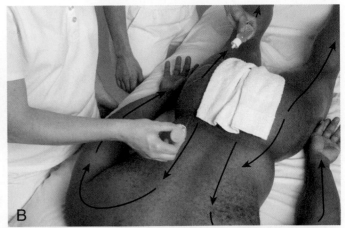

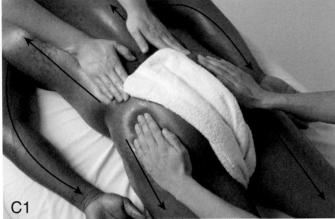

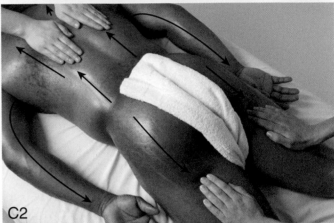

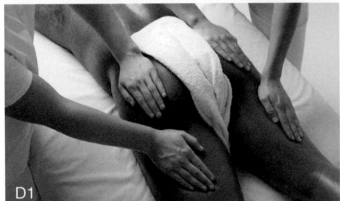

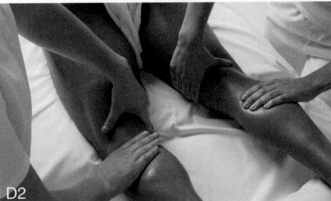

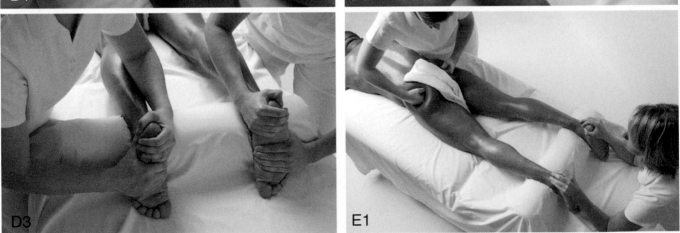

Figure 11-7 Abhyanga synchronized massage routine. (A) Ground and center. **(B)** Application of oil to the posterior body. **(C1** and **C2)** Spreading the oil in tandem. **(D1** and **D2)** Posterior leg massage. **(D3)** Hold the energy at the foot on the conclusion of the last straight sweep. **(E1** and **E2)** Gluteal massage.

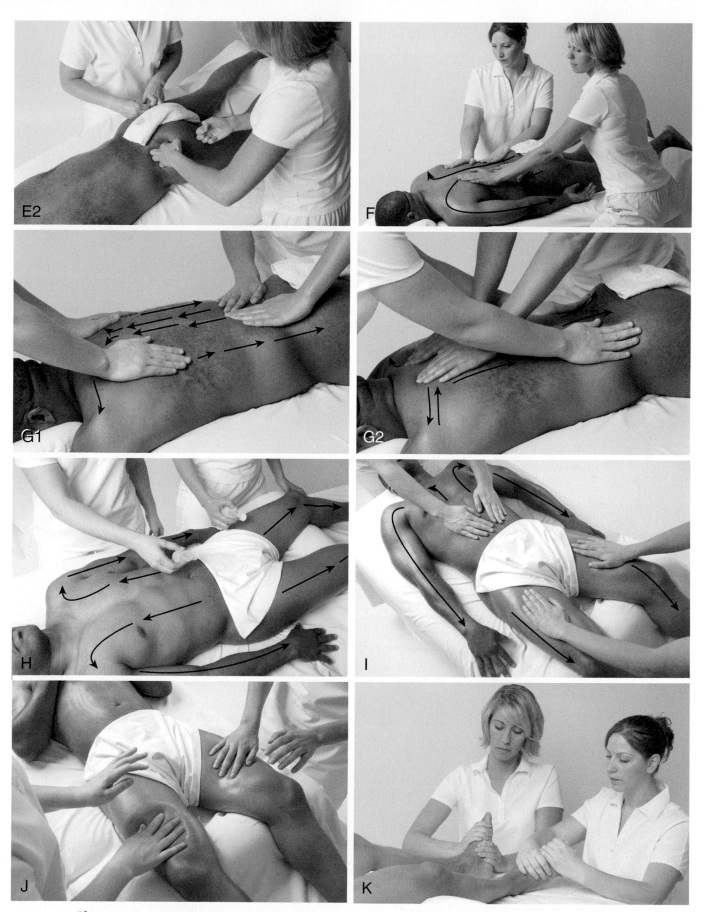

Figure 11-7 *(continued)* **(F)** Back massage. **(G1** and **G2)** Creative back massage strokes. **(H)** Application of oil to the anterior body. **(I)** Spreading the oil in tandem. **(J)** Anterior leg massage. This picture shows the tapping technique. **(K)** Foot massage.

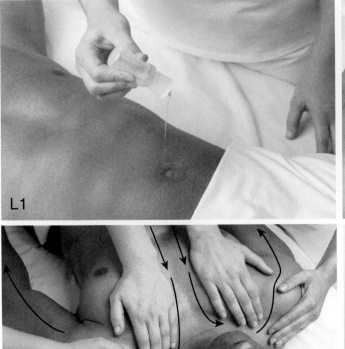

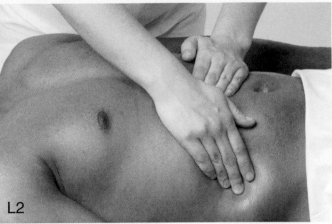

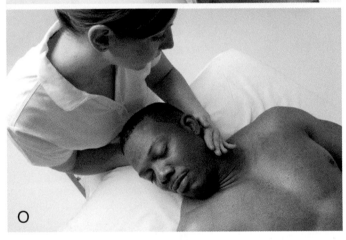

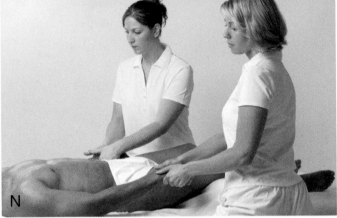

Figure 11-7 *(continued)* **(L1** and **L2)** Abdominal massage. **(M)** Upper body massage. **(N)** Arms. **(O)** Neck and face massage.

Gluteal Massage. After completing the legs, the follower holds both feet to ground the client's energy while the leader massages the gluteals. Eventually, the follower joins in on one side of the gluteal massage to make a smooth transition onto the back.

Back Massage. The therapists stand on either side of the table at the hips facing toward the head of the client. They apply the five traditional strokes simultaneously starting at the lower back, running up the back to the shoulder, and down the arm to the hand. They begin with 20 to 25 straight sweeps and hold at the hand on the last stroke. Progress from the straight sweeps to the tapping technique, followed by kneading, rubbing, and finally squeezing. Marma points can be incorporated into the routine at the discretion of the leader or treatment designer. End with another 20 straight sweeps and hold at the hand on the last stroke to end the back sequence.

As part of the back routine, the therapists can develop a number of creative tandem strokes. One idea is for each therapist to do a deep tissue stroke starting at the top of the spine and running down to the sacrum on either side of the spine.

Another enjoyable stroke is to do effleurage strokes in a rhythmic and crossing sequence as shown in Figure 11-7G.

Application of Oil to the Anterior Body. The leader turns the client into the supine position, bolsters him or her for comfort, and drapes the client with a breast drape and an anterior pelvic drape. The follower moves to the client's feet. The leader turns the client's head to one side and applies oil down the neck and across the shoulder. At the same time, the follower applies oil from the hip to the foot and up the leg to end at the hip. They repeat this procedure on the opposite side.

Spreading the Oil in Tandem. The leader spreads the oil in an even layer on the upper chest, neck, and down the arms. At the same time, the follower spreads the oil in an even layer on the lower legs.

Anterior Leg Massage. The leader moves to stand at one hip facing toward the feet, and the follower stands at the other hip facing the feet. Again, the energy is pushed out from the navel toward the feet with the five strokes performed simultaneously (sweeps, tapping, kneading, rubbing, squeezing). End with 20 to 25 straight sweeps and a hold at the feet.

Foot Massage. The leader takes one foot and the follower takes the other foot and massages them together with the same series of strokes. Foot massage strokes are described in Chapter 8. The other option is to have the leader move to the top of the table and place the hands on the client's shoulders while the follower massages the feet. At the end of the foot massage, the follower grasps both feet and holds them with their thumb on the Talahridaya (heart or center of the foot) marma. Interestingly, this is called the solar plexus point in reflexology. It is believed to pacify vata and ground and center the body.[7]

Abdominal Massage. The leader moves to the abdominal area and fills the navel with oil. The oil is worked into the abdominal area by the leader while the follower continues to press the feet and stabilize the client's energy.

Upper Body Massage. The follower moves with the leader to the upper body when the abdominal massage is complete. The two therapists stand on either side of the client and apply oil from the chest and down each arm simultaneously. The oil is spread in an even layer working from the abdominal areas up to the upper chest and down the arms to the hands with straight, sweeping strokes (20 to 25 times). If the client is a woman, the therapists "jump" the breast drape when it gets in the way of their stroke.

Massage the Arms. Each of the traditional strokes (sweeps, tapping, kneading, rubbing, squeezing) is carried out on each arm simultaneously starting at the glenohumeral joint and working down to the hand. End with straight sweeps (20 to 25 times) and a hold at the hand on the last stroke.

Neck and Face Massage. The leader moves to the head of the table and massages the neck and face, while the follower moves to the bottom of the table to ground the client's energy through the Talahridaya marma on the bottoms of the feet.

Session End

Abhyanga can be ended in a number of different ways. For example, hot, moist hand towels can be steeped in an herbal infusion and laid across the anterior body. The body is then wrapped in thermal blankets and allowed to relax or nap for a period of time after the session. Sometimes the body is simply covered with a drape and shirodhara takes place. The client can also be covered with a steam canopy or moved to a steam cabinet or steam room for the swedana treatment.

A nice way to end the treatment is to pour oil from a spoon into the ears (Figure 11-5D). Oiling the ears is called karna purana. It is practiced to relive itching or dryness in the ears, to settle the vata dosha through the sense of hearing, and to relax the mind and body. In Karna purana, a towel is placed under the client's head, and the head is then rotated to one side so that the ear can be filled with a spoonful of warm sesame oil. The area around the ear is gently massaged, and the client is encouraged to open and close the mouth two to three times. In most states, it is out of the scope of practice for massage therapists to massage inside the ears of a client, so only the outer area of the ear is massaged. The head is rotated to the other side and the procedure is repeated on the second ear. The oil in the first ear will run out onto the towel under the client's head. Massage around the second ear and ask the client to repeat the process of opening and closing the mouth. Turn the head and allow the oil to run out of the second ear. The client can then dry the ears out with a tissue.

🧴 Sanitation

The comb used to detangle the client's hair before the Indian head massage should be soaked in barbicide solution in a jar with a lid. Barbicide solutions are available from spa suppliers.

Shirodhara

Shirodhara (*shiro* means head, and *dhara* means threadlike stream) is the application of a thin stream of sesame oil on the forehead or in a pendulum-like motion that pauses for a moment each time it reaches the point between the eyebrows, sometimes called the third eye. The marma point between the eyebrows is known as Sthapani, or "what gives support or holds firm." This point is associated with the sixth chakra, Prana (primary life force), the mind, senses, and pituitary gland.[7] The purpose of the treatment is to center the mind and body, to increase relaxation and inner peace, and to settle vata disorders such as anxiety and insomnia.

In the shirodhara treatment, refined sesame seed oil is traditionally used in the shirodhara vessel, but herbal milk, seawater, buttermilk, coconut milk, medicated oils, and other products can also be used. The treatment lasts between 20 and 30 minutes and is often combined with abhyanga. The Shirodhara Snapshot and Figure 11-8 provide an overview of this service.

Snapshot: Shirodhara

Indications
Aggravated vata; insomnia; to decrease stress and mental exhaustion; to balance the body, mind, and spirit

Contraindications
Broken or inflamed skin on the forehead, low blood pressure, illness or fever, pregnancy

Supplies for the Treatment Table Setup (from the bottom to the top layer)
1) Bottom massage sheet
2) Plastic body wrap placed so that it covers the top quarter of the treatment table, falls over the top of the table, and has its ends tucked into a bowl. Place a number of Kleenex tissues in the bowl to dampen the sound of the oil hitting the plastic.
3) Bath towel set over the top of the plastic
4) Top massage sheet
5) Blanket for warmth
6) Warm packs as needed
7) Bolster
8) Rolled hand towel for positioning the head
9) Shirodhara stand and vessel
The setup for the shirodhara table is shown in Figure 11-9.

Supplies for the Work Table Setup
1) 1 quart (or more) of refined sesame oil (or other product as deemed appropriate for the individual dosha). The oil should be warmed to 100° to 104°F.
2) Thermometer
3) Rose petals soaked in full-fat warm milk or an eye pillow (optional)
4) Small cup to capture the first part of the flow of oil out of the shirodhara vessel

Procedure
1) Position the client's head for shirodhara.
2) Place a warm pack on the abdominal area.
3) Ground and center with the client and take three slow breaths.
4) Prepare the forehead by rubbing it gently with oil.
5) Open the tap of the shirodhara vessel first into a small cup and then allow it to run onto the forehead.
6) Check the stream's position or move the stream in a pendulum motion across the forehead.
7) Stop the stream of oil and gently massage the neck, shoulders, and scalp.
8) Allow the client to rest without being disturbed for a time determined by the therapist.

SESSION START

The client begins the treatment in the supine position with the head at the very top of the treatment table. He or she is bolstered as for a massage and is covered by a warm blanket. A warm pack can be placed on the belly and under the feet if appropriate. The therapist begins the treatment by gently

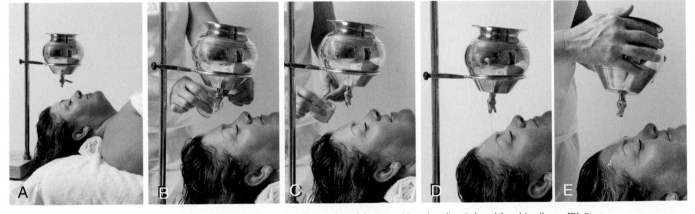

Figure 11-8   Shirodhara. (A) After massaging the neck and face, position the client's head for shirodhara. **(B)** Start the flow of oil into a small cup and adjust the stream of oil to the proper consistency. **(C)** Move the cup away so that the oil begins to flow onto the client's head. **(D)** While the oil streams onto the client's head, the therapist must be as quiet as possible. This should be a time for reflection and introspection without undue distraction. **(E)** Option: some therapists choose to hold the shirodhara vessel so that they can play it over the client's forehead freely. Some shirodhara sets are attached above the treatment table and can swing from side to side.

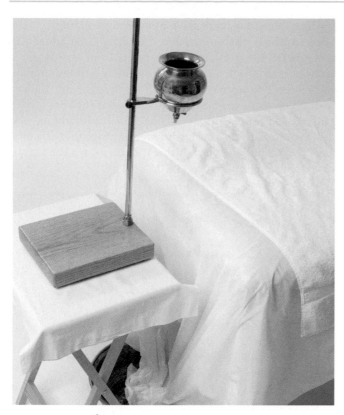

Figure 11-9   Shirodhara setup.

massaging the neck and face to relax and prepare the client for the treatment. The client will probably not move the head for the next 20 to 30 minutes, so this initial massage is important. At the end of the neck massage, the therapist positions the shirodhara equipment and takes three long, slow grounding breaths with the client.

STEP 1: POSITION THE CLIENT'S HEAD FOR SHIRODHARA

A small pillow or rolled towel is placed under the client's head in such a way that the head tips back slightly. It is not necessary for the client's head to be tipped at an extreme angle.

Rose petals soaked in full-fat milk and placed over the eyelids during the treatment feel relaxing and elegant. To prepare the rose petals, place them in a bowl of either warm or cool milk. Warm milk releases more of the rose fragrance and feels calming. Cool milk feels refreshing and leaves the tissue around the eyes looking smooth and soft.

The rose petals are crushed gently between the therapist's fingers and then placed over the client's eyes. Crushing the rose petals releases the fragrance and ensures that excess milk will not drip down the client's face during the treatment. An eye pillow can be used instead of rose petals, or the client's eyes can be left uncovered if desired by the therapist.

The warm oil is taken from the hot water bath and the temperature is tested with the thermometer. It is then poured into the vessel that is positioned over the client's head and adjusted to the appropriate height. Some therapists use a small cup to recycle oil that has run off the client's head into the bowl at the bottom of the table. The oil is poured back into the vessel to prolong the treatment.

STEP 2: SHIRODHARA

A drop of warm oil is placed on the therapist's index finger. The therapist circles this finger around the client's forehead in a clockwise direction where the oil will be drizzled. By performing these initial circles, the therapist prepares the client for the stream of oil and awakens the client's nervous system.

The therapist holds a small cup under the vessel and opens the tap so that the oil begins to flow into the cup. The stream is adjusted as it runs into the cup to a thin drizzle. After it is adjusted, the therapist warns the client so that he or she is not startled and then removes the cup so that the oil begins to flow onto the client's head.

The therapist must now check that the vessel position is correct and that the oil is hitting the target point between the eyebrows. He or she will also check that the oil flowing off the client's head runs into the bowl on the floor and not onto the floor itself. The oil should run onto Kleenex tissues in the bottom of the bowl rather than being allowed to hit the sides of the bowl, which would make noise.

The stream of oil can either be left in the same position for the entire treatment or it can be moved backward and forward in a pendulum motion across the forehead. Any movement must be steady and even, so this requires practice. As the oil starts to run out at the end of the treatment, place a cup under the stream of oil and turn off the tap on the vessel. It is important that the oil is not allowed to sputter out and drip unevenly on the client's head as it starts to run out at the end of the treatment.

An important thing to remember with shirodhara is that the less there is happening in the treatment room, the better. The client's senses will be heightened by the treatment. Any excess movement by the therapist, any chatter in the hallway, and any crinkling of plastic will all be distracting to clients while they are focusing in on their own thoughts. The darker and quieter the room can be, the better. For this reason, music is not recommended.

SESSION END

The therapist removes the rolled hand towel from underneath the client's head and the rose petals or eye pillow from their eyelids. The neck, shoulders, and scalp are massaged with very gentle strokes. The therapist can also mist over the client with an aura mist or simply allow the client to relax for 15 minutes undisturbed. It is important that shirodhara is the last service that the client receives during a day at the spa. Clients often emerge from shirodhara calm, open, sensitive, and awakened to all that is around them. If they are taken to another treatment, it is likely to overstimulate them and leave them feeling irritated and restless. The exception is a soaking tub because clients can relax quietly in the warm water and remove the oil from their hair at their leisure.

It is important to offer the client a small snack or cup of herbal tea at the end of the treatment. This helps the client return to the present time and prevents low blood sugar or shakiness. Some therapists give the client their shirodhara oil to use at home for self-oiling. This is a nice way to salvage the oil and encourages the client to bring ayurveda more fully into his or her life.

Sanitation

The traditional shirodhara vessel and bowl are copper and require careful cleaning to keep them looking attractive. Clean out the inside of the vessel with hot, soapy water; dry the vessel; and then wipe it with alcohol. Use a copper cleaner and a soft cloth on the outside of the vessel and bowl to remove fingerprints and oil.

Udvartana

Udvartana (sometimes spelled *ubvartan* or *urdvatana*) is a treatment in which herbal powders or pastes are rubbed into the body to stimulate circulation and cell renewal, smooth the skin, tone the body's tissues, support detoxification, and relax the body. Originally, udvartana was a beauty treatment that was (and still is in some treatment centers) used with a specific diet, herbal teas, incense, showers, baths, and relaxing music in a 40-day course to return the body to a state of radiant health.[4]

Ubtan is a paste made from nuts, seeds, and unprocessed flour to which oils, spices, and milk have been added. An easy spa-friendly ubtan recipe is offered in the Udvartana Snapshot, although a variety of combinations and ingredients exists. The paste is massaged into the skin and allowed to dry slightly. As the paste starts to dry, it is rubbed off with mitts, rolled towels, or bare hands. Sometimes ubtan powder (without liquids) is used during abhyanga for the kapha massage. For an overview of this treatment, see the Udvartana Snapshot and Figure 11-10.

Snapshot: Udvartana

Indications
To support detoxification, to increase circulation, to decrease stress and mental exhaustion, to smooth the skin and add a healthy glow, for relaxation or sore muscles

Contraindications
Broken or inflamed skin, high blood pressure, serious heart or circulatory conditions, illness or fever, any condition contraindicated for massage

Supplies for the Treatment Table Setup (from the bottom to the top layer)
1) Bottom massage sheet
2) Top massage sheet
3) Blanket or bath sheet for warmth
4) Bolster
5) Two hand towels to use for draping
6) Warm packs
7) Fabric drop cloth or flat massage sheet placed under the massage table

Supplies for the Work Table Setup
1) Ubtan mixed up and warming in a heating device
2) Massage oil or taila appropriate for the dosha
2) Two dry, rolled-up hand towels
3) Soda cooler
4) Hot, moist herbal infused towels
5) Aura mist

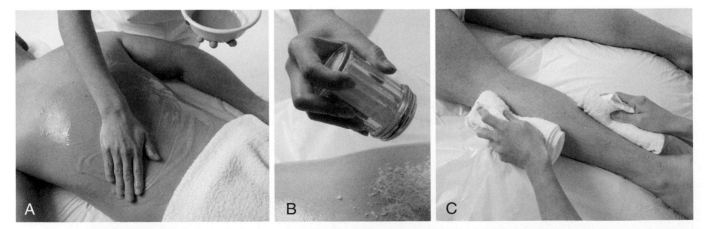
Figure 11-10   Udvartana. (A) Application of ubtan. **(B)** Option: apply dry ubtan to an oiled body from a shaker. **(C)** Buffing off ubtan.

Supplies for the Foot Soak Setup

1) Foot soak container (copper is traditional; jasmine or other flowers floating on the surface are a nice touch)
2) Comfortable chair
3) Bath towel placed under the foot soak container
4) Pitcher of extra warm water
5) Exfoliation product for the feet
6) Robe
7) Dry hand towel
8) Slippers

Procedure

1) Foot soak and Indian head massage.
2) Move client to the treatment table.
3) Oil massage of the posterior body areas (optional based on dosha).
4) Apply ubtan to the back and posterior legs.
5) Allow the ubtan to dry slightly.
6) Buff off the ubtan.
7) Apply hot, moist herbal towels.
8) Turn the client supine.
9) Oil massage of the anterior body (optional based on dosha).
10) Apply the ubtan to the anterior body.
11) Allow the ubtan to dry slightly and buff off the ubtan
12) Apply hot, moist herbal towels and cocoon the client if desired.
13) Aura mist.

Spa-Friendly Ubtan Recipes

Base 1/2 cup of chic pea powder, 1 Tbsp of mustard seed powder (additional mustard seed powder can be added for a 'warmer' treatment), 1/2 cup of milk, 1/4 cup of sesame oil, 1 Tbsp of turmeric and one of the following

Addition 1: 13 drops sandalwood, 1 drop patchouli, 1 drop rose

Addition 2: 10 drops of sandalwood, 1 drop of vetiver, 2 drops jasmine

Addition 3: 4 drops ginger, 1 drop of rose, 5 drops myrrh, 8 drops mandarin

 Sanitation

Ubtan can get messy when it is buffed off the body. It is helpful to place a clean flat massage sheet or a fabric drop cloth (like those used for interior house painting) under the massage table. This collects any ubtan that falls off the table but does not make a plastic sound while the therapist moves around the table.

SESSION START

The treatment begins with a dosha questionnaire, foot soak, and Indian head massage as described previously under the abhyanga procedure. The client is moved to the treatment table in the prone position after this opening segment.

STEP 1: OIL MASSAGE: POSTERIOR

An oil massage can be performed right before the application of ubtan if desired by the therapist or treatment designer. This adds an additional textural layer to the treatment and makes the service more oily for vatas, but the ubtan will be slow to dry out. If a massage is to be included in the treatment, it is suggested that the ubtan is mixed up with less oil than normal.

STEP 2: APPLICATION OF UBTAN: POSTERIOR

Apply the ubtan to the posterior legs and back with vigorous massage strokes. The paste will feel sticky, so the therapist should use compression strokes or circular palm friction rather than longer strokes. The paste is worked into the skin and then left to dry slightly. While it dries, the client's arms are pulled forward off the front of the massage table so that the hands can be massaged.

STEP 3: BUFF OFF THE UBTAN: POSTERIOR

As the ubtan dries, it is buffed off the client with mitts or towels. Hand towels rolled into sausages work well. The buffing feels brisk and rough, so it is quite stimulating. If this feels too forceful for the client (often this feels too coarse for vatas), the ubtan can be removed with hot, moist towels. If the ubtan does not dry out fast enough, remove most of the ubtan with hot, moist towels and then buff the remaining ubtan with dry rolled towels.

STEP 4: APPLICATION OF HERBAL TOWELS: POSTERIOR

Apply a steamy herbal towel to each leg and to the back. Allow the towels to steam the area and then use them to remove any remaining ubtan. Alternatively, a steam canopy can be used to steam the body or this step can be eliminated entirely at the discretion of the therapist or treatment designer.

STEP 5: OIL MASSAGE: ANTERIOR

Turn the client into the supine position and bolster him or her for comfort. Drape the client with a breast drape and anterior pelvic drape. Massage the anterior body briefly with oil if this step is being used by the treatment designer or therapist.

STEP 6: APPLICATION OF UBTAN: ANTERIOR

Apply the ubtan to the anterior legs, arms, and belly. While the ubtan dries, the client's feet are massaged.

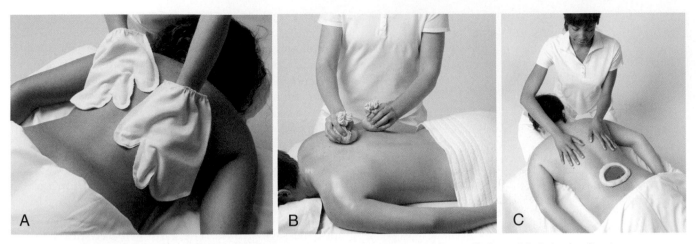

Figure 11-11 Other ayurveda body treatments. (A) Gershan. Massage with raw silk gloves. **(B)** Pinda. The client is massaged by a therapist holding muslin bags full of rice, milk, and herbs. **(C)** Kati basti, a treatment using heat and specific medicated oils to address low back pain. The oils are held on the spot by a "basti" or bladder made of dough.

STEP 7: BUFF OFF THE UBTAN: ANTERIOR

As the ubtan dries, it is buffed off the body using mitts or rolled hand towels. Alternatively, most of the ubtan can be removed with hot, moist towels and the remainder can be buffed with dry rolled towels.

STEP 8: APPLICATION OF HERBAL TOWELS: ANTERIOR

Apply steamy herbal infused towels to both anterior legs, to both arms, and to the belly. As soon as the towels have begun to cool, use them to remove any ubtan still on the skin after buffing or wrap the client while the towels are still hot so that he or she can relax in a cocoon.

SESSION END

The therapist may choose to oil the ears as described previously under the abhyanga procedure. The treatment can end at this point, or it can be followed with shirodhara or swedana.

Figure 11-11 shows some of the other ayurveda body treatments that might be adopted for use in a spa or massage clinic.

Summary

Ayurveda is a traditional medical system from India and is closely linked to Hinduism. It is based on the idea that everything in the universe is composed of five elements or eternal substances. These elements are space, air, fire, water, and earth. When the elements combine in a person, they form that person's unique dosha, or constitution. An ayurvedic physician uses a deep understanding of a person's dosha for diagnosis and treatment. In a spa setting, the focus is on the aspects of ayurveda that teach mindful living, healthful diet, and meditation as ways to achieve dosha balance. External therapies such as Indian massage, shirodhara, udvartana, and others are used to promote relaxation, gentle detoxification, general well being, and inner peace. Ayurveda is a complex system that cannot be covered comprehensively in this chapter. Important areas such as diet and meditation have been touched on only briefly. Interested therapists should review the books listed in the reference section of this chapter and the resources section at the end of the book for more information.

REFERENCES

1. Wujastyk D: *The Roots of Ayurveda: Selections from Sanskrit Medical Writings.* London: Penguin Books, 2003.
2. Warrier G, Gunawant D: *The Complete Illustrated Guide to Ayurveda: The Ancient Indian Healing Tradition.* Shaftesbury, Dorset, UK: Element Books Inc., 1997.
3. Frawley D, Ranade S. Ayurveda: *Nature's Medicine.* Twin Lakes, WI: Lotus Press, 2001.
4. Johari H: *Ancient Indian Massage: Traditional Massage Techniques Based on the Ayurveda.* New Delhi, India: Munshiram Manoharlal Publishers Pvt. Ltd., 2003.
5. Miller L, Miller B: *Ayurveda and Aromatherapy: The Earth Essential Guide to Ancient Wisdom and Modern Healing.* Twin Lakes, WI: Lotus Press, 1995.
6. Frawley D. Ranade S, Lele A: *Ayurveda and Marma Therapy.* Twin Lakes, WI: Lotus Press, 2003.
7. Morrison J: *The Book of Ayurveda: A Holistic Approach to Health and Longevity.* New York: Fireside Books, 1995.
8. Selby A: *Ayurveda.* Minnetonka, MN: Creative Publishing International, Inc., 2001.

REVIEW QUESTIONS

Multiple Choice

1. Ayurveda is best defined as:
   a. The practice of Hinduism in a spa
   b. The practice of Indian massage and spa treatments
   c. A medical system that is mainly focused on massage
   d. A medical system and a philosophy about how to live life in balance

2. In traditional ayurveda, everything in the universe is composed of five elements (panchamahabhutas). These include:
   a. Space, air, fire, water, and earth
   b. Metal, wood, space, air, and breath
   c. Space, breath, water, fire, and spirit
   d. Earth, planets, sun, fire, and forest

3. Although every individual has elements of all three doshas, one or more is dominant. This unique dosha combination is referred to as a person's:
   a. Prakriti
   b. Vata
   c. Pitta
   d. Kapha

4. It is best to eat the main meal of the day during _____ time because this is the dosha that governs digestion.
   a. Pitta
   b. Vata
   c. Kapha
   d. Prakriti

5. It is best to wake up during _____ time (by 6:00 AM) to start the day with quick and energetic qualities.
   a. Pitta
   b. Vata
   c. Kapha
   d. Prakriti

Fill in the Blank

6. Specific combinations of the _____ make up the three doshas (tridoshas) that govern the make-up of an individual.

7. Kaphas need a massage that is _____.

8. Each dosha has its own qualities. Vata qualities are dry, light, cold, subtle, and unstable. Three kapha qualities are _____, _____, and _____.

9. Pittas are aggravated when the temperature becomes too _____.

10. The most unstable of the doshas and the dosha most likely to go out of balance is _____.

Stone Massage

Chapter Outline

Key Terms

Basalt: A type of igneous rock formed from the solidification of molten magma. Because magma cools quickly on the earth's surface, it generally has microscopic crystals and a smooth texture. Basalt holds heat better than many other rock types, and ocean or river basalt has a smooth surface, so it is one of the best types of stone for stone massage.

Lamina grove: Located between the spinous and transverse processes of the thoracic and lumbar vertebrae, the lamina groove is a vertical depression filled with the fibers of the transversospinalis (multifidi, rotators, semispinalis) and erector spinae (spinalis, longissimus, iliocostalis) muscles.

Pin and stretch techniques: Techniques in which the muscle is first shortened, then "pinned" at its origin, insertion, or muscle belly, before being lengthened. The effect of this technique is to reset proprioception and lengthen chronically shortened muscles.

Proprioception: Proprioception is the kinesthetic sense in which sensory receptors receive information about rate of movement, contraction, tension, position, and stretch of tissue. This information is processed in the central nervous system, which sends motor impulses back to the muscle, causing it to contract, relax, restore, or change position.

In stone massage, both hot and cold stones can be combined with various massage techniques to produce a unique treatment that can be adapted to meet the needs of each client. Stone massage can be used for relaxation, injury rehabilitation, energy balance, deep tissue, reflexology, and many other types of massage. It can also be incorporated into spa treatments as an accent or to provide textural variety.

In a relaxation treatment, the stones are heated and usually applied with long, flowing Swedish strokes. Large, flat stones placed on points of tension increase circulation to the area and help to loosen muscle tissue. These "placement" stones also help to draw the client's awareness to an area, which supports deeper muscle release. Sedative and calming essential oils might be incorporated into the treatment to decrease stress and balance the central nervous system.

For an invigorating treatment, a hot stone can be used in one hand and a cold stone in the other, or the area is heated first with hot stones and then massaged briskly with cold stones. This "contrast therapy" feels refreshing and stimulating without being too cold or uncomfortable.

Stones are not just used for relaxation or stimulation. Like any thermal medium, hot or cold temperatures can be used where they are needed for the different stages of inflammation in the healing process. In the early stages of injury, cold stones can be used in the same way as an ice cup is used for ice massage. Heated stones can be placed proximal to the injury site to decrease muscle spasm and guarding. The uninjured areas of the body can be worked with hot stones, helping the body balance and relax. The use of alternating hot and cold stones might also be used in cases of subacute inflammation to achieve a vascular flush effect.

Later, in the late subacute and chronic stages of inflammation, heated stones can be used for specific techniques such as trigger point and cross-fiber friction, saving the therapist's hands from repetitive stress. The stones bring a comforting sense of weight and depth to the work, especially with deep tissue techniques. Essential oils used during the stone treatment help to stabilize and soothe the nervous system.

Hot stones can also be used for reflexology to activate the reflex points on the feet and hands more deeply, which affects the entire body in a positive way. Pointed stones can be used for specific techniques, and larger stones placed around the feet and lower legs provide soothing warmth.

Today, energetic bodywork systems are a synthesis of ancient practices and insights gained from contemporary sciences such as quantum physics, psychology, and medicine. Exploring these concepts gives practitioners new insights into the healing process. Many practitioners have an instinctive and deeply held belief that stones and essential oils have their own peculiar "energetic stamp." They use these "stamps" to balance the electromagnetic field to support the body's natural healing mechanisms. Hot or cold stones are often used with this approach in a number of energetic bodywork practices such as polarity therapy, chakra balancing, guided meditation, and other techniques.

Stones included in a spa treatment introduce the earth element into the treatment or help to cover a transition between one phase of a session and another. They can be incorporated when applying products or included as a separate step to warm the tissue before a product is applied. Increasingly, stones are used as a defining feature in facials, body applications, manicures, and pedicures. Their smooth surface can be used to apply the rougher textured products such as exfoliants, creating a unique sensation for the client.

Specialized approaches to stone massage begin to evolve when therapists experiment with stone techniques. In one example, a therapist wanted to use hot stone massage to bring balance and calm to emotionally disturbed children. She developed her own unique approach to stone massage that incorporated a number of different ideas, including polarity therapy with stones, aromatherapy, placement stones, vibration with the stones, and gentle clicking of the stones. Her routine calmed and captivated her young clientele, and she was able to develop a series of practical techniques that she taught parents to use at home. This is just one of the innovative ways that therapists are using stones for relaxation and healing. Therapists should not feel bound by the routine described in this chapter. Instead, they should view these techniques as a starting point, a resource for exploring their creativity.

General Treatment Considerations

CONTRAINDICATIONS

A hot stone massage increases circulation and lymph flow in the same way that a standard massage does, but because of the heat involved, the body tends to react more strongly to a stone massage. This can produce a positive result such as deep muscular release or a negative result such as accelerated detoxification and nausea. Any condition contraindicated for regular massage is also contraindicated for stone massage. Acute illness, fever, circulatory conditions, sunburned skin, broken or inflamed skin, recent soft tissue injury, advanced or poorly treated diabetes in which tissue is unhealthy and circulation is decreased, edema, thrombus, deep vein thrombosis, gout, heart disease or a serious heart condition, high blood pressure, neuropathy, high-risk pregnancy, renal diseases, rheumatoid arthritis, varicose veins (site contraindication), and intolerance to heat are all contraindicated.

STONE TEMPERATURES

Before they are used, stones are warmed up in water heated to between 120° and 140°F. The best water temperature for most clients and therapists is between 130° and 135°F. At 120°F, the stones are warn and comfortable, but they cool so quickly that it is difficult to maintain any flow in the massage. At 140°F, the stones are too hot for many clients and are too hot for many therapists to hold in their hands. It is not advisable to work with stones above 140°F at any point during the treatment because both the client and therapist may get burned. The therapist's hands will quickly grow accustomed to the heat, and soon very hot temperatures will feel only warm. For this reason, the temperature of the stones must be constantly monitored using a thermometer. Novice stone massage therapists are advised to work at lower temperatures until they have mastered stone massage techniques. As with any treatment, it is better to err on the side of caution and give a warm stone massage rather than endanger a client in any way.

THERAPIST SAFETY

The therapist should always wear shoes during stone massage because the client can move accidentally, sending one of the placement stones flying onto the floor (or the therapist's feet), or the therapist might drop one him- or herself.

DRAPING AND INSULATION FOR PLACEMENT STONES

In promotional brochures for hot stone massage, you often see photos of clients with the stones placed directly on their body. If the stones are hot enough for the treatment, they will burn the client if placed on the skin in this way. Either some form of protection from the heat is needed or the stones need to be moved rapidly until the client gets used to the temperature. Placement stones are usually placed on top of the client's drape. A large bath towel provides enough protection so that the stones do not burn the client but at the same time the client can feel the warmth of the stones penetrating through the drape.

ESSENTIAL OILS

Essential oils can be added to the massage blend used in a stone massage, but a few cautionary notes should be mentioned. It is important to remember that any essential oils that are skin irritants are probably more irritating when they are applied with heat. A blend with lemongrass and clove that works fine in a regular massage may cause serious irritation with a stone massage. Therefore, it t is best to keep the concentration of the essential oils at 2% or lower (12 drops in 1 fl oz of carrier).

Equipment and Setup

Before a therapist can deliver a stone massage, he or she must invest in some additional equipment, purchase or find a set of massage stones, and organize the treatment room so

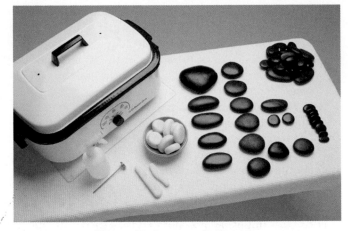

Figure 12-1   Stone equipment.

that all the items needed are within easy reach during the service (Fig. 12-1).

STONES

Basalt stones are the main type of stones used in hot stone massage because they hold heat so well. Basalt is formed from the solidification of molten magma after erupting from a volcano or else it solidifies near the surface of the earth and is exposed later by erosion or upheaval during movements of the earth's plates. It is tumbled to smoothness in river beds and on ocean shores over thousands of years.

Marble is often used for cold techniques in stone massage. In its natural state, marble feels cool to the touch because it absorbs heat rapidly. Marble must be specially cut into manmade disks for use in stone massage. Although marble stones are visually pleasing and have a unique texture, they are not strictly necessary for cold stone therapy. Cooled basalt works just as well, is easier to find, and is less expensive.

Many different companies offer training in stone massage. Most of these companies sell sets of stones that work well with their particular techniques. Most therapists use a set of approximately 55 stones, of which some are "placement stones" and some are "working stones."

Placement Stones

Placement stones are larger and rougher than working stones. They are placed on the body to heat an area and to relax the client with their weight. Placement stones consist of a sacral stone, four large oblong stones, six to eight back stones, two palm stones, two foot stones, eight toe stones, and an optional neck "pillow."

- **One sacral stone:** The sacral stone is the largest stone in the set. It is placed on the sacrum in the posterior layout or on the belly in the anterior layout.

- **Four large oblong stones:** The four large oblong stones are slightly smaller than the sacral stone and are used in the posterior layout to heat up the erector muscles on either side of the spine. In the anterior layout, they are placed up the centerline of the body and at the origins of the pectoral muscles.
- **Six to eight back stones:** The back stones are placed underneath the client in a "spinal layout" just after the client has been turned from the prone position. The stones are lined up on either side of the spine, so they should be rounded with flat surfaces and matched in size. It is important to note that the client never lies directly on these stones. Instead, the stones are covered with a towel so that they do not burn the client. The back stones can also be used during the posterior layout if the client has a long back and the four oblong large placement stones do not cover a large enough area.
- **Two palm stones:** The palm stones are placed in the client's hands after they have been smoothed with massage oil (or else they feel dry).
- **Two foot stones:** The foot stones are about the same size as a back stone with a flat side that fits easily into the arch of the foot. They are held in place on the foot by being wrapped and tied on with terry strips or with hand towels.
- **Eight toe stones:** Eight small stones are placed between the client's toes. It is a good idea to have a large set for big feet and a small set for small feet. The toe stones must be cooled before they are placed between the toes because this is a tender, bony area that is sensitive to heat. The toe stones cool off very quickly because they are small, but remember to ask the client if they are too hot as you put them in.
- **One neck pillow:** The neck "pillow" is placed under the neck when the client is in the supine position and then pulled gently up against the occiput to provide a slight traction.

Working Stones

Working stones are usually smoother than placement stones and fit comfortably in the hands of the therapist. It is useful to have a variety of sizes that can be used for different techniques. It is also helpful to have at least two stones that have a sharper point and so can be used for trigger point or reflexology techniques.

HEATING UNITS

As stone massage has become widely popular, spa and massage suppliers have developed a number of different ways to heat stones in the treatment room. Some of these heating units are designed to look more like pieces of art than a practical piece of equipment. Research the equipment options available to identify the type of heating unit that matches both the budget and the type of stone massage that will be provided. The very practical type of heating unit for stone massage is an 18-quart roaster oven (see Fig. 12-1). A smaller roaster oven or a crock pot can be used if the therapist only plans to use a few stones in the treatment.

EQUIPMENT ORGANIZATION

The heating unit is placed on top of a bath towel to absorb any water splashes as the stones are removed. A white plastic dish mat (cut to size) is then placed in the bottom of the heating unit, and the stones are arranged on top of it. The white dish mat helps the stones to stand out against the otherwise black interior of the heating unit. This makes them easier to see in the low light of the treatment room and prevents the stones from making a scratching noise on the bottom of the heating unit as they are removed.

The most efficient way to arrange the stones is to place them in the order that they will be pulled out of the heating unit. The sacral stone is placed in the upper right-hand corner of the unit with the four large oblong stones in front of it. In the next row are the back stones, palm stones, foot stones, and toe stones. The toe stones are placed in a small mesh bag so that they do not get lost under other stones during the treatment session. On the left-hand side of the roaster are the working stones in a pile. Some therapists split their working stones into four or five mesh bags that contain prearranged sizes and shapes of stones. This makes it easy to quickly pull the right stones from the heating unit.

A bowl of iced water containing four to six working stones (or marble disks) is placed on the work table. These stones will be used for the "vascular flush" or to provide a contrast to hot stones. A glass of water for the client to drink during the spinal layout is also placed on the work table.

A pitcher of cold water is placed close to the heating unit in case the stones get too hot and need to be cooled quickly. A thermometer is used at all times to monitor the temperature of the water in the heating unit. A digital thermometer is the easiest type to use because the unit can be fixed to the outside of the heating unit and read from a distance while the attached probe is placed in the water. A set of thermal gloves and a strong slotted spoon are placed to the side of the roaster. The gloves are used to pull the placement stones from the roaster during the posterior and anterior layouts. The slotted spoon (slotted so that the water can drain out) makes it easier to remove the stones from the hot water in the heating unit.

A bottle of expeller-pressed massage oil (sunflower or hazelnut work well, although many different types of cold pressed or expeller-pressed oil can be used) and an aroma mist are placed on a rolling cart along with six to eight dry hand towels. Stone massage does not work well with a massage gel or cream product. These products leave a sticky residue on the stones and turn the water in the roaster cloudy.

The massage table is laid with sheets and a large bath towel over the top sheet. The bath towel is necessary because it provides an insulating layer to prevent burning.

Sanitation

To quickly clean the stones between clients, the stones are removed from the roaster and sprayed with alcohol. The water in the roaster is dumped out and the interior of the roaster is sprayed with alcohol. At the end of the day, the stones are washed with hot soapy water and allowed to dry completely. The roaster should be rinsed out and sprayed with alcohol. If the stones become sticky or gummy, they can be soaked overnight in a covered container filled with rubbing alcohol. The stones can also be cleaned in a dishwasher (make sure that the stones are secured in the dishwasher because they may cause damage to the unit if they become dislodged and fall). Alternatively, for those concerned about the effect on the "energy" of the stones, they can be soaked overnight in baking soda, water, and lemon juice.

Core Techniques

Before working through the basic stone massage procedure, it is helpful to practice some core techniques and basic strokes. After these have been mastered, the therapist is ready to move on to a full-body stone massage.

INTRODUCTION OF THE STONES TO THE CLIENT'S BODY

After the body area has been oiled, the therapist picks up a stone in each hand and moves them briskly over the skin to begin the massage. The therapist should not place the stones directly on the skin and hold them still while asking, "Is this too hot?" The stones will be too hot and the client will be tense for the rest of the massage. The important thing to remember is to keep the stones moving briskly over the skin and keep flipping them (described below) until they begin to cool. After only three or four passes, the client will have adapted to the temperature, and the stones will be cool enough so that deeper, slower strokes can be used for the treatment work and to add variety to the massage.

STONE FLIPPING

Therapists will notice that the side of the stone that is next to the client will cool more quickly than the side of the stone that is touching the therapist's hand. To keep the stone temperature even for the client, "flip" the stone over at the end of a long stroke. When the stones are very hot, the therapist will need to flip the stone repeatedly to protect his

or her own hands (although the stone is static for the therapist, it is moving for the client). To flip the stones, pick up one end of the stone with the thumb and turn the stone over while it is in motion. With practice, flipping the stones becomes easy and natural.

STONE TRANSITIONS

The smooth transition from one stone (that has cooled down) to another (which is nice and hot) is an important part of the stone massage technique. This transition can be made in a number of different ways. The first method is to keep one stone moving and take the other hand off the body. Change the stone in the first hand and then repeat the process with the second hand (Fig. 12-2). The second method is to take the stones off a body area in a long, slow sweep; quickly grab fresh stones; and return the new stones to the same place on the body. A third method is to leave a cooled stone on the body area while picking up new stones. The cooled stone gives the client the sensation of the therapist's presence until the new stones are introduced. Finally, a fourth method is to try taking the stone off the body while an elbow or forearm continues the stroke. Use the free hand to change the stones for both hands. Whichever method is used, the aim is to minimize any disruption to the flow of the treatment when changing stones.

BAD STONE BODY MECHANICS

It is not uncommon for novice stone therapists to "death-grip" a stone during a stroke, to position their wrists at extreme angles, or to watch the stone as it moves over the body and therefore begin to hunch over the client. Although stones can feel slippery, it is best to trap the stone against the client's body with the palm and reach the fingers around the stone so that they contact and palpate the client's tissue. Some techniques do require the therapist to grip the stone. In these cases, the therapist must think about gripping without overstraining their hands. The therapist must also

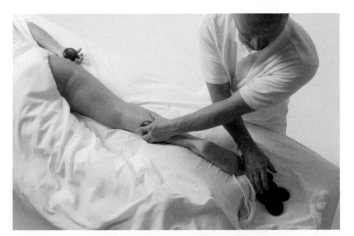

Figure 12-2 Stone transitions.

watch the position of the wrists when using stones so that they remain as straight as possible during a technique. Any technique that causes strain to the therapist's body should be reevaluated and either changed to avoid unnecessary stress or eliminated from the routine.

"ROASTER SPEED" VERSUS "BODY SPEED"

In stone massage, there are two different speeds at which the therapist works: roaster speed and body speed. A therapist with good roaster speed is fast and focused when removing stones from the roaster (heating unit). The minute the therapist's hands leave the client, they move into high gear, remove the next set of stones from the roaster, and then return to the client. As soon as the hands get to the client, they shift to a slower body speed. Their pace becomes slow and relaxing again. The therapist instantly grounds and centers him- or herself as the hands make contact with the client's body and he or she starts to massage.

REMOVING ENOUGH STONES

A common mistake of novice stone therapists is that they do not remove enough stones form the heating unit for the body area being worked on. The therapist pulls two or three stones, walks to the client, undrapes the area, and massages, and soon the stones are cold. The therapist must now walk back to the heating unit and swap the cold stones for hot stones. Instead, the therapist should remove a minimum of six to eight stones for each body area. Stones start to cool off the moment they are used on the client's body, but when they are sitting off to one side of the client wrapped up in a towel, they remain relatively hot. This way, the therapist does not need to walk away from a client to get more hot stones more often than necessary.

DRAPING

Before placing any stones, first check the client's drape. In both the supine and prone positions, pull the drape up toward the top of the client's body so that there is excess over the shoulders. Many clients have shoulders that slope downwards. This is especially true of women with larger breasts. Placement stones tend to roll or slide off these clients with the slightest movement. To avoid this and other problems, the drape is brought around the stone, creating a "pocket" to hold the stone in place. The drape is then anchored with another stone, and both the client and therapist can relax.

STONES ON THE FACE

In promotional brochures, it is common to see photos of clients with stones on their faces. A warm stone on the forehead or over the eyes feels very nice. However, if the stone is oiled with a massage blend that contains essential oils, do not place it over the eye because the eyelid is sensitive, and

the oils may also penetrate through the gap between the eyelids and irritate the eyes. The other problem is that when stones are left in place on the face for too long, the client tends to tense the neck muscles to keep the stones from sliding off. Stones used for massage on the face should only be kept on for a short time and should be warm rather than hot (around 120°F or lower) to protect delicate facial tissues from irritation.

Basic Strokes

Similar to Swedish massage, stone massage strokes often follow a progression from effleurage at the start, to petrissage, friction, deep tissue techniques, **proprioceptor** techniques, vibration, and finally tapotement. Therapists can explore their own massage techniques for inspiration. If they have a massage stroke that they particularly like, it will usually be possible to find a way to do the same technique with a stone. On the other hand, some really great moves are impossible to perform with a stone. In this case, transition out of using the stone for long enough to perform the move. Try to keep what is unique and special about your massage and just add stones to enhance the performance. This is what makes a stone massage a personal and creative experience. Basic strokes are illustrated in Figure 12-3.

LONG STROKES WITH THE STONE FLAT

Long strokes (effleurage with stones) are the basic type of stroke used in a stone massage (see Fig. 12-3A). They are used when a stone is first introduced to a body area and to transition between different types of strokes. The stones are placed flat against the body and passed up the length of the body area and down again without losing contact. If an area is particularly bony, lighten the stroke over the area. Stones glide over bony areas as long as there is enough oil on the skin. The therapist must still pay attention so that he or she does not knock the stone accidentally into a bony prominence. It also helps to palpate the tissue around the edges of the stone by keeping the fingertips on the surface of the skin. This helps the therapist to judge the appropriate depth for the stroke.

STONE PETRISSAGE

A small stone is placed in each hand so that the therapist is able to use the fingers to lift the tissue as in normal petrissage (see Fig. 12-3B).

WRINGING WITH STONES

A medium-size stone is placed in each hand and used in a cross-motion, lifting the tissue at the top of the stroke where the hands meet (see Fig. 12-3C).

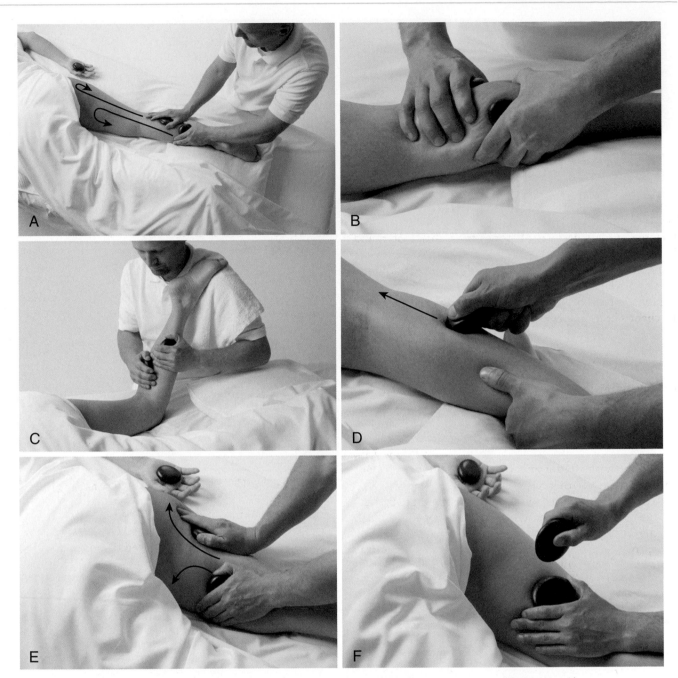

Figure 12-3   Basic stone strokes. (A) Long strokes with the stone flat. **(B)** Stone pétrissage. **(C)** Wringing with stones. **(D)** Stone stripping. **(E)** Rotation of a stone with compression. **(F)** Stone vibration.

STONE STRIPPING

The stone is turned on its side and used to strip the muscle tissue in a given area. This stroke can feel intense to the client and should only be used when deeper, more detailed work is desired (see Fig. 12-3D).

ROTATION OF A STONE WITH COMPRESSION

A medium-sized working stone is held flat against the body area and rotated in a half circle toward the outside of the body during a compression. This can be done with one hand or in alternating two-handed strokes. This stroke is

particularly useful on fleshy areas such as the hamstrings (see Fig. 12-3E).

STONE VIBRATION

Place a large stone against the body area and use a smaller stone to tap it (see Fig. 12-3F). This creates a pleasant sound and a gentle vibration. Some therapists open their massage routine by tapping on the sacral stone before massaging the legs. Another nice idea is to gently tap both edges of the neck pillow while it is positioned up against the client's occiput. This creates a vibration throughout the head and face, which feels relaxing for some clients.

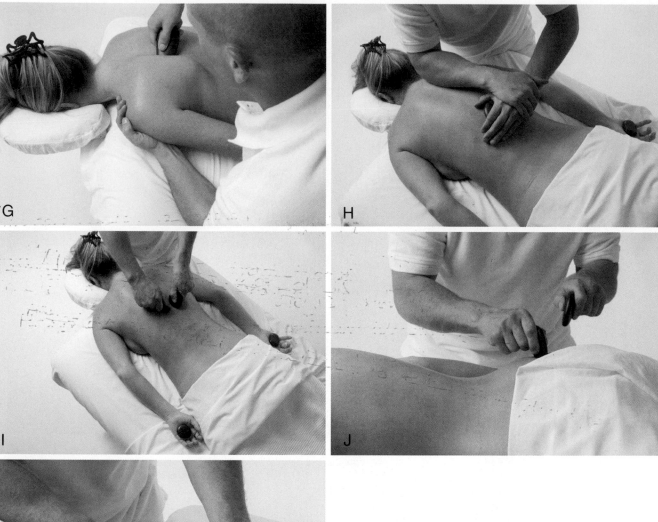

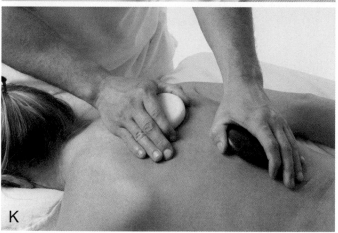

Figure 12-3 *(continued)* **(G)** Deep tissue with the edge of the stone. **(H)** Deep tissue with the flat of the stone. The stone is used to heat the area while the pressure is exerted with the forearm or elbow. The stone must be cool enough to be moved slowly. **(I)** Friction with the stones. This friction stroke is performed by running the stones down the lamina groove. It could also be performed in the same manner on any area of the body where the therapist normally uses the thumbs. **(J)** Stone tapotement. **(K)** Vascular flush with stones. In this picture, a marble stone is used to show that the stone is a cold stone. Cooled basalt could also be used.

DEEP TISSUE WITH THE EDGE OF A STONE

The edge of a stone is placed on the area to be worked, and as the client exhales, the stone is pressed into the area. This technique is particularly useful around the scapulae (see Fig. 12-3G).

DEEP TISSUE WITH THE FLAT OF THE STONE

A medium-sized stone is held flat against the body ahead of the therapist's elbow or forearm. The stone is not used

to exert pressure but is used to warm the area ahead of the elbow or forearm, facilitating a deeper release. The stone must be cool enough to be moved very slowly (see Fig. 12-3H).

FRICTION WITH STONES

Stones can be held in the hands and used in place of the thumb for friction. For example, a stone is useful for producing friction as it is run slowly down the **lamina groove** (see Fig. 12-3I).

STONE TAPOTEMENT

A stone is placed in each hand and used to apply gentle tapotement to the body (see Fig. 12-3J).

VASCULAR FLUSH WITH STONES

A hot medium-sized stone is held in one hand, and a cold medium-sized stone is held in the other hand. With the hot stone leading, both stones are run over the body area in long, brisk strokes. This feels stimulating and invigorating and is a nice way to finish a body area before redraping and moving on (see Fig. 12-3K). In a variation of this technique, the body area is heated with hot stones and then two cold stones are introduced with brisk strokes over the area. This technique can also be used as contrast therapy on an area of subacute injury. In a general massage, hot stones are then used again to finish the area off.

Stone Strokes for Specific Areas

A number of the hot stone techniques used on specific areas of the body can be described as **pin and stretch techniques**. *Pin and stretch* refers to a technique in which the muscle is first shortened; then "pinned" at its origin, insertion, or muscle belly; and then lengthened. Some therapists describe this technique as muscle striping with range of motion. Others express it as deep tissue with Swedish gymnastic. Some say it is Golgi tendon organ release with range of motion. Regardless of how the technique is described, its effect is to reset proprioception and lengthen chronically shortened muscle.

The heat from the stones seems to support proprioceptor resetting and the release of chronically held tissue. The techniques described here are meant to offer some ideas for moving beyond a typical stone routine (effleurage with a stone) into a deeper, more satisfying level of stone bodywork. Stone strokes for specific areas of the body are illustrated in Figure 12-4.

POSTERIOR LEGS: GASTROCNEMIUS AND SOLEUS PIN AND STRETCH

Lift the lower leg to a 90-degree angle and place the hand closest to the end of the massage table across the plantar surface of the foot, grasping the heel. Place a stone in the other hand and wrap the fingers around the Achilles tendon (see Fig. 12-4A). Plantar flex the foot to shorten the gastrocnemius and soleus and then dorsiflex the foot while the hand with the stone travels down the posterior leg. At the end of the gastrocnemius and soleus pin and stretch, place the foot on your shoulder while facing toward the head of

the table and then use two stones to "wring" the lower leg (see Fig. 12-4C).

POSTERIOR LEGS

Hamstring Pin and Stretch

Stand at the side of the table by the hamstring, and facing toward the head of the table, lift the lower leg so that the knee is flexed (see Fig. 12-4B). Place a medium-sized stone on the hamstrings close to the posterior knee and then lower the leg into a neutral position before bringing it up into a flexed position as the stone runs toward the ischial tuberosity with moderate pressure. As the stone reaches the gluteals, it can be circled around the greater trochanter to create a long, flowing stroke.

Double-Arm Deep Tissue Stroke

Holding a medium-sized stone in each hand, stand at the posterior knee. Push the forearms forward on either side of the posterior knee (see Fig. 12-4C) and then bring them back again. As the stones come back, they are placed onto the skin and separated. One stone goes toward the foot while the other goes toward the hip. They are then brought back together again, and the stroke is repeated.

THE BACK

Stoning the Lamina Groove

A number of strokes can be performed using the lamina groove as a guide. The two stones can be pressed into the lamina groove on either side of the spine and run slowly with moderate pressure toward the sacrum (see Fig. 12-3I). The therapist can also stand on one side of the client and place the edge of a stone in the groove on the opposite side of the spine. Press downward and then flare the stone outward (see Fig. 12-4D). This is a small movement that nevertheless feels intense. Novice therapists should work slowly and carefully while building their palpation skills. Running stones quickly or roughly over the spinous processes feels uncomfortable for the client and may cause an injury.

Latissimus Pin and Stretch

Shorten the latissimus by bringing the arm behind the back into extension and internal rotation. Pin anywhere along the lateral body from just above the waist to the axilla with a warm stone (see Fig. 12-4E). Ask the client to inhale. On the exhalation breath, bring the client's arm out, around, and forward into flexion. A running pin can begin close to the axilla and run down toward the posterior superior iliac spine as the arm is brought into flexion.

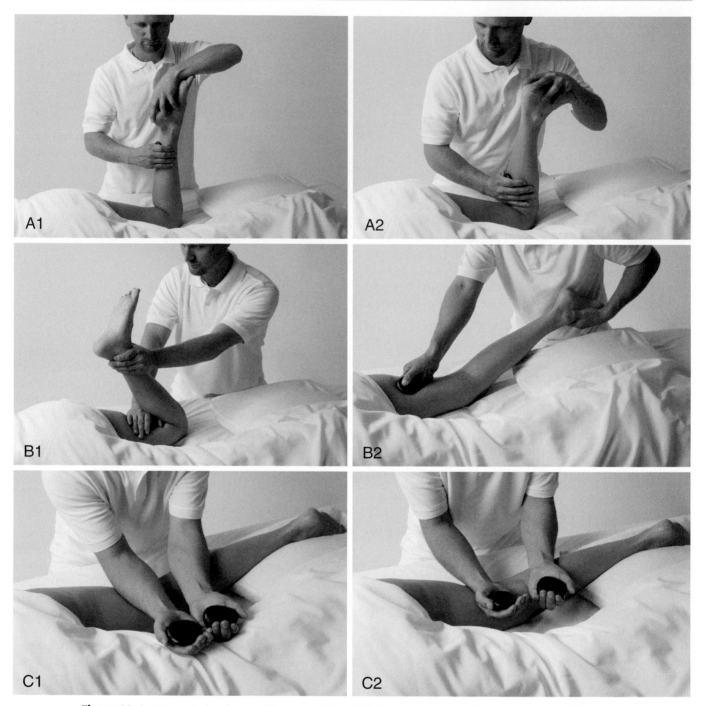

Figure 12-4   Stone strokes for specific areas. (A1 and **A2)** Gastrocnemius and soleus pin and stretch. **(B1** and **B2)** Hamstring pin and stretch. **(C1** to **C5)** Double-arm deep tissue stroke with stones. **(D)** Lamina groove "flare." **(E1** and **E2)** Latissimus pin and stretch.

ANTERIOR LEGS

The bony anterior lower leg can be a tricky place for stone massage. The stones are kept on either side of the tibia, where they access the many attachment sites for the extensors of the ankle and toes. In a nice technique for the peroneus muscles, the lower leg is held in medial rotation and a hot stone is worked up the lateral side of the leg (see Fig. 12-4F). A stone can also be held on one side of the tibia while the foot is passively dorsiflexed and plantar flexed.

Quadriceps Pin and Stretch

The client's leg is dropped off the side of the table (see Fig. 12-4G). The ankle is held in one hand and a stone in the other. The stone is pushed with moderate pressure into the rectus femoris just above the patella. As the therapist

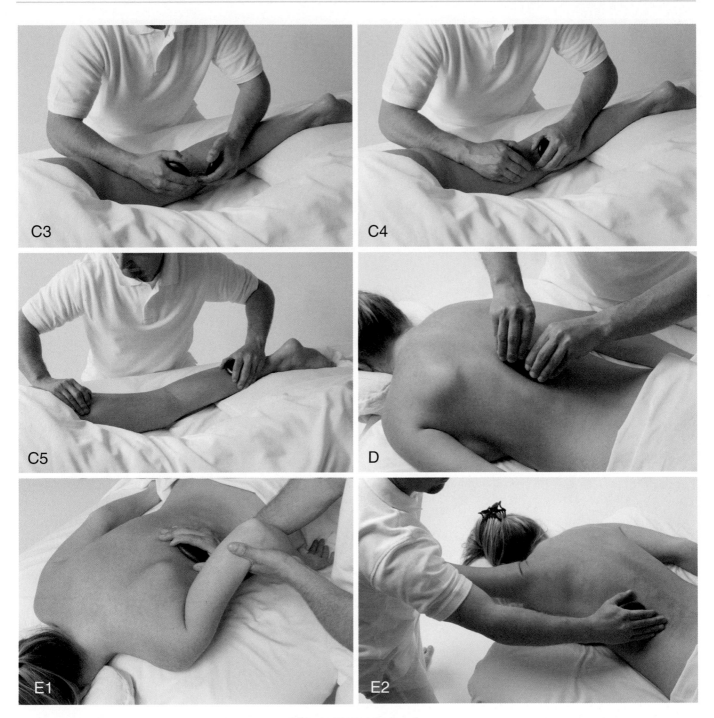

Figure 12-4 *(continued)*

extends the lower leg and then returns it to a flexed position, the stone is pushed toward the anterior inferior iliac spine.

Tensor Fasciae Latae and Iliotibial Tract Stretch with Stones

With the knee flexed, place the foot on the lateral side of the opposite leg (see Fig. 12-4H). Press the stone into the iliotibial tract superior to the lateral knee and run up the lateral leg while the bent knee is gently pressed across the opposite leg.

This stretches the fasciae latae and iliotibial fascia. The stone can be lowered posterior to the greater trochanter and taken into the lower back to finish the stroke.

ARMS

The Triceps

Range of motion is important in the arm massage because it facilitates a better release in the muscles and feels flowing and interesting to the client. The triceps can be accessed by

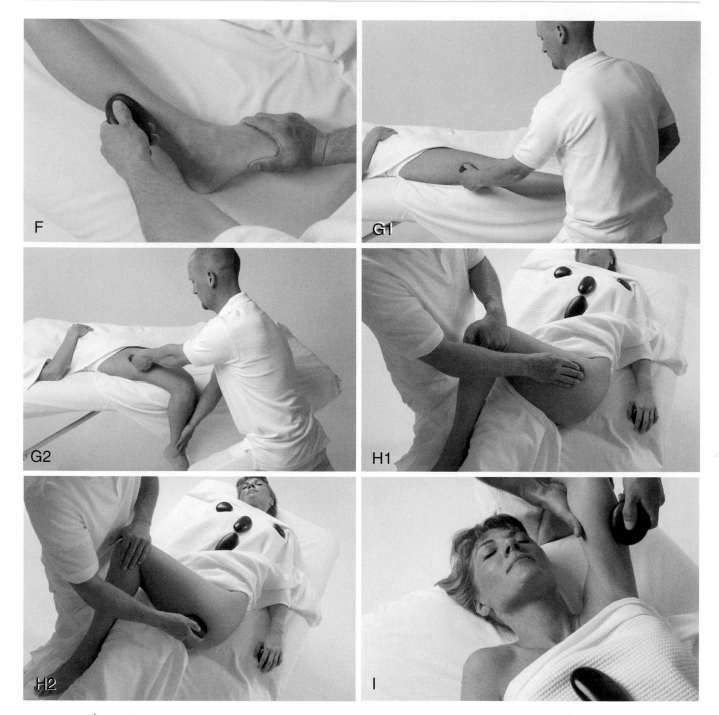

Figure 12-4   *(continued)* **(F)** Stone massage on the peroneus muscles. **(G1** and **G2)** Quadriceps pin and stretch. **(H1** and **H2)** Tensor fasciae latae and iliotibial stretch with stones. **(I)** Stone massage on the triceps.

lifting the arm over the head and "locking" the hand gently against the treatment table with the thigh (see Fig. 12-4I). The stone is passed from the medial to the lateral side of the triceps across the biceps. To finish the stroke, the therapist stretches the arm behind the client and passes the stone down the lateral side of the lower back.

Flexor or Extensor Pin and Stretch

A passive pin and stretch is achieved when the therapist holds the client's hand and flexes and extends the wrist while they use a smaller sized stone to provide a running pin up either the flexors or extensors (see Fig. 12-4J and K).

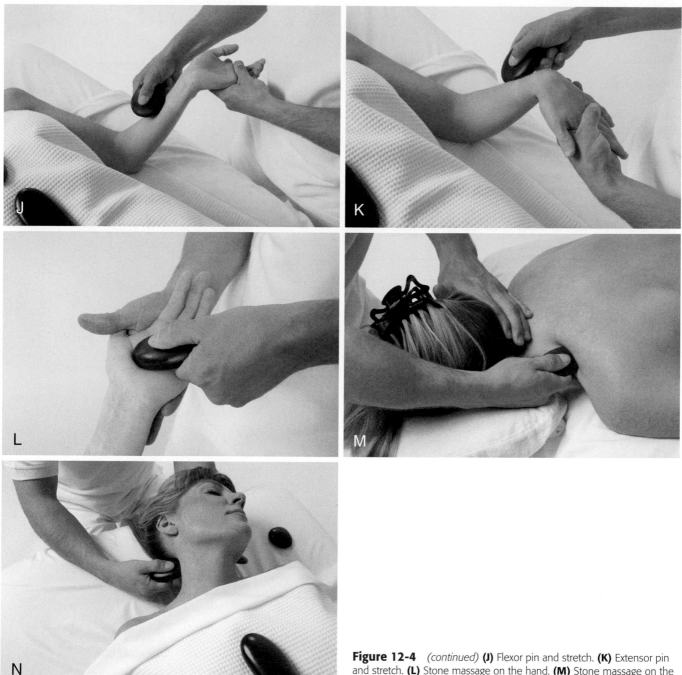

Figure 12-4 *(continued)* **(J)** Flexor pin and stretch. **(K)** Extensor pin and stretch. **(L)** Stone massage on the hand. **(M)** Stone massage on the neck: prone. **(N)** Stone massage on the neck: supine.

HANDS

Stones do not feel particularly good on the posterior surface of the hand, so it is better to incorporate a warm stone to hold the hand while the fingers are massaged. The palm can be massaged with a stone using reflexology point work (see Fig. 12-4L).

THE NECK

Prone

The upper fibers of the splenius capitis, the trapezius, and the suboccipitals can be accessed when the therapist sits at the head of the table and brings the stones up the lamina groove and out toward the mastoid process (see Fig. 12-4M).

To reach the suboccipitals, a deeper, more specific pressure must be used.

Supine

Stone massage on the neck works best when the client's head is kept in gentle and constant movement. This opens up the neck so that the stone can flow without becoming stuck in flesh. On the anterior neck, the stone should be kept in a flat position for the client's safety. On the posterior neck, the edge of the stone can be used to access the suboccipitals, splenius capitis, and trapezius at the occiput (see Fig. 12-4N).

A Basic Full-Body Stone Massage Procedure

The treatment snapshot offers a quick overview of a complete full-body 90-minute stone routine. Figure 12-5 shows the stone positions for the posterior and anterior placements of the stones. Therapists can adapt this routine and cut it down to 60 minutes by removing certain body areas (e.g., the abdominals) and simplifying stone placement (e.g., eliminate tying stones on the feet). Some therapists choose not to use placement stones and simply use a set of stones

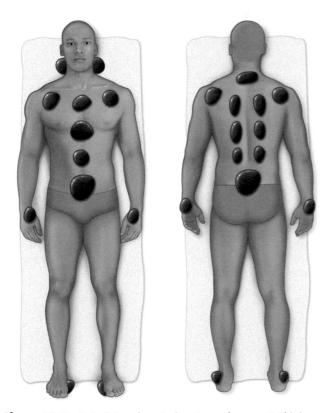

Figure 12-5   Anterior and posterior stone placement. This image represents some options for placement of stones in the anterior and posterior position. Figure 12-6 shows the specific techniques for placement on the feet, the spinal layout, and anchoring a stone in a pocket. A drape has not been used in this image so that the therapist can better see stone placement. A drape should always be used to protect the client from burns.

to "open" the body area with effleurage strokes before progressing on to their regular massage routine. Timing options are shown in Table 12-1.

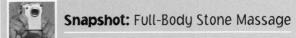

Snapshot: Full-Body Stone Massage

Indications
Muscle soreness, stress, chronic musculoskeletal condition, low energy, to promote relaxation

Contraindications
Heart condition, high-risk pregnancy, vascular conditions, illness or fever, acute conditions, inflammatory conditions

Supplies for the Treatment Table Setup (from the bottom to the top layer)
1) Bottom massage sheet
2) Top massage sheet
3) Bath sheet (drape)
4) Bolster

Supplies for the Work Table Setup
1) Heating unit placed on top of a bath towel and with white plastic dish mat inside
2) Stones arranged in the unit and covered in water
3) Insulated gloves and/or a slotted spoon
4) Bowl of ice with four to six medium-sized basalt stones or marble disks inside
5) Thermometer
6) Pitcher of cool water
7) Massage oil
8) Aroma mist
9) Glass of drinking water
10) Six to eight hand towels
11) Rolling cart (optional)
12) Bowl of soapy water in which to soak toe and foot massage stones after they are used (optional)

Procedure
1) Place the posterior stones.
2) Massage the legs.
3) Remove the back stones.
4) Massage the back.
5) Turn the client supine and sit up the client.
6) Place the spinal layout. Client lies down.
7) Place the anterior layout.
8) Massage the anterior legs and feet.
9) Remove the upper chest stones and neck pillow.
10) Massage the arms.
11) Massage the abdominal muscles (optional).
12) Massage the neck and face.
13) Remove all stones and end with an aura mist.

SESSION START

Upon entering the treatment area, bolster the client while he or she is lying in the prone position. Pull the drape up high over the client's shoulders so that there is enough to wrap a stone in a "pocket" to avoid it slipping. Check the

Table 12-1	Suggested Timing Options for a Stone Massage Session
DESCRIPTION	**TIME ALLOTMENT (MIN)**
90-MINUTE SESSION	
1. Posterior layout	6
2. Posterior legs	14 (7 each)
3. Back	15
4. Turn the client supine and sit up the client	2
5. Spinal layout	3
6. Anterior layout	3
7. Anterior legs	12 (6 each)
8. Feet	10 (5 each)
9. Abdominal area	4
10. Arms	12 (6 each)
11. Neck and face	8
12. Session end	1
TOTAL	**90**
60-MINUTE SESSION	
1. Posterior layout	6
2. Posterior legs	10 (5 each)
3. Back	13
4. Turn client (omit spinal layout)	1
5. Modified anterior layout (place a belly stone and neck pillow only and omit stones on the feet or hands)	3
6. Anterior legs and feet (combine the feet with the anterior legs)	12 (6 each)
7. Arms (omit abdominal massage)	8 (4 each)
8. Neck and face	6
9. Session end	1
TOTAL	**60**

temperature of the stones and adjust the heat as needed by either turning up the roaster or pouring in cold water.

STEP 1: POSTERIOR PLACEMENT

The placement stones are then removed from the heating unit using insulated gloves, tongs, or a slotted spoon. Place each stone in order up the sides of the spine as follows (see Fig. 12-5A):

1. Place the sacral stone over the coccyx of the client rather than directly over the sacrum. This will provide a slight fascia traction that stretches the tissue.

2. Place stones on either side of the spine directly above the sacral stone all the way up the length of the back. Place the four large placement stones on the lower back and place the back stones on the upper back. These are the same stones that will be used in the spinal layout after the client has been turned later on.

3. The foot stones are wrapped in a towel and tied around the arch of the foot. To do this, fold a towel in half across its length and slip the stone into the pocket that is created by the folded towel. The towel is then tied around the client's foot with the stone placed directly over the arch (Fig. 12-6).

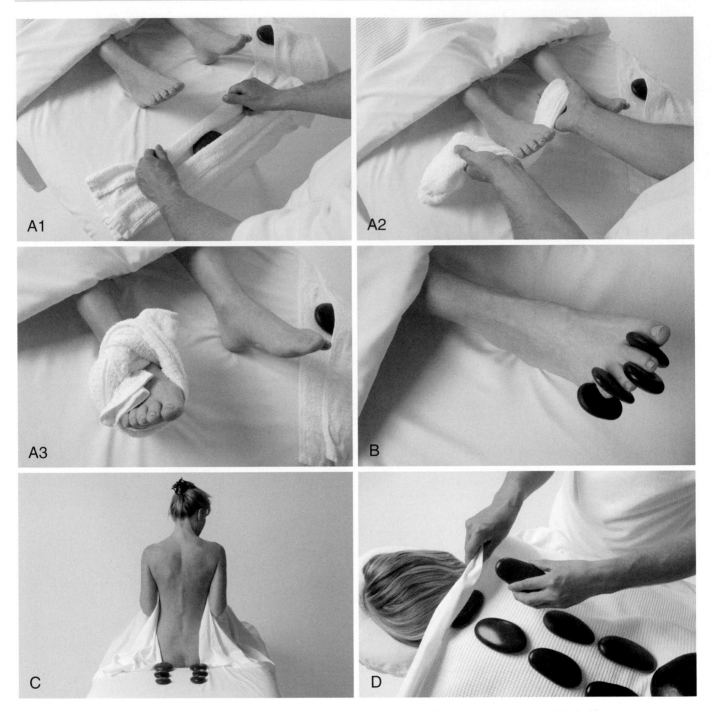

Figure 12-6   Placement specifics. (A1 to A3) Tying a stone on the foot. **(B)** Toe stone placement. **(C)** Spinal layout. **(D)** Posterior layout. Anchoring a stone in a pocket.

4. The two palm stones are oiled and slipped into the client's hands by lifting the drape and placing the stone in the palm. If the stone is too hot, the client may not be able to hold it, so a washcloth can be placed across the client's hand for protection.

5. Once the stones have been placed on the client, the therapist is ready to "open" the massage section of the treatment. Take a moment to ground and center by "activating" the sacral stone and the stone at the midback. To "activate" the stones, press down on each stone to increase the client's perception of weight and depth. As you press down, take three deep breaths with the client. This creates a nice transition between the placement of the stones and the massage. Some therapists tap four to six times ceremonially on the sacral stone with a smaller stone to open the session.

STEP 2: MASSAGE THE POSTERIOR LEGS

The stones for the first leg are removed from the heating unit before the client's leg is undraped (six to eight stones of various sizes or one mesh bag of working stones). The stones are placed in a towel on a moveable cart so that they are easy to reach.

The leg is undraped and oil is massaged into the skin. More oil is used than with a normal massage so that the stones glide over the skin more easily. Hot stones are then introduced using a variety of strokes. If the stones become cool during the massage, they should be changed for a fresh set of hot stones. All the stones that are not on the body should be placed back in the heating unit to reheat.

At the end of the posterior leg massage, a cold stone vascular flush can be performed by taking a hot stone in one hand and a cold stone in the other and running both stones over the area with effleurage strokes. The area is spritzed with an aroma mist and the stones are placed back in the heating unit to reheat. The first leg is redraped, and the therapist moves onto the second leg.

STEP 3: MASSAGE THE BACK

After both posterior legs have been massaged, remove the placement stones from the back and put them in the heating unit to reheat (these stones will be placed on the anterior body when the client is turned into the supine position).

The working stones for the back are removed from the heating unit and placed close to the therapist for easy access. The back is undraped and oil is massaged into the skin before the stones are introduced. Range of motion techniques such as the latissimus pin and stretch (described previously) and deep tissue techniques bring variety to the back massage. At the end of the back routine, finish with a stone vascular flush. An aroma mist is spritzed over the client and the stones are put back into the roaster.

STEP 4: TRANSITION TO THE SUPINE POSITION AND SPINAL LAYOUT

Before the therapist turns the client, it is a good idea to quickly reorganize the work area. Any stones left on the work surface are placed back into the heating unit to reheat. If any stones remain on the client's body, they should be removed and reheated at this point.

Remove the back stones from the heating unit and then ask the client to turn over. When the client has been turned over, ask him or her to sit up after removing the bolster. Offer the client a glass of water before starting to place the spinal layout on the massage table. To set up the spinal layout, place a towel behind the sitting client by tucking the edge close to the gluteals. Place six to eight back stones (de-

pending on the size of the client) on the towel, covering the massage table as shown in Figure 12-6C. A towel is placed over the top of the back stones and tucked in around the bottom stone. This is very important because if the stones are uncovered, they may burn the client as he or she lies back down.

Support the client as he or she lies back down onto the spinal stones. Place one hand on the client's shoulder and the other on the client's hip before rocking the client gently back and forth. If the client feels that any of the stones are in an uncomfortable position, adjust them so that the client feels comfortable before laying out the anterior stones and bolstering the client.

STEP 5: ANTERIOR PLACEMENT

After the therapist has made sure that the spinal layout is comfortable for the client, the therapist puts a bolster under the client's knees and lays out the anterior stones. The anterior placement is shown in Figure 12-5A.

1. The sacral stone is placed over the navel to act as a belly stone.
2. Two large placement stones are positioned up the centerline of the body.
3. The two remaining large placement stones are placed above the origin of the pectoralis minor muscle on either side of the body.
4. The feet are wrapped with fresh foot stones and a toe stone is placed between each of the toes. It is important to cool the toe stones sufficiently because they can feel uncomfortably hot in the bony, unprotected area between the toes.
5. Two fresh palm stones are oiled and placed in the client's hands. Some clients like to bring their hands around the edges of the blanket and rest their hands over the belly stone (sacral stone) instead.
6. The neck stone is placed in the crook of the neck and then pulled toward the occiput to traction the neck slightly. This stone can be used either hot (wrap it in a towel before placing it under the neck) or cold.

Before beginning the anterior massage, take a moment to activate the two pectoralis minor stones and take a few breaths with the client. This helps to create a smooth transition into the second half of the massage. Some therapists gently tap ceremonially four to six times on both ends (at the same time) of the neck pillow with small stones to begin the anterior routine.

STEP 6: MASSAGE THE ANTERIOR LEGS

The stones (six to eight stones of various sizes) for the first leg are removed from the heating unit and placed in a towel on a moveable cart so that they are easy to reach. The client's leg is undraped and oil is massaged into the skin with the hands. Hot stones are introduced to the area with a variety of strokes. At the end of the posterior leg massage, a cold stone vascular flush can be performed before the area is spritzed with an aroma mist and redraped.

STEP 7: FOOT MASSAGE

Remove six to eight stones from the heating unit to massage the feet. For ideas on foot massage techniques and reflexology, review Chapter 8. Some therapists prefer to massage the foot while massaging the anterior leg. If so, it helps to remove the toe stones first. Other therapists choose to delay the placement of the toe stones until after the foot has been massaged. In this case, the therapist removes the toe stones as the end of the neck and face massage. Note that the toe stones cool quickly and as soon as they cool, they often feel uncomfortable to the client, so they should not be left in place for too long.

 Sanitation

The used toe stones and foot stones are not put back in the roaster. Instead, they are put to one side of the heating unit or directly into warm, soapy water to soak until the equipment is cleaned and reorganized for the next client.

STEP 8: ABDOMINAL MASSAGE (OPTIONAL)

Abdominal massage with hot stones feels soothing and deeply relaxing and is a nice addition to the stone massage routine. The abdominal area is undraped and oiled with the hands. Hot stones are applied in a clockwise, circular motion. For a massage that aims to relieve chronic lower back pain, hot stones are very useful for supporting abdominal release during psoas work. However, therapists who are not experienced in palpation of the psoas should not try to use a stone for this purpose.

STEP 9: ARM AND HAND MASSAGE

The upper chest stones, neck stone, and palm stones are removed to facilitate mobilization of the arm during massage. If the stones are left in place, they may roll or shift uncomfortably as the arm is moved.

The arm is undraped and oil is massaged into the skin before hot stones are introduced. Range of motion techniques and gentle stretching add variety to the stone massage. The hand is massaged together with the arm. This is perhaps one of the more difficult areas in which to use stones. Reflexology-like pressure point techniques work well, but stone massage does not feel particularly good on the posterior side of the hand. It is best to massage the posterior side of the hands without a stone. To finish the area off, cold stones are used in brisk effleurage strokes and the area is spritzed with an aroma mist. New stones are removed from the heating unit for the second arm.

STEP 10: NECK MASSAGE

Stone massage for the neck feels best when the neck is mobilized during the work. This opens up the area and allows the stones to move freely in a flowing arc. The stones are used only in flat positions on the anterior neck to protect the client. In the posterior areas, an edge may be used to work deep into the suboccipitals and upper trapezius.

STEP 11: FACE MASSAGE

The face is massaged with warm (120°F) or cooled stones. Light upward strokes with the edge of the stone allow the therapist to avoid the use of oil on the face. Ideas for face massage techniques are described in Chapter 3. As the facial massage comes to an end, a warm stone can be placed on the forehead. This stone remains in place while all of the other stones, with the exception of the spinal layout (which the client is lying on), are removed.

SESSION END

The therapist may choose to end the massage with a full-body aura mist that fills the treatment room with a refreshing scent. The belly stone and forehead stone are removed last, and the client is asked to get up carefully because the spinal stones are still in place underneath the client.

Some spas and clinics give the client a small stone to take home after their stone massage. This is a nice way to say thank you to the client and to remind them to come back and get another treatment.

SAMPLE TREATMENTS

A hot stone relaxation massage can be described in many different ways: Body Stone Balance, River Rock Massage, Desert Stone Massage, Serenity Stone Massage, Lava Stone Therapy, and Hot Stone Therapy are just a few of the names that can be used.

Body Stone Balance: 90 Minutes

Promotional Description

Experience the elegance of a hot stone massage and restful botanicals combined together in a treatment that delights the senses and soothes the soul. The warmth of the stones relaxes tight muscles and eases pain, and the scent of fruits and flowers calms the nervous system and returns the whole body to balance.

Treatment Outline

Follow the treatment steps for the relaxation stone massage.

Essential Oil Blends

The therapist can choose to use one of the blends described here for the massage oil and one blend for the body mist to provide an interesting smell-scape for the client.

Symmetry

2 fl oz of carrier product, frankincense (5 drops), mandarin (10 drops), rose (1 drop), sweet birch (3 drops), clove (1 drop)

Body Boost

2 fl oz of carrier product, grapefruit (10 drops), neroli (2 drops), myrrh (6 drops), helichrysum (1 drop)

Botanical Balance

2 fl oz of carrier product, lavender (10 drops), patchouli (4 drops), rosemary (3 drops), sweet orange (14 drops)

Fatigue Fighter

2 fl oz of carrier product, rosemary (4 drops), geranium (2 drops), lemon (15 drops), cardamom (8 drops)

Solar Stone Glow: 90 Minutes

Promotional Description

The warmth of the sun is felt in the luxurious weight of hot stones placed strategically on the body. The stones, like liquid heat, glide over the skin and relax tight muscles. After the massage, a sensuous polish is applied to the skin, leaving a radiant glow and a soul alight.

Treatment Outline

Follow the treatment outline for the relaxation stone massage with the following addition. Massage the area with stones and then add a body polish product to the skin. Work this in with the stones and then remove the polish with hot towels. It is important that the polish has an emollient base to protect the skin from overexfoliation. The therapist should only use light strokes with the stones during the polish phase.

Summary

In stone massage, both hot and cooled stones can be combined with various massage techniques to produce a unique treatment that can be adapted to meet each client's needs. Stone massage can be given for relaxation, injury rehabilitation, energy balance, deep tissue, and reflexology work. It can also be incorporated into other spa treatments as an accent or to provide textural variety. Similar to regular massage, hot stone massage increases circulation and lymph flow. Because of the heat involved in the treatment, the body tends to react more strongly to stone massage. This usually results in a deep muscular release, deep relaxation, and a decrease of stress. Specialized approaches to stone massage often evolve as therapists begin to experiment with the stones using them to replicate and extend their existing massage techniques. Stone massage techniques can be used in a variety of situations and will introduce the earth element into any treatment.

REVIEW QUESTIONS

Multiple Choice

1. Placement stones are used to:
   a. Warm a body area by being placed on the client
   b. Facilitate deeper breathing when placed on the belly
   c. Draw the client's awareness to an area of tension to facilitate relaxation
   d. All of the above

2. Working stones refer to:
   a. Stones that are used for deep tissue techniques only
   b. Stones that are placed on areas of tension
   c. Stones used in the late subacute stage of inflammation for cross-fiber friction techniques
   d. Stones that are held in the therapist's hands during a massage technique

3. A stone vascular flush refers to:
   a. A hot pack held down with stones
   b. A cold pack held down with stones
   c. One hot stone and one cold stone run over a body area at the same time
   d. All of the above

4. Stones included in a spa treatment introduce the:
   a. Sea element
   b. Sky element
   c. Water element
   d. Earth element

5. Hot stones should never be heated hotter than:
   a. 120°F
   b. 130°F
   c. 135°F
   d. 140°F

Fill in the Blank

6. List three contraindications to hot stone massage:
   _____, _____, and _____

7. List three indications for hot stone massage
   _____, _____, and _____

8. The therapist should always wear _____ during the treatment in case the client moves suddenly, sneezes, or coughs and sends the placement stones flying.

9. Hot stones should never be placed directly onto the client's _____. Instead, a drape should be used to provide some insulation.

10. Essential oils can be used with hot stone massage at low concentrations. This ensures that the oils will not cause _____ with heat.

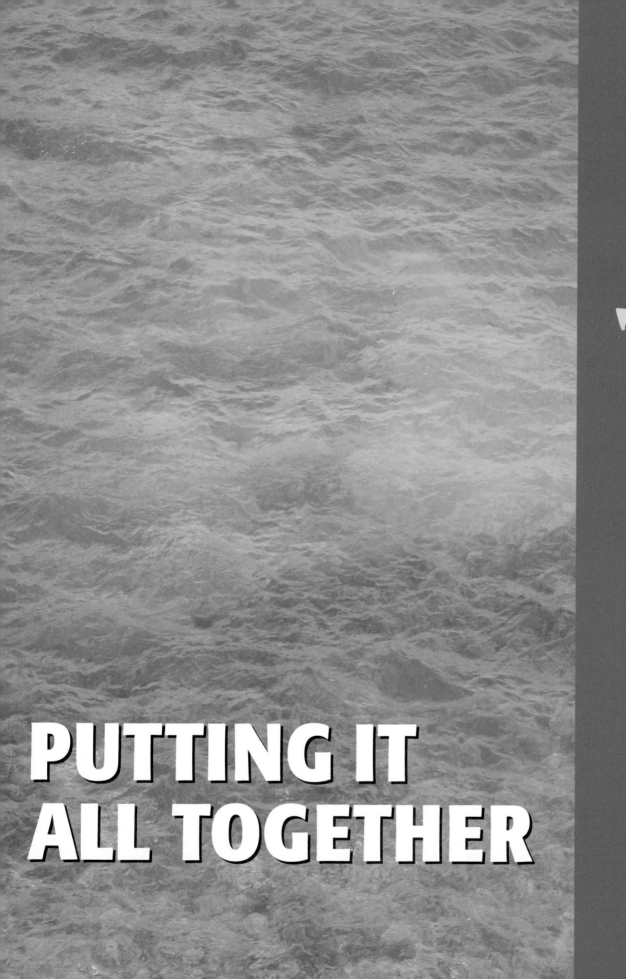

PUTTING IT ALL TOGETHER

Treatment Design and the Signature Spa Treatment

CHAPTER 13

Chapter Outline

INDIVIDUAL TREATMENT DESIGN
    The Therapeutic Goal
    Finding Inspiration Through a Treatment
    Concept
    Treatment Texture
    Enhancing Treatments
    Transitions
    Product Planning
    Client Management
    Retail Sales as Part of the Treatment
    Treatment Planning Forms
    Considerations When Pricing Services

THE SIGNATURE SPA TREATMENT

SUMMARY

Key Terms

Menu: A spa menu is like a menu at a restaurant. It lists all of the services that a client could "order" when visiting.

Signature spa treatment: A special treatment that is only offered by one spa. It is designed to highlight the spa's unique features and particular strengths.

Spa philosophy: The fundamental beliefs that an individual or business holds about health, wellness, and beauty. The spa philosophy might also include a consideration of the clients that the therapist would like to work with and the environment where he or she wants to practice.

Spa program: Collectively, all of the different services that are offered at a spa.

Treatment concept: An abstract idea that helps both to organize the different parts of a treatment and to send a specific message to the client.

Textural elements: The word "texture" describes the varied sensations the therapist creates during the treatment by paying attention to what the client sees, hears, smells, tastes, and feels.

Imagine for a moment that body treatments are pieces of performance art. With careful planning, a spa experience can be very similar to classical theater. Each moment of a play (treatment) is broken down, examined, staged, practiced, smoothed, and memorized by the artist (therapist). On opening night, the audience (client) is unaware of the intense planning that went into the piece (treatment). Instead, the audience is dazzled by what they see, moved by different sensations, revitalized by what they smell, and intrigued by what they hear. The play (treatment) feels alive, spontaneous, free flowing, and effortless, when, in fact, it has a carefully designed structure. If the director (spa designer) has successfully achieved his or her vision, the audience (client) leaves feeling revived and satisfied.

All spa businesses, regardless of size or financial status, can achieve "art" with their services. A big spa with a large budget might hire a spa consultant who will do the planning and train the staff for them. A smaller massage clinic or day spa is more likely to do it all themselves. Each designer has his or her own method for achieving the spa's goals. The process is dynamic, layered, and exciting. At times, it can feel overwhelming because most plans need revision and flexibility. The goal of this chapter is to encourage therapists to reflect on the artistic elements of spa treatments and to provide a framework for the creative design of original spa services.

Individual Treatment Design

The process of designing an individual spa service frequently begins with a reflection on the **spa's philosophy**. A spa philosophy is defined as the fundamental beliefs that the individual or business holds about health, wellness, and beauty. The treatment designer wants to uphold the spa's philosophy with each treatment created for the spa. Often, a complete **spa program** is adopted before the individual treatments are planned (Table 13-1). This allows the designer to balance the services on the **menu** so that one area does not dominate another (e.g., the spa ends up with three body polish treatments and only one body wrap treatment). The spa philosophy, spa program, and spa menu are discussed in greater detail in Chapter 14, which relates closely to this chapter.

The development of each treatment goes through the same design process. First, the therapeutic goal of the treatment is decided and matched against the spa's philosophy. A concept may be adopted to inspire the **textural elements** that add richness and depth to the service. Core treatments are matched with smaller enhancing services before appropriate spa products and retail opportunities are identified. Finally, the treatment is practiced many times so that the designer can smooth transitions, recognize and eliminate problems, and determine how clients will be managed from the time of their arrival at the spa until their departure.

THE THERAPEUTIC GOAL

It is helpful if the goal of the treatment is clearly defined before beginning the design process. Treatment goals can be physiological (e.g., decreased muscle pain), psychological (e.g., increased contentment), spiritual (e.g., an increased sense of connection to nature), mental (e.g., decreased mental exhaustion and confusion), or a combination of these effects in a more holistic treatment. Holistic treatments are

Table 13-1	Overview of the Design Process	
1. THE FIRST DRAFT MENU	**2. DESIGN THE INDIVIDUAL TREATMENTS**
■ Identify the spa's philosophy. ■ Identify the target client. ■ Determine the spa program. ■ Identify specific services.	■ Define the therapeutic goals of the treatment. ■ Find inspiration. ■ Plan textural elements. ■ Plan enhancing treatments. ■ Plan transitions. ■ Plan product and retail tie-ins. ■ Create a signature treatment.
3. PLAN CLIENT MANAGEMENT	**4. THE MENU REVISION**
■ Greeting and pretreatment. ■ Client management during the treatment. ■ Presentation of retail items. ■ Payment and rescheduling.	■ Check for balance and continuity. ■ Write strong promotional descriptions. ■ Determine what you will charge for each treatment.

* The spa philosophy, spa program, and spa menu are discussed in greater detail in Chapter 14 which relates closely to this chapter. This chapter is focused predominantly on part 2 of the design process: design of the individual treatments.

designed to consider all aspects of a client's mental, physical, and spiritual health.

A treatment usually tries to achieve three to six therapeutic goals, with some goals being more important than others. For example, in an herbal detoxification wrap, the primary goal of the service is detoxification, so the body should perspire profusely. The client may feel so hot that he or she is uncomfortable to the point of being mildly agitated. Some degree of relaxation needs to be sacrificed to achieve an effective level of detoxification. If relaxation as well as detoxification is the goal, the therapist would be more likely to base the treatment design on a lymphatic dry brush and deep tissue massage. These treatments encourage the body to eliminate wastes but are more relaxing to receive than a detoxification wrap.

FINDING INSPIRATION THROUGH A TREATMENT CONCEPT

A **treatment concept** is an abstract idea that helps to connect all of the different aspects of the treatment so that together they convey a specific message to the client. Both

the treatment concept and the spa's philosophy must be carefully coordinated so that they do not conflict. The inspiration for a treatment concept can be drawn from any aspect of life, but in this chapter, art, world culture, spirituality, mysticism, simplicity, and food and drink are explored.

Art as Inspiration

What would a treatment based on Claude Monet's painting *Les Tuileries, Esquisse* (The Tuileries Study, 1876) be like (Fig. 13-1)? The Tuileries is a French garden that is the most central park in Paris. Designed by Le Notre (the gardener of Louis XIV) in 1664, it is a place filled with shady walks, fountains, and elegant statues. The painting by Monet was composed using soft greens and a gentle orange haze, as if the sun were ready to set. A designer would want the spa treatment to capture the early evening feel of the painting. This is a time when people are finished with work and lounge in a café sipping iced coffee before heading home. Paris is famous for being one of the most refined and fashionable cities in the world. The treatment would want to borrow that feeling of sophistication and the edgy,

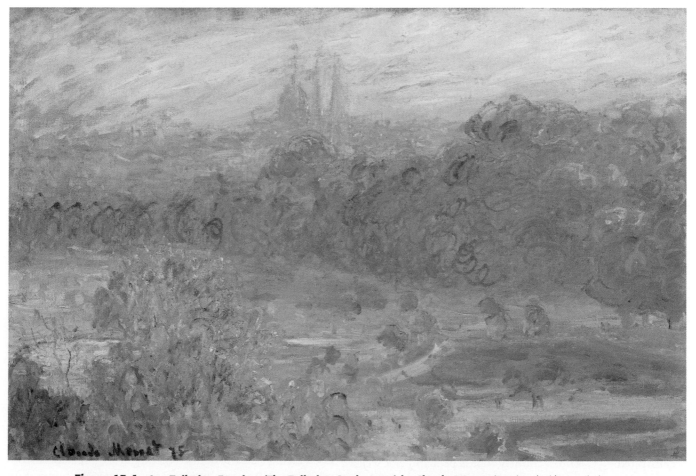

Figure 13-1 *Les Tuileries, Esquisse* **(The Tuileries, Study, 1876) by Claude Monet.** (Reprinted with permission from The Bridgeman Art Library.)

free-spirited grace of young Parisian women. This is not a treatment in which the therapist would stack stones on the client or burn incense. It should be a treatment in which the client can enjoy traditional elegance in the form of a rose petal foot bath, a paraffin dip for the hands, a European firming face massage, an emollient body polish, and a firming breast mask.

Compare this treatment with one inspired by the novel *One Hundred Years of Solitude* by Nobel Prize winner Gabriel Garcia Marquez. Marquez weaves a magical tale of the Buendia family living in the mythical town of Macondo. Birth, death, love, sadness, rage, passion, joy: all of the human emotions are explored and leave the reader with a deeper understanding of what it means to be alive. This one is more difficult, but it seems reasonable that a treatment based on *One Hundred Years of Solitude* would have spiritual and emotional aspects and would require a variety of contrasting textures. This treatment might include a vigorous eucalyptus loofah scrub, a thick application of alabaster kaolin clay with tingling oils such as rosemary and bay laurel, a relaxing hot stone massage, and Lomi Lomi stretches. Paintings, books, songs, poems, and movies each give a different feeling and help the designer to generate ideas to develop a treatment.

World Culture as Inspiration

Many spas draw on different world cultures to formulate their philosophy and inspire their treatments. The Mii Amo Spa at Enchantment Resort in Sedona, Arizona, uses the red rock landscape and Native American traditions of the Sedona area as an inspiriation.[1] Treatments that link to these concepts include the Blue Corn Polish and Sedona Clay Wrap. The "Connect with Spirit" section of the menu offers the Mii Amo Meditation in which clients are "smudged" with a sage stick at the beginning of the service. "Smudging" is a traditional Native American practice in which smoke from a branch of sagebrush or juniper is wafted over a person to purify and protect them.

Eastern and particularly ayurvedic influences are currently very popular in the spa industry. This is probably because Eastern cultures have well-designed and time-honored healing systems that are already valued by Westerners. Eastern culture also has a particular environmental style that consists of clean lines and simple, elegant beauty. This style is appealing to the senses and allows the treatment creator to use a room design that supports the concept of the treatment.

Although Eastern culture is popular, any culture can be used as a starting point to stimulate fresh ideas and offer new insights for treatment design. The designer must simply find out something about the country and let the information guide the treatment choices. The example below was inspired by Gabon, a country that is probably not well known to most Americans. This unfamiliarity gives it an intriguing appeal.

Treatment Name: Eshira: The Night Ceremonies. Located on the west coast of Africa, most of Gabon is covered in dense equatorial rain forests, although the coastal plain is characterized by narrow lagoons and estuaries. The Gabonese consist of 40 Bantu tribes, which are divided into four different tribal groups. The Eshira are a Bantu group who hold "Night Ceremonies," which are meant to bring the tribe together into "only one heart," through singing, dancing, and the use of hallucinogenic plants. The Eshira people trade in many natural products that may be useful in a spa treatment. These include bananas, cassava, cocoa, coffee, palm oil, rice, and sugar cane.[2]

The Night Ceremonies are about celebration, feeling connected to the earth, and reinforcing relationships. The treatment is carried out in a darkened room, lit only by candles. It begins with rain forest night sounds and then evolves into a 30-minute massage choreographed specifically to an uplifting and rhythmic piece of African music. The massage should fit the music perfectly and evoke the spirit of African dance (tribal unity). The music then transitions back into the sounds of a rain forest. During the rain forest segment, the body is polished with palm oil, sugar, and cocoa powder. This is then either removed with steamy towels or in a Vichy "rain" shower. While the feet are being massaged (relationships), heated stones are placed over specific areas of the body to invoke earth energies. The music then transitions back into the African music and "dance massage" for the final 30 minutes of the treatment. The service ends with an aromatic mist of rain forest scents.

Spirituality and Mysticism as Inspiration

Some spas embrace a mystical philosophy and tie their services into a broad-based spiritualism. This is sometimes handled in a serious way and sometimes in a funky, offbeat way. Serious treatments may include services such as Reiki, guided meditation, yoga, shirodhara, and psychologically oriented aromatherapy. Spas may consider using mythology, ancient goddesses, or sacred places to inspire unique treatments.

For a more offbeat, mystical concept, the spa might base the design of all of their services on the zodiac or on forms of divination such as tarot cards, rune stones, or Ogham symbols. It is a fun idea. Consider designing all of the spa's services on the zodiac; each of the treatments could be tailored to one of the sun signs. If you are a Pisces, you would probably receive a seaweed treatment because Pisces is a water sign. Capricorns are ruled by the earth element, so they would probably opt for a mud treatment or hot stone massage. Geminis would get an aromatherapy treatment to balance their split personalities! It is important to remember that this type of spa fits a niche market. This can hurt or help a spa depending on the location and the type of clientele. Having a clearly defined niche can set a spa apart from other spas in the area but may also restrict the population to which the spa can market its services.

Simplicity as Inspiration

Many spas design their treatments to be as straightforward as possible. The treatment names and descriptions are not particularly evocative, but the client is left in no doubt about what they will receive. In the most generic examples, the treatments are called by their common names such as herbal body wrap, mud wrap, seaweed soak, full-body paraffin mask, body polish, and so on. On the more creative side, a straightforward designer may use the body treatments listed above but add names that suggest their use in specific conditions, such as travel fatigue fighter (seaweed soak), dry skin boost (paraffin mask), stress tonic (mud wrap), body soft (body polish), and so on. In the United States, these straightforward themes are often made to sound more sophisticated by using European place names. For example, an herbal body wrap becomes the Swiss herbs wrap. A seaweed soak may become the Brittany sea algae soak, and a mud mask might become the Italian fango wrap. These basic treatments are very different from the "world spa" already discussed.

Food or Drink as Inspiration

Occasionally, spas develop a treatment based on a type of food or drink in a way that is surprisingly interesting. Consider these treatment names: Orange Sorbet, The Champagne Sparkler, The Manhattan, Crème Brulé, Hot Cider Twist, Strawberries and Cream, Chocolate Mousse, Lime Margarita. A treatment called the Champagne Sparkler conjures up images of cocktail dresses, smooth radiant skin, and bubbly vivacity. A treatment called the Manhattan inspires the same metropolitan appeal, and a treatment named after a chocolate mousse is likely to be decadent, smooth and contain chocolate, which smells wonderful and softens the skin. The Lime Margarita sounds upbeat and sassy and could be expected to include a salt glow.

It is clear that the treatment designer can draw inspiration from a variety of sources and that brainstorming a new treatment is a lot of fun.

TREATMENT TEXTURE

The treatment concept often influences the different treatment textures that are chosen for the service. A good spa treatment includes an assortment of "textures," or layers of varied sensation that enrich the overall experience. To do this, the designer needs to consider what the client smells, feels, hears, sees, and even tastes. This does not mean that the therapist should go to extremes of either hot or cold; rather, it means that the therapist should pay attention to the different textures in products and use those textures to increase the clients' awareness of tactile sensations during the treatment so that they enjoy the treatment more. For example, research indicates that there are four main types of skin receptors that respond to hot, cold, pain, and pressure. But our experience of the world goes beyond these simple sensations because combinations of receptors allow us to feel in vivid and varied detail. Consider all the nuances of sensation. Pain can feel dull, or it can shoot down a nerve path. It can burn or feel like a twinge or pinch. When a kitten licks our skin, it has a wet, scratchy feel. The velvety softness of a horse taking a sugar cube off our hand feels completely different. In *A Natural History of the Senses*,[3] Ackerman explains that:

> Any first time touch, or change in touch (from gentle to stinging, say), sends the brain into a flurry of activity. Any continuous low-level touch becomes background. When we touch something on purpose—our lover, the fender of a new car—we set in motion our complex web of touch receptors making them fire by exposing them to a sensation, changing it, exposing them to another. The brain reads both the firings and the "stop-firings" like Morse code and registers smooth, raspy, cold.

In a spa treatment, the application of each unique product or technique, along with its special texture, awakens the mind and body to the novelty of sensation. The rough scratch of the dry brush; the smooth, all-encompassing warmth of heated mud; the tingly shiver of mint lotion; the delicate flicker of cool mist over a hot forehead; the rapturous scent of orange blossoms: each of these becomes a word in the complex language of enjoyment.

What Will the Client Smell?

Beverley Nichols writes that: "To be overcome by the fragrance of flowers is a delectable form of defeat."[4] Good smells have been used by ancient and modern cultures all over the world for spiritual, emotional, and therapeutic purposes. In a spa treatment, they provide a powerful point of interface between the mind and body by affecting the psyche, nervous system, and immune system.[5] They link a client to the cultural context of treatments that are developed around a foreign theme or ethnicity. They transport the client to the landscape of the treatment, whether it is the desert or ocean, a field, a flower garden, an alpine forest, or an orange grove.

In Chapter 5, the sense of smell and the possible effect of aroma on mood and emotion are discussed, as are the ways in which the client's enjoyment of a service is enhanced through a smell-scape. The concept of a smell-scape encourages the therapist to think carefully about what he or she wants a client to smell during a spa service. The therapist should also change the smells during the treatment to create greater olfactory interest. The smells may be tied to a particular place as in an Eastern-inspired treatment. In this case, the designer uses aromas that are characteristic of the East such as mandarin, ginger, vetiver, and spikenard. The smells might be familiar and comforting like grapefruit, pine needle, and nutmeg, or they could be unexpected and exotic like Peru balsam (it has a velvety, powdery, vanilla-like but darker smell). The important thing is that the smells communicate something about the treatment to clients and facilitate their immersion in the "world" of the service (Table 13-2).

Table 13-2	Themes, Smell-Scapes, Accents, and Associations*	
THEME	**SMELL-SCAPE**	**ACCENTS OR ASSOCIATIONS**
Summer	Citrus oils, floral oils, tropical aromas, spicy oils	Joy, brightness, warmth, openness, strength, the sun, light, tan skin, the beach, ice cream, lemonade, water sports, seaweed treatments, buff and bronze treatments, sunburn treatments
Winter	Peppermint, clove, nutmeg, cinnamon, apple cider, fir needle, pine needle, frankincense	Hibernation, going within, recuperation, the end of a cycle, flannel, hot chocolate, winter sports such as skiing, warm cocoons and body wrap treatments
Spring	Light floral scents, herbaceous scents	New beginnings, opportunities, childlike enthusiasm, renewal of energy, gentle rain, gentle breezes, hydrotherapy treatments such as a Vichy shower
Autumn	Woody scented oils, earthy oils, warm or homey aromas	Slowing down, preparation for quiet and reflection, midnight, the moon, hot cider, apples, dried leaves, wind, warm cocoons and detoxification treatments
Ocean or sea	Camphor, chamomile, eucalyptus, gardenia, helichrysum, jasmine, lemon, geranium, sandalwood, vanilla, ylang ylang	Wisdom, inner peace, harmony, emotional balance, intuition, the subconscious, the moon, guided meditation, seaweed treatments, marine fango treatments, hydrotherapy with seawater, buff and bronze treatments
Desert	Sage, juniper berry, spicy oils	Simplicity, purification, transformation, change, openness, aloe gel, cactus syrup (which can be used in cocoons or as a masking product), sisal fiber cloth for exfoliation, Sedona clay, other desert clays
Forest or alpine	Fir needle, bay laurel, sweet birch, cedarwood, cypress, juniper, pine, spruce, Canadian balsam, cade, oakmoss	Growth, strength, wisdom, shelter, protection, exploration, adventure, flannel, hot cider, foot treatments aimed at hikers, any treatment offered at a ski resort or winter resort
Garden	Floral oils, herbaceous oils	Tranquility, peacefulness, cultivation of manners, refinement, inner beauty, fertility, abundance, botanical products, iced tea, herbal tea, shortbread, tea cake, gentle treatments aimed at relaxation
Jungle or tropical	Ambrette seed, amyris, copaiba balsam, peru balsam, tolu balsam, West Indian bay, cascarilla bark, cassie, clove, elemi, ginger, lime, nutmeg, oakmoss, opopanax, black pepper, rosewood, schinus molle, tagetes, tonka bean, turmeric, vanilla	Instinct, exhilaration, adventure, courage, wildness, impulse, travel, exotic fruits (e.g., mango, papaya, coconut, pineapple), body polish treatments, natural product cocoons
Eastern	Star anise, benzoin, bergamot, calamintha (Himalayas), calamus, camphor, ylang ylang, cardamom, cassia, cinnamon, clove, costus, sweet fennel, galangal, gardenia, ginger, grapefruit, jasmine, lemon, lemongrass, litsea, mandarin, mastic, orange, neroli, palmarosa, patchouli, rose, sandalwood, spikenard, liquidambar, turmeric, vetiver	Peace, harmony, spiritual practice, mindfulness, elegance in simplicity, balance of body, mind, and spirit, cycles of creation, purification, detoxification, meditation, jasmine tea (India), green tea (China), ayurvedic treatments, Chinese herbal treatments

Table 13-2 | *(continued)*

THEME	SMELL-SCAPE	ACCENTS OR ASSOCIATIONS
Mediterranean	Lemon balm, basil, bay laurel, bergamot, cumin, cypress, inula, sweet fennel, helichrysum, hyssop, labdanum, lavender, lemon, sweet marjoram, mastic, myrtle, neroli, orris, rose, rosemary, clary sage, sage, santolina, thyme, lemon verbena	Connection, relationships, exchange of ideas, travel, exploration, culture. The Mediterranean sea is a part of the Atlantic Ocean almost completely enclosed by land. On the north side is Europe, on the south is Africa, and on the East is Asia. In ancient times, the Mediterranean was a byway for trade between the peoples of the region, including the Egyptians, Romans, Greeks, Phoenicians, and Middle Eastern people. Herbal treatments (many herbs are indigenous to the region), seaweed and clay treatments
South or Central American	Cabreuva, Peru balsam, tolu balsam, cardamom (El Salvador, Guatemala), cascarilla bark, guaiacwood, jaborandi, lime, orange, palmarosa, black pepper, rosewood, schinus molle, tagetes, tonka bean, tuberose, vanilla, lemon verbena	Central and South America are regions of environmental and cultural diversity. The environment ranges from the lush tropical rain forests of the Amazon to the high altitude desert of the Andes. This area is the home of the Incas and Mayans, innovative and advanced cultures. It is also a place where the influences of the indigenous peoples are mixed with Spanish, Portuguese, and African people. Any type of treatment could be developed with a Central or South American concept.
Egyptian	Chamomile, cumin, frankincense, calendula, sweet marjoram, myrrh, rose, spikenard	Culture, beauty, innovation, preservation, timelessness, abundance. The Egyptians had an advanced understanding of aromatic plants and how to use them for beauty, spiritual connection, and preservation of tissue. Other associations include gods and goddesses, lotus flowers, art, any treatments aimed at renewal.
Earth element	Earthy aromas, musky aromas, woody aromas, green aromas	Home, survival, the mother, solid and steadfast, heavy, weighty, core, true self, stone massage, clay, mud, peat treatments, natural elements cocoons
Air element	Citrus oils, oils with a light or fresh aroma, oils with a powdery aroma	Breath, mental processes, communication, wisdom, understanding, wit, light treatments, dry treatments, treatments that include movement
Fire element	Spicy oils, carnation absolute, atlas cedarwood, cinnamon, clove, frankincense, myrrh, neroli, rosemary	Passion, creativity, transformation, purification, death and rebirth, truth, spicy foods, lemon and ginger tea, detoxification treatments, hot stone massage
Water element	Camphor, chamomile, eucalyptus, gardenia, helichrysum, jasmine, lemon, geranium, sandalwood, vanilla, ylang ylang	Emotion, intuition, the female, the flow of life, rebirth, subconscious, inner clarity, receptivity to new ideas, hydrotherapy treatments, seaweed

* Associations with different themes, words, ideas, or places are subjective and should not be taken as fact. This table is meant to provide one example of ways to investigate themes during treatment design. It is meant to remind therapists to have fun and explore ideas before settling on one way of working. The treatments indicated under some of the associations are just suggestions and should not limit the therapist in any way. For example, there is no reason that a treatment inspired by winter could not be paired with a buff and bronze treatment. Perhaps the whole idea of the treatment is to invoke summer in the midst of cold and snow (e.g., "Missing the sun? Our buff and bronze treatment will leave you relaxed and feeling sunny. . . ."). Table 5-4 provides lists of oils in basic scent categories and should be used in combination with the smell-scapes provided here.

When providing a smell-scape, the therapist should make every effort to use products with natural as opposed to synthetic fragrances or to scent plain products in house with high quality, therapeutic-grade essential oils. Synthetic fragrances do not come from aromatic plants, fruits, or flowers. Clients often develop adverse reactions (e.g., headaches, sore throat, sneezing, coughing, and emotional irritation) to synthetic fragrances and may avoid all strong aromas as a result.

What Will the Client Feel?

Therapists who pay attention to the texture of a spa treatment usually plan every tactile sensation that the client experiences. As soon as the client is on the treatment table, the therapist will want the client to be enveloped by warm, soft textures. This is not easy if the client is lying on plastic during the treatment. One idea is to put a Fomentek (large hot water bottle) under a pillowcase (to insulate it) under the plastic sheeting. A soft bath towel can also be placed horizontally across the top and bottom of the table to anchor the plastic sheeting and provide a soft place for the upper body and feet to rest. Regardless of the type of treatment bedding used, it can and should be warm before the client gets onto the table.

With the exception of those products that are meant to be applied cool, every product should be warmed just before it is applied. Cold mud, cold lotion, cold anything is jolting and distracting. Cool temperatures alternating with very warm temperatures can feel refreshing and invigorating under the right circumstances. Think about the tactile sensations experienced in a dry room salt glow. First, the client is massaged with warm oil using soothing Swedish strokes. Salt is then applied in rhythmic circular strokes. This feels scratchy and rough but very pleasurable and invigorating. A hot towel (it should be nice and hot, not lukewarm) is placed on the body area and left for a few seconds to steam the skin. It is then pressed into the skin by the therapist (which increases the sensation of heat) and pulled in a straight line from the proximal to distal areas of the body to remove the salt.

To add a new sensation, the therapist can mist the area with a toner. This feels bracing and stimulating, and if the right product is used, it will balance the pH of the skin. Another texture can be added by applying an aloe gel after the body mist. Aloe gel goes on in a satiny smooth layer. It will not make the client sticky, and it gives a final textural sensation before the therapist moves on to the next body area.

Although this may all seem like common sense, it is easy to use an inappropriate product in a treatment. For example, in an herbal detoxification wrap, the client feels very hot and continues to perspire after being removed from the thermal blankets. A massage with oil at this point would feel unpleasant, but a body mist with cool water followed by the application of a light cucumber, aloe, or seaweed gel will decrease body temperature and replace moisture without making the skin feel clogged. Usually, an exfoliation comes first in a treatment, but there is no reason that a therapist could not end an herbal wrap with an invigorating and cool-ing grapefruit scrub. This will cool the client, contribute to the treatment goals, and give a pleasing textural variation.

One of the problems with the delivery of spa services in a wet room is that the area is often completely covered in tiles and feels cold. Vichy showers can splash on a client's face if the Plexiglas face guard is not adjusted properly and sometimes the first blast of the water from the showerheads is jolting. All of these things affect the pleasure of the experience, so therapists must plan treatments carefully to minimize these disruptions.

What Will the Client Hear?

When planning a treatment, the auditory environment is also important to consider. The wrong sort of music is likely to be disturbing and irritating to the client. Most therapists have probably encountered "spa" or "massage" CDs that were downright alarming. One on the market features wolves howling incessantly in every song. It would be difficult for a client to relax if he or she felt like prey!

The right music can evoke strong feelings and enhance the service. In the treatment inspired by the Eshira tribe from Gabon (The Night Ceremonies treatment), the music is a central and pivotal element. The treatment begins with a massage choreographed to African music. As the music changes into rain forest sounds, the treatment also moves on to the body polish section, a new tactile experience. When the music changes back to an African rhythm, the treatment moves with it, and the body is massaged again. Pairing music with specific massage strokes and product applications creates a powerful and evocative service. This is spa theater!

There is no need to feel restricted about the types of music that can be used. The music does not have to be of the minimalist and often chime-ridden background "spa" variety. Instead, it should always be chosen to fit the mood of the treatment. An example is a buff and bronze treatment that was delivered at a beachfront spa in New Jersey that had a funky style of décor, treatment names, and staff attire. Instead of regular "spa music," the therapist played the Beach Boys during the service. This is a perfect and creative complement to an autotanning service and encouraged clients to take pleasure in the fun of the moment.

What Will the Client See?

The visual texture of the treatment is probably the most difficult aspect to achieve because it requires that the décor of the treatment room is changed to match the services being offered. Sometimes all of the treatments can be carried out in rooms with a common décor style as in an ayurvedic spa, which would use cultural flourishes from India, or a desert spa that uses Native American designs. The form of visual texture used usually depends on the therapist's skill and attention to detail. Details can include flowers floating in the foot soak basin or tucked into the fold of the linens on the treatment table, decorative Japanese lanterns lit for an

Eastern-inspired treatment, or the splash of a brightly colored throw for a treatment inspired by summer. At the very least, the treatment room should be clean and organized with the spa products attractively displayed on the work table.

What Will the Client Taste?

The Bantu tribe (the tribe of people who inspired the Eshira Night Ceremonies treatment) believes that handing food between two people creates a "clanship of porridge." Food is celebratory. Children commemorate their birthdays with ice cream parties, cake is eaten at weddings, special friends are invited over for meals, and the first threads of true love are often experienced over a romantic dinner. When carefully chosen food items are used in a spa treatment, an ancient subconscious message is sent to the client. As Diane Ackerman writes in *A Natural History of the Senses*:

> Our friends offer us food, drink. It is a symbolic act, a gesture that says: This food will nourish your body as I will nourish your soul. In hard times, or in the wild, it also says I will endanger my own life by parting with some of what I must consume to survive. Those desperate times may be ancient history, but the part of us forged in such trials accepts the token drink and piece of cheese, and is grateful.

With culturally inspired treatments, the use of a traditional food item helps to envelop the client in the world of the service. This might be as simple as a cup of green tea served from a Chinese tea set before an Eastern-inspired treatment or a complementary chocolate on Valentine's Day or at the end of a couple's massage. Similarly, the therapist could plan a sports drink to be served at the end of a sore muscle sports wrap. In the summer, clients can leave the seaweed treatment with a colorful Popsicle to remind them of the "at the beach" feel of the service. Therapists are reminded to keep it simple enough to be manageable but to hold in their minds the intention of the offering: to welcome; to nourish on a spiritual level; and to show care, thoughtfulness, and appreciation.

ENHANCING TREATMENTS

Enhancing treatments are accent pieces that add value to the service and make it feel special. They are not large enough to constitute a service on their own, but when added to the main treatment, they act as moments of particular "radiance." In a basic massage, a therapist who pays attention to detail might add one or two enhancers. The therapist might perhaps place a hot, steamy rosemary towel on the client's back before beginning the back massage. The therapist may repeat this process with a hot, steamy rosemary towel on each foot before the foot massage and on the face before the face massage. This feels wonderful, smells wonderful, and is an unexpected treat. The steamy towel enhancer is simple enough not to cut into the client's massage time, but special enough to stand out in the client's mind as a valuable part of

the treatment. The simple addition of hot towel steams and aromatherapy mists to a treatment often increases client loyalty and may become so popular at a clinic that they are adopted as standard practice in every massage.

Small food items can be used to provide accents to a treatment, as mentioned previously, or to help smooth transitions from one section of a service to the next. It is sometimes necessary for the client to receive a service from one therapist and then move to a second therapist for the rest of the treatment. In such cases, the client can be moved to a chair in the treatment room and served with a small plate of simple appetizers while the first therapist makes sure that the second therapist is on schedule and ready to take over the client's treatment. For long treatments or for treatments that accelerate detoxification, a drink is as much a necessity as a nicety. The same is true for spa packages in which the client is undergoing a series of treatments. Some time must be planned for the client to stop, rest, and have a snack.

Non–spa-oriented activities can also be planned to accompany a service and enhance the treatment. In the discussion of the spa treatment concept, the idea of using a Zodiac sign to inspire a treatment was described. A creative designer might arrange for the client to receive his or her horoscope printed on nice paper, rolled up, and tied with nice ribbon at the end of the service. In an upscale spa, the designer might pair sterling silver charms with treatments. Each treatment could have its own charm, which the client receives at the end of the service. These little extras are not strictly necessary, but they add to the overall experience of the client and the perception of the spa.

TRANSITIONS

Transitions are the moments between the steps of a treatment. There are small transitions such as the transition between the application of a product (e.g., an exfoliant) and its removal with hot towels, and larger transitions such as the movement of the client from the treatment table to the Swiss shower. Transitions are the parts of the treatment that are the most likely to feel disjointed if they are not carefully planned. For example, if the removal of a product with hot towels has not been carefully planned, the therapist may find that he or she has to walk over to the hot towel cabbi to get a towel out for the removal. A better option is to have some hot towels in a soda cooler that can be carried around the table with the therapist. This way, the therapist simply reaches down and grabs a towel and then progresses to the next step of the service.

One of the most difficult transitions in a dry room is the removal of plastic from underneath the client after a cocoon. First, the treatment product has to be removed quickly so that the client does not get cold. At the same time, the plastic sheeting that is under the client must be rolled up and removed. The messy product cannot be allowed to get onto the clean sheet that is under the plastic. This is not something that can be done smoothly without practice.

Another aspect of the transition to consider is the communication that needs to occur between the client and therapist. The therapist should practice the language that he or she will use to move the client between the different steps of the treatment. Clients are often in a deeply relaxed state and become confused if the therapist does not explain things clearly and concisely. This is important because poor communication can result in the need to have the client adjust position on the treatment table. If the client is told exactly how to position on the treatment table, it will save the client from feeling that he or she has to move in one direction or another to accommodate the treatment.

PRODUCT PLANNING

Every product that is used in a spa treatment needs to be carefully chosen and evaluated for its suitability. To find spa products, therapists might do searches on the Internet and review spa supply websites. They might also visit other spas as part of their market research and find out what products those spas use. A number of spa suppliers can be found in the resources section at the back of the book.

Before ordering a product, it is a good idea to call the supplier and ask for an ingredient list if one is not readily available. Assess the ingredients and check the information on each provided in an ingredient dictionary such as the *Skin Care and Cosmetic Ingredients Dictionary* by Natalia Michalun.[6] If the product is acceptable, it should be ordered in its smallest size (sometimes a sample size can be ordered) and tested by the therapist to ensure that it works well before large quantities are ordered.

Designers are often faced with the dilemma of not being able to find suitable spa products for their original treatments. In this case, they have to modify an existing product or make a new product in house. Both options can work but are not ideal because they require extra time and planning by the spa staff. More and more suppliers are offering base products that spas can modify to fit their needs. Some offer premade essential oil blends for quick smell-scapes. Although this is a positive move that allows for greater creativity in treatment design, spa suppliers often use a substandard aromatherapy product. Designers are advised to check their essential oil sources carefully or preferably buy their essential oils from an aromatherapy supplier that sells therapeutic-grade oils instead.

CLIENT MANAGEMENT

Good client management leads to good client retention, so client management activities should be built right into the plan for the individual service. The client's path through the clinic or spa must be premeditated, and every effort must be made to pamper the client from the moment he or she first contacts the spa. The receptionist must be friendly, upbeat, and knowledgeable. He or she needs to know all about each of the services that the spa offers and should have received each service on the treatment menu at least once. This way, the receptionist will be ready for any question that the client may have about the treatment. The receptionist should also practice describing a treatment in a way that is captivating yet clear and concise. If the receptionist describes a salt glow simply as a treatment in which "salt is rubbed on the body," he or she will obviously need to be coached in order to express the intention and feeling of the treatment more clearly.

The spa should plan what happens when a client walks through the door. How will the client be greeted? Some spas have a changing room with lockers for the client's belongings, where clients can change into a robe and slippers before beginning a treatment. The client may then be taken to a quiet room and served herbal tea while his or her feet rest in a foot soak and the health history intake form is completed. In a smaller clinic or spa, the client may simply be given the necessary paperwork on a clipboard and asked to wait in the reception area. The main thing is that the client should be treated warmly, professionally, and efficiently.

Pampering activities include offering a beverage while the client fills in paperwork, providing a snack during longer sessions, and allowing the client to relax at the end of a session instead of feeling pressured to get up and move on. Pampering might begin with a complementary foot soak or paraffin dip with every service. The treatment table should be warm and inviting with good-quality linens and special treats such as thick fleece padding and a heated gel face cradle lining. Warm packs, eye pillows, inviting scents, and relaxing lighting add to the sensation of luxury.

After the treatment has started, the client should never be left alone. If the client is wrapped, receiving hydrotherapy, or sitting in a sauna or shower, the therapist should always be within earshot. To leave a client is not only unprofessional—it is dangerous. For this reason, the therapist must be completely prepared for the session before it begins. The use of checklists for equipment and products ensures that the therapist is not hunting for the finishing lotion halfway through the treatment.

How the session ends is as important as the session itself, and it must be planned just as carefully. In one example, a client had a facial at a well-known and highly regarded spa that flawlessly handled sales of the retail line and the process of paying for the service. After the treatment, the client was taken to the spa "shop" where café tables were set up in a softly lit room. Spa products on glass shelves lined the café's exterior. Other clients sat enjoying herbal teas or lemonades and glancing through the spa's product brochures and fashion magazines. The client was offered a glass of lemonade with a small plate of bread, cheese, and fresh fruit and then handed a product brochure. After a few moments, an elegant young woman walked up and asked if the client had any questions. She addressed the client by name and informed her that her esthetician had mentioned that she had very sensitive skin and would respond well to a particular product. A sample was offered, and the line was so well described that instead of buying just the night cream, the client bought the whole sensitive skin care line.

The purchase was placed in an attractive bag, and a bill was brought to the table and presented in a leather folder (just as the bill would be presented at a fine restaurant). The client put her credit card in the folder and enjoyed her magazine and lemonade while the elegant young woman took the credit card to the front desk for processing. The client left the spa having spent far more than she intended, but very happy with the service.

Although most massage clinics and even many day spas do not have the space or staff available to handle the payment as described above, there is much that can be learned from such an experience. How the spa presents the retail items available and how the staff handles the payment for the service in a way that is relaxing and elegant are very important. Having to stand in line to ask the receptionist a question about a particular product or waiting to pay for your service is not ideal. The spa must develop a clear plan for handling clients and communicate this plan to its staff. The staff should practice moving clients from the reception area, to the treatment room, and then to the retail area. Work out how to smooth the payment process. Some clinics stagger treatment room schedules so that they are 15 minutes apart. This way, the receptionist only has one client at a time to deal with. This seems an easy and workable option for most clinics or spas.

RETAIL SALES AS PART OF THE TREATMENT

In Chapter 14, retail sales are discussed as an important contribution to the financial stability of the spa business. Retail sales must be handled in such a way that they do not mar the relaxation experienced during the treatment. If a client feels pressured to buy something that they do not want or need, the whole spa experience will be ruined. Instead, sales of spa products should be built into the treatment itself so that it feels like a natural extension of the treatment and is not jarring.

To take advantage of retail opportunities during the course of a treatment, therapists must have a solid knowledge of the services and product lines offered by the spa, their benefits, and most importantly, a commitment to hearing the needs of their clients. The products that they attempt to sell the client should be matched carefully to the treatment that the client is receiving and to the client's perceived needs. For example, a client visiting the spa for a slimming and contouring treatment will probably be interested in home care cellulite products that continue the results achieved by the spa treatment. A pregnant woman would probably not be interested in the home care cellulite cream, and the therapist should not attempt to sell it to her. Clients often express their needs while receiving a treatment. The attentive therapist can support the client's healing process by guiding him or her toward products or services that will meet these needs. For example:

- While providing a massage to a client, the therapist learns that the client loves essential oils and would like some custom blending. The therapist suggests that the client visit the resident aromatherapist, who will create the blends that she needs. The therapist also shows the client the line of essential oils and home care blends that the clinic provides and helps the client to make an informed purchase.
- At the end of a buff and bronze treatment, the treatment designer has built in time for the therapist to show the client bronzing home care products and to offer tips on getting a good result at home.
- During a massage, a client expresses doubt that seaweed has any benefits for his body or skin. The knowledgeable therapist outlines some of the research that has been done on the benefits of seaweed and introduces the client to a sea soak product offered for home care in the clinic gift shop. The therapist also shares her experience in receiving the seaweed wrap offered at the clinic and encourages the client to give it a try.
- A massage therapist learns that a client is often sore from working out. The soreness passes after 2 or 3 days but interferes with the client's other activities. The therapist recommends a home care soaking product offered in the spa gift shop that is specifically designed for sore muscles.
- During a foot treatment, the client mentions to the therapist that it is her husband's birthday and that she has run out of gift ideas. The therapist mentions that the hot stone massage offered at the spa is a big favorite with men and that gift certificates are available at the front desk.

In each of these examples, the client was given the time and attention to help him or her make an informed decision about the purchase of a product or service. The therapist also increased his or her income by receiving a commission on the sale.

The most important point is that advice should be offered that is directly linked to the client's needs. This advice should be offered in a professional manner without any pressure so that the mood of the treatment session is not disturbed. The retail process should feel like a natural extension to the treatment itself.

TREATMENT PLANNING FORMS

After the treatment designer has considered all of these areas, he or she is ready to formalize his or her ideas and begin the planning process. The treatment planning form and the example treatment that follows help designers to get started. A blank form is provided in the appendix section at the back of the book. It is best to start with too many ideas and narrow them down in the later stages of development. The first planning form should be used in a brainstorming session, and the second form is worked through to streamline the ideas. The next step is to try to deliver the treatment itself. Complications during delivery lead to changes in the treatment and a third copy of the planning form. The final planning form can be added to the spa's operations manual as a guide for staff members (Figs. 13-2 and 13-3).

TREATMENT PLANNING FORM (with directions)

TREATMENT NAME: Sometimes the treatment will start with a catchy name and sometimes the name will come later in the planning process		
THE SPA'S OVERALL CONCEPT What is the spa's main focus? Is it relaxation? Is it spiritual? Is it health and fitness? Is it skin care and beauty?	**THE SPA'S PRIMARY STRENGTH** Describe the spa's primary strength. For example, the spa may focus on reflexology and its primary strength may be foot treatments.	**THE TREATMENT INSPIRATION** Describe the source you used to inspire the treatment and determine the treatment concept.
THE TREATMENT CONCEPT Very briefly describe the overall concept of the treatment.	**PROMOTIONAL DESCRIPTION** Describe this treatment as you would in the menu. New ideas for a treatment often come when the promotional language is developed.	
TREATMENT GOALS List three to six goals for the treatment. Are the goals physiological, psychological, or both?	**INDICATIONS** List three to six situations for which this treatment would be indicated.	**CONTRAINDICATIONS** List three to six situations for which this treatment would be contraindicated.
CORE TREATMENTS List the core treatments (focus points) that will take place during this service. There may be one focus point or many depending on the size and scope of the service.	**ENHANCERS/EXTRAS** List the enhancers and extras that will be used to round out or accent elements of the treatment.	**RETAIL OPPORTUNITIES** List retail items or opportunities that could be paired with this service.
TEXTURAL ELEMENTS		
SMELL-SCAPE List the scent combinations that will be used to create olfactory texture for the treatment.	**MUSIC/SOUND** List the music or sounds that will be used to add auditory texture to this treatment.	**VISUAL ELEMENTS** List any special visual elements that will be used to enhance this treatment.
SUPPLIES AND EQUIPMENT		
PRODUCT CHOICES List the products that will be used for the treatment and any modifications that must be made.		**SPECIAL EQUIPMENT** List the special equipment that will be required to deliver this treatment.
TREATMENT/TRANSITION/CLIENT MANAGEMENT STEPS		**NOTES**
List the treatment steps, transition steps, and client management steps required in the delivery of this treatment.		Make notes as new ideas occur to you.

COMMENTS: The therapist uses the comments section to briefly describe how the first or second run-through went. These comments will be read directly before the second or third run-through so that improvements can be made to the treatment.

Figure 13-2   Treatment planning form with directions.

TREATMENT PLANNING FORM (example)

TREATMENT NAME: IKEBANA FLOWERS RITUAL

THE SPA'S OVERALL CONCEPT	THE SPA'S PRIMARY STRENGTH	THE TREATMENT INSPIRATION
Eastern bodywork and spiritual practices. To date, the spa has not focused on indulgence, slimming, or a relaxation treatment.	Japanese stone massage and a reputation for exceptional bodywork. Even though this is the spa's strength, the focus with this treatment is to find greater balance in the service menu by adding a relaxation and slimming treatment.	Ikebana is the art of Japanese flower arranging (history dates back 7 centuries). In Ikebana, the main aim is to use as few stems and leaves as possible in composing elegant contours that highlight the flower's beauty.

THE TREATMENT CONCEPT

A flower ritual to achieve relaxation, contour, elegance, and harmony.

PROMOTIONAL DESCRIPTION

Inspired by the centuries-old art of Japanese flower arranging, this treatment strives to realize beauty, gracefulness of body, and inner harmony. These ideas are achieved through a massage with fragrant oil, an elegant body polish, and alabaster clay and rose petal mask. Warm Japanese river stones applied to areas of tension complete this flowers ritual, leaving tranquility, perfection of form, and radiance as its result.

TREATMENT GOALS	INDICATIONS	CONTRAINDICATIONS
Increase relaxation and inner peace, firm and contour the body's shape, gentle detoxification	Stress and feelings of disharmony, to feel beautiful and refreshed	Broken or inflamed skin, conditions contraindicated for massage

CORE TREATMENTS	ENHANCERS/EXTRAS	RETAIL OPPORTUNITIES
Massage and full-body polish, kaolin and rose petal mask of the back and breasts, hot stone face massage	Flower-filled foot soak, hot stones placed on the body during the mask phase of the treatment	Sell the Ikebana body polish products (unmodified) as a skin-smoothing trio

TEXTURAL ELEMENTS

SMELL-SCAPE	MUSIC/SOUND	VISUAL ELEMENTS
Single floral scents such as jasmine, rose narcissus, and neroli balanced by Eastern spices such as ginger and turmeric with lemongrass accents.	Simple Japanese flute music will be played very softly throughout the treatment. Chimes will sound once at the beginning of the treatment and once at the end of the treatment.	The treatment room will be lit with Japanese lamps and small candles. The client will enter and see the foot soak prepared with flowers floating on the top of the water. A single flower will be placed on the treatment table.

SUPPLIES AND EQUIPMENT

PRODUCT CHOICES

Body polish: Bamboo and lemongrass body polish modified with a hint of jasmine absolute to introduce the flower theme. Green tea body wash modified with ginger, rose, and mandarin essential oils. Seaweed-based finishing gel modified with a few drops of narcissus and mandarin.

Massage: Warm sesame oil with a few drops of neroli and sweet orange essential oil for the face massage. The massage oil for the body will also include turmeric to add a spicy base note.

Kaolin clay, green tea infused water and ground rose petal mask; this will need to be created in house because it could not be adapted from an existing product.

SPECIAL EQUIPMENT

Hot stones and heating unit

Bamboo and rattan table to hold products

A large Japanese bowl would be ideal for the foot soak.

It would be nice if the client could wear a kimono instead of a robe during the foot soak.

Figure 13-3   Treatment planning form sample.

TREATMENT/TRANSITION/CLIENT MANAGEMENT STEPS	NOTES
1. Greet the client and take him or her to the treatment room. Instruct the client to change into the kimono and slip his or her feet into the flower foot soak. Pour the client a cup of green tea from a Japanese tea set sitting on a small rattan table next to the client's chair. While the client relaxes, conduct the intake interview and describe the treatment to the client. Highlight the Ikebana body polish trio, describe the product benefits, and mention that they are carried for home use in the spa gift store.	*Get a Japanese tea set for the foot soak.
2. Exfoliate the client's feet while they are in the foot soak. Remove the feet from the soak and dry the feet. Explain to the client how he or she should position on the treatment table. Leave the room and collect the hot towels needed for the treatment.	*The mask dried out before it could be applied. It cannot be mixed up and kept warm before the treatment. Hot water will need to be mixed into the mask directly before it is applied.
3. Return and bolster the client. Place a warm pack on the client's feet and place one hand on the sacrum and one hand at the top of the spine. Ask the client to take three deep breaths. Remove the hands from the client's back and ring the chimes once to signify the start of the treatment.	*Add lemongrass to the hot towels to add more olfactory texture.
4. Treat each body area with the following series of steps: 1) Massage the area with the warm sesame or essential oil combination using long, flowing strokes. 2) Apply a small amount of cleanser to the hands and work into lather with hot water. Apply this to the client's body area with long strokes. 3) Apply the body polish directly over the body wash without removing the wash (to save laundry and time). 4) Remove both with a hot towel. When each of these steps has been completed on the posterior body, turn the client into the supine position. Rebolster the client and repeat the massage and exfoliation steps on the anterior body.	*Mixing the mask took too long, and the practice client opened her eyes and looked at me to see what I was doing. I need to find a way to smooth that transition. I will try a hot, steamy towel placed on the face during the second practice run.
5. Mix the clay and rose petal mask. Remove eight hot back stones from the heating unit. Remove the bolster and ask the client to sit up (give the client a glass of spring water to drink to cover this transition). Place hot stones under the client and cover him or her with a bath towel. Place a piece of body wrap plastic over the bath towel. These two steps must happen very quickly or else the transition takes too long. Place plastic gloves on both hands and apply the clay mask to the client's back in a thick layer using one hand. Remove the dirty glove and ask the client to lie back down. Check that the position of the stones is comfortable. Remove and place them in the client's hands.	*Problem: The towels have lemongrass on them, and the lemongrass might irritate the client's facial skin. Try using only one drop of lemongrass placed in the bottom of the soda cooler to decrease a chance of irritation.
6. Apply a thick layer of clay to the upper chest, breasts (optional), and belly of the client with the other hand, which is still gloved. Remove the glove and cover the mask with a piece of plastic sheeting followed by a bath towel. Remove five large placement stones and two palm stones from the heating unit and place them on the belly, anterior charkas points, and the bilateral origins of the pec minor muscles. Oil the palm stones and place them in the client's hands.	
7. Remove eight small stones from the heating unit and sit at the top of the table. Use the stones in a face and neck massage (20 minutes) with the warm aromatic sesame oil. At the end of the face massage, remove the excess oil with facial toner and cover the face with a cool towel. Mist high over the client's face with a rose and mandarin spritz blend.	*The spinal layout stones were placed too high on the first run-through. They interfered with the neck massage. Use six stones instead of eight and end the layout at the bottom of the rhomboid muscles.
8. Remove the stones from the anterior body and use the plastic body wrap to pull some of the clay off the client. Remove the rest of the clay with hot towels. Apply the seaweed finishing gel to the belly, around the breasts, and upper chest. Cover the client and apply finishing gel to the arms and hands. Undrape each anterior leg and apply the gel to the legs. Standing on one side of the client, gently (but quickly) remove the stones from under the client by reaching the hands under the towel and pulling the stones out the sides. Repeat on the other side of the client. Unbolster the client and ask him or her to turn over. Rebolster the client.	*Problem: If the client is very large, the therapist will not be able to get the stones out from underneath him or her.
9. Apply finishing gel to the posterior legs and back with soothing massage strokes. Redrape the back and place a hand on the sacrum and a hand at the top of the spine. Ask the client to take three deep breaths. Ring the chimes once to signify the end of the treatment. Unbolster the client and tell him or her to take as much time as needed to get up from the treatment table. Wait for the client outside the treatment room.	
10. Escort the client to the reception area and offer a glass of water. Check to see how the client feels after the treatment. Inform the client of any areas of tension you found during the massage, or of skin care or body products that might specifically suit the client's needs. Show the client to the spa gift shop if appropriate. Process the client's payment and invite him or her to return.	

COMMENTS: After the first run-through of the treatment, I have identified the areas that need improvement. The main concern is the transition from the massage (the climax of the treatment) to the removal of both the stones and the clay. The practice client commented that the removal of the anterior stones and clay was fine but that it felt strange to her that I reached under her to remove the spinal layout stones. We agreed that it would have been odd to sit her up for a second time to remove the stones. She felt that the initial warmth of the spinal layout was very enjoyable and that she wouldn't remove that part of the treatment even though the transition is a bit awkward. The practice client also commented that she enjoyed all the scents used in the treatment but was disappointed when she found out that the retail products were not scented in the same way as the treatment products. This is a bit of a problem because I could not find products that fit my flower rituals theme and feel that I need to modify the product to make it work. Perhaps some other retail tie-in could be created.

Figure 13-3   (continued)

CONSIDERATIONS WHEN PRICING SERVICES

Part of the development process is deciding what to charge for a treatment. This can be a fairly complex process. In general, the spa or clinic should consider the surroundings first. A full-service day spa with elegant décor and extra support staff can simply charge more than a small massage clinic for the same service. The spa or clinic should also check what competitors with similar facilities are charging and charge a similar amount for their services. When a massage clinic adds spa treatments to its massage menu, it is recommend that spa treatments are priced at about $25 to $40 more than the rate charged for the same amount of massage time. If a 1-hour massage is $50, a 1-hour spa treatment should cost between $75 and $90. The exact difference should be determined by the cost of the products used to deliver the treatment and by the prices offered by the competition for similar treatments. Whereas salt glows can cost as little as $2 to deliver, a Parafango treatment can cost as much as $12 to $15. The product cost will have to be factored into the final cost of the treatment. Figure 13-4 shows an example of how to determine the cost of delivering a treatment. This information will help treatment designers to price the treatments and make accurate budget projections.

The Signature Spa Treatment

A **signature spa treatment** is a special service that is exclusive to the spa where it is being offered. It is developed to highlight the spa's unique features and particular strengths. For example, some spas have access to a local product that has healing associations (e.g., a special botanical ingredient, local mud). The use of this product in a treatment will become the spa's "signature." A spa in a desert setting may offer a cactus syrup wrap using syrup that is produced from the cacti that grow in the region. If the spa uses a local healing mud, it will probably base their signature treatment on the use of this special mud. The spa may also remind its clients that this type of mud application is not available anywhere else. In Seattle, a center of coffee culture and the home of Starbucks, there is a coffee shop on almost every street corner. A number of spas in Seattle developed signature treatments based on coffee in the late 1990s. These coffee treatments appealed to Seattleites' sense of humor and also just happened to be firming for the skin.

The Golden Door Spa in California has a unique and beautiful custom-made labyrinth designed to create a calming and spiritual environment (Fig. 13-5).[7] A labyrinth is a purposeful but meandering path that leads the walker from the edge of the circle to the center of the circle and then back to the edge again. The Golden Door labyrinth consists of a smooth stone path inlaid against the textured surface of a

circle. Set in a natural environment of trees and grass, the labyrinth is lit at night by candles arranged around its edge. This labyrinth was inspired by historical labyrinths that were used to focus the mind and create inner peace. Even though the labyrinth is not an actual body treatment, it could still be considered a special "signature" service.

A good signature treatment captures the overall philosophy of the spa or clinic's approach to health and well being. Spas sometimes call their special treatments "rituals" because the treatment consists of a series of carefully considered actions performed in a specific order. Signature "rituals" tend to combine core treatments (e.g., wrap, polish, massage) with enhancing add-ons such as paraffin dips, hydrotherapy soaks, foot baths, saunas, steam baths, or mini facials. In a standard emollient wrap, the client receives just the wrap and perhaps some small enhancers such as an herbal eye pillow or face massage to round off the session. In a signature "ritual," the body wrap is just one part of a more complex service. The client might start in the sauna, receive a body polish, enjoy the emollient wrap, finish with a massage or facial, and end in the meditation room. In many ways, a signature treatment is similar to a spa package in that it combines a number of different treatments in a single session.

In addition to the unique treatments offered by individual spas, some spas offer signature treatments that are based on a particular product line. Cosmetic companies often create body and facial treatments based on their own skin care products (e.g., Aveda, Decleor). They then provide training to spas on the benefits of their product line and how to use the products in specially designed treatments. Spas offering "signature" treatments using these products effectively act as marketing agents for the company by introducing the public to the skin care line and increasing retail sales of the product.

A signature treatment is a marketing tool used to identify what the spa does best for the clients. All establishments from the small local spa to the larger deluxe day spas, resorts, and international spas can benefit from introducing a signature treatment. This is why the spa's main concept should be carefully considered when developing a signature service. For example, a spa whose motto is "the ultimate desert retreat" will not want its signature treatment to be named "the alpine forest escape." It seems simple, but a search on the Internet shows that a lot of spas have missed this point. This may be because these spas want to do something really different, but they should instead focus on their strengths and do what they are especially good at. A massage clinic that specializes in automobile injury treatment may offer a number of rehabilitation-orientated spa services. Perhaps the spa normally offers a detoxifying herbal body wrap, a balancing aromatherapy wrap, eucalyptus steams, cryogenic sore muscle wraps, and reflexology foot spa treatments. Such a clinic would not want to offer a cellulite treatment for its signature service. This would not appeal to this spa's existing clients, and it would take the focus

STEP 1: Determine a General cost of Overheads

A general cost of overheads can be approximated by adding up all of the costs of running the business each month and then dividing it by the average number of treatments offered or, even better, the number of treatment hours delivered in a month. This will tell you what it costs (in terms of overheads) to deliver a treatment. This amount will vary based on how many actual treatments were delivered in a particular month because some of the running costs will be fixed.

Item	Approximate cost per month
Laundry	$400
Office costs (Internet, office supplies, phone, and so on)	$700
Receptionist(s)	$2880
Rent and utilities (the monthly cost to rent space, electricity, water, and so on)	$1500
Marketing and promotion	$1000
TOTAL	$6480/1440 treatments = $4.50 per treatment

STEP 2: Determine the Product Cost for the Treatment

To determine the product cost for the treatment, the therapist must calculate a unit price for the product and how many units of each product will be required to deliver the treatment. Please note that the prices listed here are appoximate and do not represent an industry standard or norm.

Product/Item	Bulk Price	÷	Bulk Quantity	=	Unit Price	X	Product Quantity	TOTAL
Exfoliation product	$32.00		16 oz		$2.00 per oz		1 oz	$2.00
Gel seaweed	$100.00		1 gal (128 fl oz)		$0.78		5 oz	$3.90
Cosmetic sponges	$25.00		100 per pack		$0.25		2 sponges	$0.50
Plastic body wrap	$129.00		600 feet		$0.21 per foot		6 feet	$1.26
Skin toner	$28.00		16 oz		$1.75		0.5 oz	$0.87
Moisture lotion	$98.00		1 gal (128 fl oz)		$1.30 per oz		2 oz	$2.60
Cellulite cream	$20.00		8 oz		$2.50 per oz		0.25 oz	$0.62
Lavender essential oil (added to moisture lotion)	$27.00		6 mL (one mL = approx 20 drops)		$4.50 per mL = $0.22 per drop		7 drops	$1.54
Rosemary essential oil (added to moisture lotion)	$19.00		6 mL		$3.16 per mL = $0.16 per drop		2 drops	$0.32
								$13.61

STEP 3: Determine the Total Cost of Delivering the Treatment

Add in the compensation amount to the therapist to determine the total cost to deliver the service.

Item	Cost
Overhead	$4.50
Product cost	$13.61
Compensation to therapist (arbitrary amount that does not reflect an industry standard)	$30.00
TOTAL	$48.11

The spa should charge at least $95.00 for this service

Figure 13-4   The cost to deliver a spa treatment.

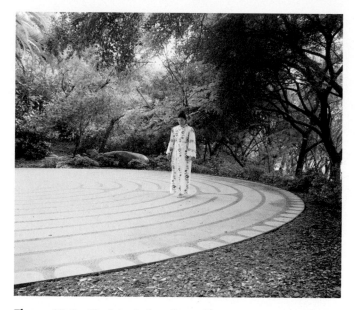

Figure 13-5   The labyrinth at the Golden Door Spa in California.
(Photographer: Rachel Weill. Photo courtesy of the Golden Door Spa, Escondido, CA.)

off what they do best—rehabilitation. Instead, this spa's signature treatment could be a European fango treatment for arthritis or a Parafango treatment for chronic pain conditions and fibromyalgia. Similarly, a salon that is well known for its skin care and esthetics treatments will not want to highlight a treatment for the muscular system.

Summary

Treatment planning is required for every service that is delivered at a spa or a massage clinic. Even basic services such as salt glows require careful consideration. The therapeutic goals of the treatment must be matched to appropriate spa products. The best application method, enhancers, and product removal techniques used will be chosen based on the facility's restrictions or its particular strengths. The environment created in the treatment room—the sights, sounds, and smells that the client experiences—and the way a client is managed during the treatment all require thought. If the treatment is the spa's signature service, it must be clearly developed to express the spa's overall philosophy and approach to health and well being.

REFERENCES

1. Mii amo, a Destination Spa at Enchantment Resort. Available at http://www.miiamo.com
2. Warne S: *Gabon, Sao Tome and Principe.* Chalfont St. Peter, Buckinghamshire, UK: Bradt Publications, 2003.
3. Ackerman D: *A Natural History of the Senses.* New York: Vintage Books, 1995.
4. Pert C: *Molecules of Emotion: The Science Behind Mind-Body Medicine.* New York: Touchstone Books, 1999.
5. Nichols B: *Down the Garden Path.* Cambridge, UK: Timber Press, Inc., 2005.
6. Michalun N, Michalun MV: *Skin Care and Cosmetic Ingredients Dictionary,* 2nd ed. Albany, NY: Milady, Thomson Learning, 2001.
7. The Golden Door Spa. Available at http://www.thegoldendoor.com

REVIEW QUESTIONS

Multiple Choice

1. A good signature treatment will:
   a. Be exclusive to the spa at which it is offered
   b. Highlight a spa's unique features and particular strengths
   c. Promote a line of products or draw attention to a particular amenity
   d. All of the above

2. A spa ritual is best defined as a:
   a. Series of carefully considered actions that are performed in a precise order to lead to a specific state of being
   b. A treatment designed from accepted Eastern practices
   c. A treatment that must have a specific spiritual focus
   d. A spa package that always includes hydrotherapy

3. When designing a signature treatment, the spa or massage clinic will want to:
   a. Focus on doing something really different to "shake up" its current clientele
   b. Focus on using a widely known skin care product because skin care signature treatments sell better than any other type
   c. Focus on a treatment that highlights the spa or clinic's particular strengths, using a treatment that expresses the facility's philosophy of health and wellness
   d. Focus on opulence and price the treatment very high to generate a higher income clientele

4. A treatment concept is:
   a. Either skin care or body care oriented; it is rarely both
   b. Used only in the promotional descriptions of the treatment to the client and has no bearing on the product choices that are made
   c. Must consider the therapeutic goals of the treatment and is used to promote retail sales
   d. Is an abstract idea that helps to coordinate all aspects of a treatment so that it conveys a particular feeling, philosophy, or mental picture to the client

5. An enhancer is best defined as:
   a. The finishing point in a treatment in which the body is misted with an aromatherapy blend
   b. Accent pieces that are not large enough to constitute a service on their own but make the overall service special
   c. The middle section of a treatment in which a paraffin dip, foot bath, or light snack is used to cover the transition to the next section of the treatment
   d. Any type of hydrotherapy treatment that is added onto a service

Matching

Match the smell-scape to the treatment concept

Smell-scape:		Treatment concept
6. Grapefruit, rose	_____	A. Eastern
7. Juniper, fir needle	_____	B. Summer
8. Lavender, rosemary	_____	C. Alpine
9. Frankincense, sandalwood	_____	D. Botanical
10. Ginger, lemongrass	_____	E. Mystical

Careers in Spa

Chapter Outline

Key Terms

Back bar: Spa products often come in two sizes. The larger size is called the back bar and is used by the therapist during the treatment. It is not sold to clients and is not subject to the same labeling requirements as products sold to the public. The smaller size is sold in the retail area for clients to use for home care. It must meet the Food and Drug Administration's labeling requirements for cosmetics.[1]

Marketing: The activities that a business carries out to attract new clients and keep existing clients.

Operations manual: A policy and procedure guide for the spa staff. It lists important information such as contact phone numbers, dress code, and opening and closing procedures.

Price point: The price the public will pay for a retail item. The business must choose how much of a markup they will add to retail items. This markup becomes the price point.

Retail sales: The spa or clinic may choose to buy spa-related items or skin care products at wholesale prices from distributors. They then mark up these items (average: 40% to 50%) and sell them to the public. This provides the spa or clinic with an additional income stream.

Target market: The client group or groups on which the business focuses much of its marketing campaign. Target markets are defined by demographic and lifestyle indicators. The business designs its spa treatments and other services to meet the needs of the target market.

The ability to deliver an exceptional and satisfying spa treatment is a unique skill that combines many elements of holistic practice. Many opportunities and possibilities exist in both the massage and spa industry for massage therapists who are trained in spa therapy (Fig. 14-1). The goals of this chapter are to describe some of these areas, provide tips on finding a suitable first spa job, and provide some useful activities for therapists who want to add spa treatments to their private practice or massage clinic. Many factors must be considered in the launch of a full-service day spa. If this is the goal, the owner or therapist is referred to *Day Spa Operations* by Erica Miller[2]. *Business Mastery* by Cherie M. Sohnen-Moe[3] is also a valuable resource for all health care providers who want guidance on the development of a thriving business and career.[4]

Identify Your Spa Philosophy

There are many ways in which massage therapists might get involved in spa. They may decide to incorporate spa treatments into their private practice or massage clinic; work in the spa industry by offering massage and body treatments at an established spa; continue to develop their skills with

additional training and become spa consultants, spa product representatives, spa educators, or spa directors; or even open a full-service day spa complete with a wet room, esthetic services, nail services, and hair salon. Whatever path is chosen, it is important for each therapist to define his or her personal spa philosophy.

To do this, therapists must first examine the fundamental beliefs that they hold about health, wellness, and beauty. They must also clearly identify what type of clients they want to work with and the environment in which they want to practice spa therapies. These beliefs and the way in which they are ultimately expressed, either in a job interview or in a spa program, reflect the individual's spa philosophy. The self-assessment tasks below are meant to provide a framework for therapists to think about their career in such a way that it leads them to useful and focused actions toward success.

SELF-ASSESSMENT

The first step to identifying a spa philosophy is self-assessment. It is helpful to ask the following questions and answer them as truthfully as possible:

1. What is my personal definition of health and wellness? What actions do I need to take or services do I need to provide to work toward achieving this?

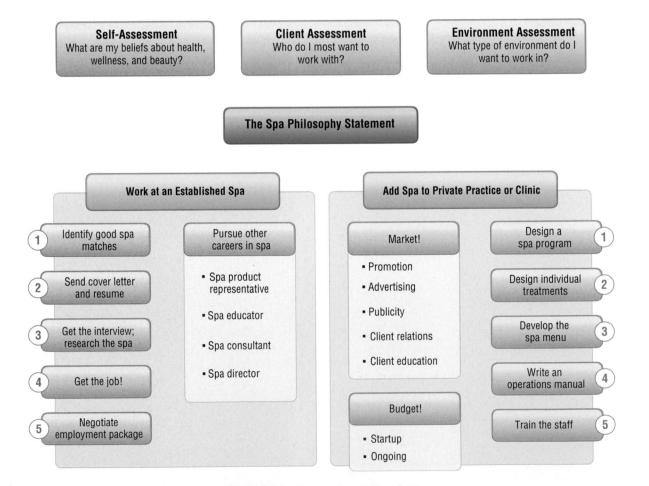

Figure 14-1   Careers in spa flowchart.

2. What is my personal definition of beauty? What actions do I need to take or services do I need to provide to work toward achieving this?

3. What is the image that I want to portray in the spa or massage industry? How will my actions, attire, and personal beliefs contribute to this image?

4. Am I happy with what I am already doing, or do I want to change the spa or massage industry? If so, what do I need to do to achieve this?

5. What are the skills and personal attributes that I possess that set me apart from other therapists and make my treatments special?

During the exercise above, a therapist may have found that he or she began to visualize him- or herself working in a particular environment. Envisioning the future is an important part of long-range planning. If negative or doubtful thoughts came up, it is important to acknowledge those thoughts but to continue to work toward achieving a clear spa philosophy.

CLIENT ASSESSMENT

The second step in identifying a spa philosophy is to determine the type of client that the therapist is interested in working with. This does not mean that services will be refused to other groups; it simply means that this is the particular group (or groups) that most interest the therapist and so some effort must be put into attracting and meeting the needs of this group. Possible target groups can be broken down into broad categories such as men, women, teens, children, athletes, pregnant women, individuals starting self-improvement programs, seniors, students, dieters, or those looking for a spiritual experience. A business planning a promotional campaign will take it a step further to identify **target markets** or rather the client groups on which they want to focus their promotional efforts.

In business marketing, the target market is determined by paying attention to demographic indicators and to lifestyle indicators. Demographic indicators include age, income level, occupation, gender, geographic location, and education level. Lifestyle indicators include philosophical beliefs, social customs, health care needs, specialty activities, and personal priorities. For example, client A is a woman (gender) with a bachelor's degree (educational level) who earns an income of $40,000 a year as a school teacher (occupation). She is also a yoga enthusiast (specialty activity) who practices Buddhism and organic gardening (philosophical beliefs). She has fibromyalgia (health care need) and is a single parent of a small child (personal priority). This client would most probably be attracted to a spa featuring a well-known yoga instructor with meditation classes and onsite childcare. Client B is a 60-year-old man (age, gender) who works as an executive in a financial firm (educational level, income, occupation). He recognizes that stress is affecting his health (health care need) and is focusing on staying fit and healthy as he ages (personal priority). He considers himself an atheist (philosophical belief) and does not like advertising that makes unsupported or unscientific claims. Client B is more likely to attend an upscale massage clinic with treatments that target men. He might well be put off by any mention of treatments that are of a spiritual nature.

Think about the target markets that interest you and try to understand these markets by investigating the relevant health care needs, specialty focus, concerns, and goals of the target group. Next assess the skills and services that you provide, and your personal beliefs in relation to the needs of these potential clients. Most often, therapists will find that they want to work with clients who hold similar beliefs to their own, but not always.

ENVIRONMENT ASSESSMENT

In step three, the therapist explores the type of physical environment in which he or she would like to work. It is important that this matches the therapist's personal beliefs about health and wellness, the type of client he or she wants to work with, and the type of services he or she wants to provide. For example, a therapist interested in providing cultural treatments aimed at promoting global understanding and spiritual awareness would probably not find her ideal spa match at a resort spa targeting clients who want the latest innovations in skin technology. On the other hand, a therapist interested in expanding his or her understanding of skin care and working with the latest hydrotherapy equipment might find that the resort spa mentioned above is a perfect match. To complete this section of the assessment, the therapist can imagine the environment in which he or she would like to work, being as specific as possible. It is also helpful to include a description of the treatments that might be offered at the imaginary spa.

THE SPA PHILOSOPHY STATEMENT

A personal philosophy statement can be put together based on the information gathered in steps 1–3. This helps therapists when looking for an appropriate job in the spa industry or in designing the spa program for a business. In steps 1–3, therapists may have found that there were some inconsistencies and mismatches between their personal feelings about health and wellness, the type of client with which they want to work, and the physical environment in which they want to work. In this case, therapists must ask themselves if they are being realistic, and if not, what changes they need to make. For example, a therapist may find that he or she is very interested in skin care and beauty treatment. In this case, he may want to go back to school to become a licensed esthetician so that he or she can offer a wider range of services without violating scope of practice restrictions. A philosophy statement should be a working document evolving and changing with the therapist. Evaluate the sample spa philosophy statements in Table 14-1 and imagine the type of environment, beliefs, and clients they relate to. These statements are distilled down to a catchy advertisement-like hook. This makes them useful as a type of positive affirmation to keep the therapist on task with career advancement.

Table 14-1	Sample Spa Philosophy Statements

Pampering, Pleasure, and Perfect Skin

Supporting Success—Maintaining Balance

Ancient Wisdom—Modern Approaches

A Haven from a Hectic Workplace

Ultimate Beauty—Ultimate Luxury

A Pure Body is a Strong Body

Jumpstarting a Healthy Lifestyle

Specialists in Helping the Athlete Achieve a Competitive Edge

Rest, Reflection, Renewal

Life Outdoors Leads to Inner Peace

Work at an Established Spa

Massage is the most popular treatment offered at spas, and spas employ more than 151,000 individuals in the United States.[2] There are plenty of opportunities for the therapist who wants to work in the spa industry at an established spa. Before beginning to search for spas that match their personal philosophy statement, there are some industry standards of which therapists should be aware.

First, working conditions can vary widely from spa to spa. Some spas require long hours and provide little flexibility, but others try hard to work out a good schedule with the therapist. Spas usually pay a flat fee for each treatment performed regardless of the price the client is paying for the service. Established spas tend to be facilities where the emphasis is on structure that creates harmony and tranquility. Dress and appearance are important, so therapists should choose a spa that fits their image. The treatments are often expensive, and both the client and spa director expect therapists to be highly knowledgeable about the indications and contraindications of the treatment and the products they are using. Spas expect therapists to be both healers and salespeople. Although many therapists resist this, sales of retail products are an important means of ensuring the financial success of the business. Most spas compensate therapists for making sales of retail items as part of their employment package.

There are many benefits of working in the broader spa industry, including exposure to many different services and new belief structures, products, and approaches. Working in spas with a team of health care professionals to formulate systematic and comprehensive approaches to wellness can be exciting and inspiring. This experience compels some massage therapists to become cross-trained in both massage and esthetics so they can offer a wider range of services. It may also inspire them to specialize in massage modalities such as lomi lomi, Thai, craniosacral, and stone massage.

The first step to finding a job in the spa industry is identifying suitable spas. The Internet is the fastest way to find spas locally and abroad. Spa Finder is a company that helps consumers plan spa vacations. Through its website (http://www.spafinder.com), therapists can find out about an assortment of spas by category, services, and price range. The site provides links to spa websites so that treatment menus and mission statements can be examined. Often spa sites have a job opportunity link that lists openings and application procedures. If the therapist does not have access to a computer, the local yellow pages will usually list spas in the area.

Before applying for a job at a spa, research and become knowledgeable about the spa's product lines, services, body treatments, facility, and philosophy. It is not a bad idea to visit the spa as a client to get a feel for the environment, the skill level of its therapists, and the general working conditions. Unless the spa has a specific job application procedure, prepare a resume and cover letter and address the package to the person in charge of hiring therapists. Call the spa to get the correct name and spelling of this person's name if it is not on the website.

GUIDELINES FOR WRITING A BASIC RESUME

A resume is an individual summary of a person's background, experience, education, training, and skills (Fig. 14-2). It is used by an employer to determine if an applicant has the experience that is appropriate for an open position. A well-written resume is a first step to securing a job interview. The most effective resumes are those that are:

- **Brief and concise:** A resume should be one page, if possible, or two pages at the most. If the resume is long or complex, the reader may skip parts of the resume or put it aside entirely.
- **Positive:** A resume should emphasize positive elements in your record and use action verbs such as *planned, organized, collected, initiated, assessed*, and so on to show employers what you have accomplished.
- **Relevant:** The information on the resume should be written in such a way as to make it meaningful to the employer and pertinent to the specific position.
- **Readable:** Care should be taken to present the information neatly, so that it is easy to gather information at a glance. For this reason, the applicant should pay attention to the type of font and the font size that are used, to the balance of information on the page, and especially to spelling and correct punctuation. Avoid abbreviations of words or incomplete sentences.
- **Honest:** A fabrication on a resume can lead to dismissal if it is found out after you are employed. Be honest about your experience and make certain that dates and time frames are correct.

Jane Anybody   214 Any Street #202
                                              Any Town, Any State   98000
                                                     (303) 222-3232
                                              janeanybody@internet.com

OBJECTIVE: To obtain a position as a massage therapist at a leading spa where I can use my skills
in massage, body treatments, aromatherapy, and reflexology.

EDUCATION: Massage Diploma, June 2005
Any Massage College, Any Town, Any State
800 Hours, Combined GPA 3.66

Spa Certificate, June 2005
Any Massage College, Any Town, Any State
200 Hours, Combined GPA 3.66

Reflexology Certification, October 2005
Any School of Reflexology, Any Town, Any State
300 Hours

Aromatherapy Certification, January 2006
Any School of Aromatherapy, Any Town, Any State
300 Hours

EXPERIENCE: Student Massage Clinic Coordinator, January 2005–June 2005
Any Massage College, Any Town, Any State

As part of the work-study program, I answered phones, assisted clients, and
managed client files. I implemented a new policy for tracking client files that is now
being used at the school's three campuses.

Walk for Breast Cancer Massage Coordinator, May 5, 2005
Any Massage College, Any Town, Any State
Initiated and coordinated an onsite massage event at the Walk for Breast Cancer
Event in Any Town, Any State. As the event coordinator for Any Massage College, I
met with event planners, organized the site where massage would be provided,
coordinated volunteer massage therapists, and managed the flow of clients at the
event.

ASSOCIATIONS: American Massage Therapy Association (AMTA)
Associated Bodywork and Massage Professionals (ABMP)
National Association of Holistic Aromatherapy (NAHA)

REFERENCES: References are available on request.

Figure 14-2   Sample resume.

Parts of a Basic Chronological Resume

While there are many types of resume, a chronological resume is easy to write and illustrates an individual's progression in a given field. New graduates without a lot of work experience should list their educational information first. Individuals with relevant work experience should list their educational information after their job experience.

Contact Information.   This includes the applicant's name, address, phone number (or numbers), and e-mail address. Nicknames and surnames such as "Senior," "Junior," or "II" should be avoided, and all words in the address should be spelled out completely (e.g., "Street," "Avenue").

Career or Job Objective.   An objective tells potential employers what sort of work you are hoping to do. Be specific about the type of job you want and be sure to tailor your objective to the specific position or employer.

Education.   Include the name and location of the institution and the date of the degree, diploma, or certificate. List the most recent education experience first and include your grade point average if it is higher than 3.0. Describe the main area of study (e.g., massage and spa), list the hours of training if they exceed the state minimum, and mention any academic honors or awards. Massage therapists should also include continuing education workshops under the "Education" heading, but these should be listed after the main educational experience despite their chronological order.

Work Experience.   In reverse chronological order with the most recent job first, include the work experience that has taught you skills. List the title of the position, name of the organization, location of the work (town, state), dates of employment, and a description of your work responsibilities. If the experience is not an actual job, list it under the heading "Experience" as in the sample resume (see Fig. 14-2).

Other Information.   Depending on the specific job for which you are applying, you may choose to include leadership experience in volunteer organizations, special certifications or accreditations, membership in professional organizations, special accomplishments, computer skills, or foreign languages.

References.   Do not include your references on the bottom of your resume. Instead, note that "References are available on request." Ask people if they are willing to serve as references before you give their names to potential employers.

GUIDELINES FOR WRITING A COVER LETTER

The cover letter introduces you to the employer and arouses their interest so that they read your resume (Fig. 14-3). This interest will hopefully lead to a job interview. Each letter should be carefully written to address the specific employer and the specific job. The letter will be written in paragraph form (avoid bulleted lists) and be conversational yet formal in tone.

Section One: Opening

The first section of the cover letter should briefly state the job you are applying for and how you learned about it. Any personal contacts you have in or with the company should be mentioned here. You should also state your general qualifications for the job.

Section Two: Body

The body of the letter should expand upon your qualifications for the specific position. For example, if the spa is well known for its aromatherapy treatments, the therapist should illuminate his or her aromatherapy training and experience. If the spa is particularly focused on Eastern influences, the therapist should highlight his or her understanding of ayurveda treatments, Shiatsu, or Tai massage. Pick out the most relevant qualifications listed in your resume and discuss them in detail to demonstrate your particular suitability for the job.

Section Three: Conclusion

To conclude the letter, request an interview (or some other response, as appropriate) and include the times when you can be reached. Thank the reader for his or her time and consideration.

Follow up with a phone call a few days latter to ensure that the package has been received and to speak to the relevant person, if possible. This initial discussion is important. It provides the therapist with the opportunity to outline his or her credentials, special skills, and knowledge of the spa's philosophy and services. If an interview is requested, refine your interviewing skills by anticipating certain types of questions and practicing clear, concise, and knowledgeable answers. Inquire if you will be asked to provide a sample of your work. If the answer is no, dress as professionally as possible (i.e., wear a business suit). If the answer is yes, dress professionally but in such a way that you can still deliver a massage or body treatment. The massage or bodywork segment of the interview should last no longer than 30 minutes unless the spa is paying you for the treatment. An experienced spa director can determine the applicant's skill level very quickly based on the applicant's quality of touch, professional communication, and control of product.

PREPARATION FOR THE INTERVIEW

In an interview, the employer will appraise your suitability for a specific position and for their company as a whole. Your self-confidence, the way in which you express yourself, your level of professional dress, and the validity and content of your answers to questions will influence the employer's evaluation. The interview is also a time for you to gather information about the company's policies and determine if this is a job that matches your personal spa philosophy and career goals.

200 Any Street, Suite 300
Any Town, Any State 98000
janeanybody@internet.com

February 5, 2006

Mr. Eric Sanders
Recruiting Coordinator
Express Spa
Any Town, Any State 79000

Dear Mr. Sanders:

Your advertisement for massage therapists in the January issue of *Spa Spectrum Newsletter* caught my attention. I was drawn to the advertisement by my strong interest in aromatherapy and reflexology, areas where Express Spa has a well-known focus.

Although I have only recently finished my education in massage, spa body treatments, aromatherapy, and reflexology, I have had the opportunity to work in a high-pressure, customer service oriented team environment as the student massage clinic coordinator for Any Massage College. I am seeking a career with a recognized and respected spa that will allow me to integrate my understanding of wellness and relaxation while building my practical skills in aromatherapy and reflexology.

I would very much like to meet with you to discuss your open positions for massage therapists. If you wish to arrange an interview, please contact me at the above e-mail or by telephone at (303) 222-3232.

Thank you for your time and consideration.

Sincerely,

Jane Anybody

Jane Anybody

Figure 14-3   Sample cover letter.

To prepare for the interview, it is helpful to roleplay with a friend or associate who will ask you questions and help you evaluate your strengths and weaknesses. During the roleplaying session, assess the manner of your speech (e.g., speaking too fast as if you are rushed) and your body language. For example, eye contact is extremely important during an interview because averting the eyes might be interpreted as a lack of self-confidence or as dishonesty. Smiling too much looks unnatural, but a tight mouth could be read as disapproval or as a judgmental personality. Crossed arms convey defensiveness, and a slouched position sends a message that you might be lazy or disinterested. Avoid gesturing too much with your hands, which can be distracting, and do not touch your hair or face during the interview.

Anticipate questions that might be asked during your interview and prepare answers that are brief but thorough. Decide what questions you would like to ask during your interview and practice politely interjecting them during different points in your interview. Asking pertinent questions is important because the answers will help you decide if this is a good match for your personal career goal.

Practice Interview Questions

1. Describe the experience and skills that you possess that you feel directly relate to this particular position.
2. What is it about working at this company that particularly interests you?
3. What is your weakest point? Note: Some think that it is best to identify a weak area honestly but then focus on a plan for self-improvement (e.g., "I have a tendency to be overly sensitive when criticized. I'm working on listening closely to constructive criticism, not becoming defensive, and then working to make positive changes."). Others believe that it is best to mention something that will be perceived as a strength (e.g., "I'm something of a perfectionist" or "I'm a bit of a workaholic.").
4. What is your strongest point?
5. What do you hope to be doing 5 years from now?
6. What is your greatest accomplishment?
7. Why should we hire you?
8. Describe a problem or conflict you have had in a previous job or at school and explain how you solved it.

Good Questions to Ask During the Interview

1. What are the company's challenges and current goals?
2. Is a detailed written job description available for this position?
3. Are there opportunities for advancement?
4. To whom would I report?
5. Why is this position open?

Show up early to your interview and treat everyone cordially, including the receptionist or assistant. When introductions are made, offer to shake hands and make it a firm handshake while looking the employer in the eye and smiling. Remember the employer's name and use it when speaking to him or her during the interview. Do not smoke directly before the interview or chew gum or drink a beverage during the interview. Bring an extra copy of your resume, a copy of your school credentials or transcripts, and a reference sheet. At the conclusion of the interview, express your appreciation for the interviewer's time and show enthusiasm for the job.

THE EMPLOYMENT PACKAGE

Before a job offer is made, discuss the employment package, schedule, dress code, training procedure, and additional duties. Some spas require therapists to train without pay, and others pay therapists while they train. Some require therapists to carry out a number of additional housekeeping activities such as sanitizing wet room equipment or doing the laundry, and other spas provide support staff to handle such duties. It is important to understand the expectations of the spa director or manager before accepting the job. Table 14-2 outlines some questions that the applicant may want to ask to clarify the employment package. Although therapists should always behave in a calm, professional, and flexible manner, they should ask for what they need in terms of scheduling and the employment package. It never hurts to ask for more money, especially for therapists who have other skills or credentials in addition to their massage certificate or license. After these items have been discussed, consider the job in relationship to any specific needs, personal philosophy, and career goals. Sometimes a job is an ideal fit, and sometimes it is not an ideal fit but provides a stepping stone toward the ultimate career goal.

Other Careers in the Spa Industry

Other careers in the spa industry include positions such as the spa educator or product representative, spa consultant, massage (or esthetics) manager, or spa director.

SPA EDUCATOR

There are many different types of spa educator. For example, spa product representatives are individuals who have been hired by a product line manufacturer to educate the spa staff at spas where their products are used and distributed. Some spa product companies develop treatment outlines so that particular products are used in each of the steps of a predesigned treatment. The product representative travels to spas, provides training on the benefits of the company's product line, and instructs the spa staff in the

Table 14-2	Evaluation of the Employment Package
Compensation	How will you be compensated for your work? Will you receive an hourly fee and commission on treatments that you perform, or will you receive a flat rate for each service?
Scheduling	Who will determine your work schedule, and how are schedule changes made when necessary? How will your shifts be covered if you become sick or have a personal emergency?
Extra duties	Will you be expected to perform housekeeping duties between appointments? Who does the laundry? Who deep cleans the hydrotherapy equipment?
Staff meetings	Will you be compensated for staff meetings? Are staff meetings mandatory? When and how often are they scheduled?
Dress code	What is the dress code? Are uniforms provided, or are you expected to purchase the uniform?
Inappropriate client behavior	How does the spa define inappropriate client behavior? If you are uncomfortable working with a particular client, will the spa require you to work with that person? When is a client refused service, and who informs the client that he or she is being refused service?
Performance reviews and wage increases	Are there annual staff performance evaluations, and are wage increases tied to the outcome of the evaluations? Are bonuses given on overall performance or on meeting certain company goals (e.g., highest retail sales for the month)?
Training	How will you learn the spa's services? When will you be expected to train? Will you be compensated for training? Does the company contribute to outside training such as continuing education workshops to help you maintain your massage credentials?
Professional exchanges	Are you allowed to trade services with other professionals at the spa? Are you required to pay for the products and laundry when participating in trades?
Discounts	Do you receive discounts on services or products provided by the spa? Can you get discounts for family members?
Retail sales	How will you be compensated for retail sales? Are there quotas for sales of retail products? What happens if you do not reach your quota for a particular month?
Health plan	Does the company provide a medical insurance plan or life insurance?
Liability insurance	Does the company provide liability insurance to cover clients who may be injured in a treatment, or are therapists required to provide their own liability insurance?
Termination of employment	What is the procedure for termination of employment? Where can you work after you terminate employment? (Some companies have noncompete clauses in their contracts that may prevent you from working in a certain radius of the spa or working for a direct competitor.)

delivery of the treatment using the specialized products. Another type of spa educator is a spa representative who is also an expert in a particular area such as aromatherapy, ayurveda body treatments, reflexology, or hot stone massage. They offer their services to a spa and provide training in the area of their expertise to meet the spa's needs. Spa educators who are not representatives may focus on the development of spa curriculum for massage schools, beauty schools, or continuing education workshops.

SPA CONSULTANT

A spa consultant usually combines the skills of a therapist with those of a business person. Often talented therapists will work their way up in the industry and learn the business through personal experience. Sometimes the consultant is a businessperson who has specialized in the spa industry. Many spa owners start their own spas because they have a strong vision of the type of environment and services they want to offer. These individuals might hire a spa consultant to review their service menu, make suggestions for additional treatments, or plan a specific marketing campaign.

At the other end of the spectrum is the large corporation that hires a highly trained individual to handle all aspects of the spa startup. In this case, the spa consultant would conduct a market assessment and financial feasibility assessment and help the spa to identify their philosophy and target client groups. In addition, the consultant might give some input on the floor plan and select the equipment and product lines that will be used. The consultant may also develop an operations manual, job descriptions, hire the initial spa staff, create the spa menu, and oversee the training of the therapists and staff. Lastly, the consultant will probably identify or give some input on how the spa should position itself in the marketplace and build its special identity with the public.

SPA DEPARTMENT MANAGERS

At larger spas, there is often a massage manager who oversees the massage therapists, an esthetics manager who oversees the estheticians, and a salon manager who oversees the cosmetologists and nail technicians. Organized and ambitious massage therapists might work their way into the massage manager position and then later into a spa director position based on their ability to learn management and business skills.

SPA DIRECTOR

A spa director is responsible for ensuring that the spa runs smoothly, efficiently, and profitably. The director is in charge of pay systems and the payroll and oversees the spa's accounting practices to ensure that proper records are kept. The spa director handles the marketing and promotion of the spa and puts practices into place that ensure good customer retention. This person usually hires and oversees staff training, stays abreast of spa trends and regulatory requirements, and makes changes to the service program if necessary.

Although the next section focuses on information pertinent to small business owners, reading this section will give spa employees a better understanding of the challenges that face the spa where they work and their management team.

Add Spa Treatments to a Private Practice or Massage Clinic

Although beautiful luxury surroundings and a full-service wet room can only enhance the spa experience, they are not strictly necessary when introducing spa treatments to an existing massage practice. Several body treatments can be added with a minimum of equipment. Some clients actually avoid spas because they perceive them as too expensive or fussy. The spa-oriented massage clinic bridges the gap between the traditional massage clinic and a full-service spa and directly appeals to the spa-shy client. There are many benefits to adding spa treatments but also some potential drawbacks. It is important for therapists to consider all aspects of their business before they invest in the additional equipment.

One benefit of adding spa treatments to a massage practice is that it allows therapists to provide their clients with more options. Spa treatments combine very well with massage and can be used together very effectively, even for serious musculoskeletal injuries such as whiplash and carpal tunnel syndrome. Many of the products used in spa treatments have some of the same physiological effects as massage and help the body to detoxify through increased circulation and lymphatic flow. Products such as seaweed and mud, for example, have a long history of therapeutic use in Europe because of their anti-inflammatory, anti-arthritic, and pain-relieving qualities.

Adding spa treatments to a massage practice also helps therapists to protect their hands and bodies from repetitive stress because many spa treatments are less taxing to deliver than a full-body massage. This allows therapists to offer more sessions in a day and increase their income with less effort. Therapists can usually charge more money for the same amount of treatment time and sell spa-related retail items to generate a second income stream for the business. Finally, and perhaps most importantly, spa treatments are fun. They provide a creative outlet for therapists that helps them to alleviate burnout and boredom.

Although the benefits of adding spa treatments are numerous, there are some aspects of spas that massage therapists should consider before they purchase equipment. Spa treatments require more setup and cleanup time than massage. This means that a therapist will have to plan additional time in between clients to prepare or change over the treatment room. If the therapist also employs a number of other therapists, he or she will need to consider how the employees are compensated for setup and cleanup time. Additional inventory will need to be managed and storage found for towels, products, and equipment. The need to remove body products with hot towels means that there will be more laundry. Spa products are usually sold in large-size bottles (often referred to as the **back bar** to differentiate them from the same product sold in smaller sizes to the client). Although the cost of delivering a particular treatment may be relatively low ($2 to $14), the initial outlay for initial product can be high. Although many products can be stored for a long time without damage to their therapeutic value, other products must be used up before they become old or dry out.

Some spa products such as seaweed or taila (the medicated oils used in ayurveda) can have a strong scent, which may be disturbing to the other massage clientele. Often, clients are intrigued by these unique scents and ask questions that help to sell them the treatment at a later date. Sometimes they are put off by unfamiliar scents, and if they are very sensitive, they may take their business elsewhere. If this is a problem, consider offering spa treatments on a particular day of the week (spa Saturdays) or at specific times (spa lunches).

Sometimes spa treatments sell best to pairs of clients, either family members or friends. In these cases, two treatments need to be delivered at the same time and sometimes two sets of equipment are required (e.g., two sets of massage stones and stone heating units). Obviously, two therapists who know how to perform the treatment need to be scheduled at the same time, and they have to deliver the treatment in a similar fashion. The last thing the owner wants is for the clients to compare their treatments and find that one therapist was more accomplished than the other.

After spa therapists have considered their spa philosophy, weighed the pros and cons of adding spa treatments to their business, and determined that spa is right for them, they are ready to design their spa program.

THE SPA PROGRAM

The spa program refers to the services that will be offered at the business and the way in which they are delivered. For marketing purposes, the owner or therapist should match the final spa program to the perceived health care needs, specialty focus, and goals of the intended target client or clients.

The spa program may be small and specific with treatments that enhance or provide benefits in synergy with massage, or the clinic owner can branch out and hire additional spa staff to offer a more diverse program. Table 14-3 provides an overview of popular services, their therapeutic benefits, and the most likely professionals to deliver the service. In a full-service facility, the spa aims to offer a wide range of treatments, including manicures and pedicures, facials, hair services, depilatory services, makeup application, hydro therapy treatments, body treatments, life coaching, meditation, nutritional programs, fitness programs, and more. A massage clinic owner will probably plan a program composed predominantly of body treatments. If the aim is for a broader spa experience, the owner can still keep it manageable with the addition of esthetic services such as facials, waxing, manicures, and pedicures. Table 14-4 gives an example of three programs that might be adopted by a moderately sized massage clinic. The first and second programs are designed to be delivered by a clinic employing only massage therapists. The third program assumes that massage therapists, an esthetician, and a nail technician are part of the staff. A sample spa menu for the first program appears in Figure 14-4.

As the clinic owner or therapist develops his or her spa program and reflects on his or her personal spa philosophy,

it is useful to look on the Internet at the programs of other spas. In this way, the owner or therapist develops an awareness of industry trends and also can draw inspiration from established spas. The example of the spa program described below shows how one therapist used an "out-of-the-box" concept to make spa therapy work in her private practice.

A Sample One Person Spa Program

The massage therapist in this example was able to offer her clients an exclusive spa experience by keeping the menu simple. With the exception of a part-time receptionist who schedules appointments from her home, this is a one-woman show. In this case, the owner or therapist is specifically interested in ayurvedic body treatments (discussed in Chapter 11). She leased a space that includes a reception-retail-consultation area and a single treatment room that opens onto a bathroom with a soaking tub. Because the space is small, she was able to decorate it according to ayurvedic principles and with attention to detail, creating a unique environment for her clients. She works with one or two clients a day, one in the morning and possibly one in the afternoon, and she is open from Tuesday to Saturday, giving her Sunday and Monday off. Her program and price are the same for every client. The session begins with an ayurveda consultation and a cup of hot jasmine tea. This is followed by an herbal foot soak, Indian head massage, and full-body dosha massage. Ubtan (an herbal paste) is applied to the skin and buffed off with dried towels before a classic shirodhara treatment and firming face massage are delivered. After the shirodhara treatment, the client is left to nap for 20 minutes while a bath is prepared. To end the service, the client soaks in a tub filled with flowers and herbs before his or her hair is shampooed to remove the oil from the shirodhara treatment. At the end of the service, the client is escorted back to the reception–retail–consultation area, where the therapist makes specific recommendations about ayurvedic products that would be good for the client. After the client has purchased some products and departed, the owner has lunch and then cleans the treatment room and bathroom in preparation for her second client. Because her program is the same for every client, she is able to maintain a small product inventory and refine the delivery of the service so that every detail is considered. In the beginning, she only offered her ayurvedic package on Saturdays, but as news of her unique service spread, she increased the number of days on which she offered the treatment, and now this is the only treatment that she offers.

Ayurveda is not the only type of treatment that works well in this type of program. Therapists with small workspaces could offer many types of program using the one described above as a model. For example, a program could be based exclusively on specific types of treatments such as aromatherapy (e.g., "Sensual" Escape), fangotherapy (e.g., Mud Madness!), or botanicals (e.g., Herbal Remedies). Another option is to combine a small number of

Table 14-3	Overview of Some Popular Spa Services*	
SPA SERVICE	**BENEFITS**	**LIKELY INDUSTRY PROFESSIONAL**
Hydrotherapy Specialized showers, steams, baths, saunas, and other applications using water	The benefits of the treatment are based on the temperature of the treatment, length of the treatment, and the effects of the specialized apparatus that is used in combination with water.	Physicians, physical therapists, massage therapists. Estheticians use specialized baths and showers in the removal of products or to improve the health and condition of the skin.
Full-body exfoliation Loofah scrubs, full-body polish, salt glows, sugar glows, dry skin brushing, almond scrub, others	Stimulates circulation and lymph flow, stimulates vital energy of the body, relaxation, revitalization, deep cleans, removes dead skin cells, softens and refines the skin's texture, beautifies the skin	Massage therapists, estheticians. Exfoliation has benefits for both skin and body. Whereas massage therapists focus on the benefits for the body, estheticians focus on the benefits for the skin. Estheticians can also deliver enzyme peels.
Autotanning Buff and bronze, spray-on tans, spray tan booths	Depending on the treatment steps, the treatment may stimulate circulation and lymph flow and relax muscles. Autotanning treatments are most often delivered to darken the skin's color so that the client appears tan.	Massage therapists, estheticians. Spray tans and booths can be facilitated by unlicensed or uncertified individuals in some states.
Body wraps A wide variety, including herbal, seaweed, fango, cryogenic, slimming, detoxifying, aromatherapy, others	The benefits of the treatment depend on the type of products and techniques that are used during the service.	Massage therapists, estheticians, depending on the desired effects of the application and on the promotional description of the service
Thalassotherapy Treatments using seawater, marine algae, sea air, and diets high in sea products	Thalassotherapy has been used for a wide range of conditions. In general, it revitalizes and detoxifies the body and beautifies the skin.	Massage therapists, estheticians, physical therapists, physicians, depending on the desired effects of the application and on the promotional description of the service
Fangotherapy Treatments using therapeutic mud, clay, and peat	Fangotherapy has been used for a wide range of conditions but especially arthritis, musculoskeletal conditions, and to beautify the skin.	Massage therapists, estheticians, physical therapists, physicians, depending on the desired effects of the application and on the promotional description of the service
Spot treatments Cellulite, back, bust, others	The benefits of the treatment will depend on the type of products and techniques that are used during the service.	Estheticians, massage therapists
Foot and hand treatments (not pedicures or manicures Treatments that do not include trimming the nails or cuticles	Pain relieving, relaxing, revitalizing, stimulate circulation, increase range of motion, can be used to treat soft tissue pathology such as plantar fasciitis, relaxing, deep cleans, softens and reconditions the skin on the hands or feet, beautifies the hands or feet	Massage therapists, certified reflexologists (some states), estheticians. Massage therapists and reflexologists focus on treatments that relax the body and decrease foot pain. Estheticians focus on the beautification of the skin of the hands and feet.
Pedicures Treatments that include trimming the nails and cuticles	Relaxing, improves the overall health and appearance of the feet, beautifies the feet	Nail technicians, cosmetologists, estheticians (some states)
Manicures Treatments that include trimming the nails and cuticles	Relaxing, improves the overall health and appearance of the hands, beautifies the hands	Nail technicians, cosmetologists, estheticians (some states)

Table 14-3 (continued)

SPA SERVICE	BENEFITS	LIKELY INDUSTRY PROFESSIONAL
Massage Swedish, Shiatsu, manual lymphatic drainage, craniosacral, lomi lomi, Thai, sports, deep tissue, others	The effects of the massage are based on the types of techniques that are used. In general, massage stimulates circulation and lymphatic flow, relaxes the body, and decreases soft tissue imbalance.	Massage therapists, physical therapists. Sometimes specialized training and certification are required to deliver certain types of massage.
Stone massage	Warms tissue, stimulates circulation, decreases tension in hypertonic muscles, decreases adhesions, relaxes the body	Massage therapists
Ayurveda-inspired body treatments Abhyanga, dosha wrap, dosha massage, ubvartana, Indian head massage, shirodhara, pinda abhyanga, pizzichilli, garshan, others	To relax the body, stimulate circulation, revitalize the body, facilitate detoxification of body tissues, bring balance to the body, promote spiritual awareness, create a space for reflection and renewal	Ayurvedic physicians, massage therapists
Ayurveda-inspired beauty treatments Facials, shirodhara, ubvartana, dosha skin wraps, scalp treatments, pedicures and manicures, others	To beautify the intended area using ayurveda principles and products	Ayurvedic physicians, estheticians, cosmetologists, nail technicians
Natural and Traditional Forms of Medicine Ayurveda, Chinese traditional medicine, acupuncture, naturopathic medicine, herbal medicine, others	To bring the body into balance, to treat a specific condition, or as a preventative to disease	Ayurvedic physicians, traditional Chinese medicine practitioners, acupuncturists, naturopathic doctors, herbal medicine practitioners
Facials	To deep clean, smooth, refine, soften, and condition the facial skin and treat certain skin conditions on the face. To improve the appearance and beautify the skin. To slow the signs of aging.	Estheticians, cosmetologists (some states)
Face and scalp massage	To relax the muscles of the face and scalp, decrease overall tension, firm and tone the muscles of the face, stimulate the skin and increase local circulation, aid in product penetration, loosen trapped debris in the follicles, facilitate product application to the face or scalp	Massage therapists, estheticians, cosmetologists
Hair removal services Physical depilatories (wax), chemical depilatories (powder, cream, others), electrolysis, electric current tweezers	To remove unwanted hair from the body. Electrolysis is a form of permanent hair removal; depilatories remove the hair temporarily.	Estheticians, cosmetologists. Electrolysis is performed by a licensed electrologist.
Nails Includes nail art, gel nails, acrylic nails	To beautify the hands and the feet, improve nail health, embellish the nails for esthetic purposes	Nail technicians, cosmetologists (some states)
Hair services Cutting, styling, highlighting, coloring, perming, straightening, conditioning, and so on	To improve the health or appearance of the hair, stimulate the scalp and promote healthy hair growth	Cosmetologists

Table 14-3 *(continued)*

SPA SERVICE	BENEFITS	LIKELY INDUSTRY PROFESSIONAL
Makeup application	To improve the appearance of the face or camouflage a skin condition or injury such as scarring from burns	Estheticians, cosmetologists
Nutrition Nutrition assessment or programming, healthy cooking	To assess the nutritional viability of a client's diet and to make recommendations that lead to better nutritional health, to support healing from a specific condition using diet	Nutritionists, fitness trainers
Fitness Fitness assessment or programming, personal training	To assess the fitness level of the client and make recommendations that lead to better physical health; to motivate clients to reach their physical goals	Fitness trainers, strength and conditioning specialists
Mind and spirit therapies Hypnotherapy, group counseling, counseling, psychotherapy, guided meditation, life coaching, yoga, others	To support the individual in finding inner peace and contentment; to guide personal transformation, create relationships and connections, generate resource states for better living	Psychotherapists, psychologists, counselors, hypnotherapists, yoga instructors, spiritual instructors, life coaches, others

* As discussed in Chapter 1, the laws, regulations, and scope of practice for professionals working at a spa vary widely from state to state. It is important for therapists to review the laws in their state before providing any treatment. They should also check that a given treatment is covered by their liability insurance. Because products and treatment techniques often provide benefits for both the revitalization of the body and the beautification of the skin, the promotional description of the treatment may become the determining factor in who delivers the service. In general (although not in every state), massage therapists focus on the effects of a treatment for soft tissue and the body, and estheticians focus on the effects of the treatment for the health and beautification of the skin. This table is meant to provide a general overview. It is not comprehensive in terms of treatments or the industry professionals who might deliver them.

different treatments, working toward achieving a specific spa philosophy. If the spa philosophy is "cleanse the body, expand the soul," the program might include a detoxification treatment and a guided meditation session. A one-person program based on "reflect, relax, renew" could include any treatment that was relaxing.

In the development of the final spa program, the main things to consider are the type of client, the limitations of the workspace, and the budget. After a draft of the program has been developed, a draft spa menu should be written up and the individual treatments designed (discussed in Chapter 13). After the treatments have been designed, the menu of services should then be revised and finalized.

THE SPA MENU

The menu is an important promotional item that outlines the spa program and describes each of the services that are offered at the facility (see Fig. 14-4). The menu should be designed and written in such a way that it upholds the overall spa philosophy. As a key promotional tool, it is taken

away with clients, mailed to clients, posted in the front window of the business, and sometimes sent out in a mass mailing to attract new business. It should be designed with care and printed professionally on high-quality paper. Usually, the menu includes the name of the business, a description of the spa philosophy or mission statement, an address, a phone number, and the hours of operation. Some menus are designed to be short and concise, and others provide lengthy and detailed descriptions. If spa treatments are new to the facility, a longer, more detailed menu is advised. Clients will want to know what each treatment includes and what benefits they can expect.

It is important to consider a few items before writing up a draft menu and designing each treatment. First, the treatments on the menu need to be balanced in such a way that they support, rather than compete, with each other. A therapist would not want to offer three body wraps that all have the same therapeutic goal of decreasing muscle soreness. This will confuse clients because they will not know which is the best treatment to schedule if they all do the same thing. Some spas offer many different versions of the same treatment, but they clearly define different treatment goals

Table 14-4 **Three Sample Spa Programs**

CORE SPA PROGRAM FOR A MASSAGE CLINIC	LARGER SPA PROGRAM FOR A MASSAGE CLINIC	LARGER SPA PROGRAM FOR A MASSAGE CLINIC WITH AN ESTHETICIAN AND NAIL TECHNICIAN ON STAFF
Massage Swedish massage Deep tissue massage Hot stone massage Pregnancy massage **Body Treatments** Salt glow: Three choices (Zen, citrus, floral) Full-body seaweed wrap Herbal detoxification wrap Parafango treatment for back pain Buff and bronze Aromatherapy consultation and massage **Reflexology Foot Spa Treatments** Treatment aimed at decreasing foot pain Treatment aimed at tired feet Treatment aimed at stress reduction	**Massage** Swedish massage Aromatherapy massage Deep tissue massage Hot stone massage Custom massage Indian head and face massage and shirodhara **Body Treatments** Full-body seaweed wrap Parafango treatment for back pain Herbal detoxification wrap Ubvartana treatment Salt glows: Three choices (citrus, alpine, floral) Loofah scrub: Three choices (eucalyptus, sage and lavender, peppermint and sweet orange) Buff and bronze **Reflexology Foot Spa Treatments** Treatment aimed at decreasing foot pain Treatment aimed at revitalizing tired feet Treatment aimed at stress reduction **Couples Romance Package (Mediterranean Theme)** Foot soak and foot massage (goat cheese, brusheta, and sliced tomato snack) Mediterranean herbs wrap Aromatic hot stone massage with essential oils of rosemary, lavender, sage, and lemon	**Massage** Swedish massage Deep tissue massage Thai massage Lomi lomi massage Hot stone massage **Body Treatments** Full-body seaweed wrap Full-body fango wrap Parafango cellulite treatment Slimming herbal body wrap Athlete treatment with sports massage and application of cryogenic product Salt glow Flowers ritual foot soak, body polish, and scalp conditioning massage Buff and bronze Skin softening emollient wrap **Facials** Signature facial (matched to skin type) Deep-cleansing facial with extractions Anti-aging facial for mature skin Gentleman's facial Teen's facial (aimed at problem skin) **Depilatory Services** Face (lip, chin, eyebrow) Legs and bikini Arms (underarm, forearm) Bodybuilder's wax (back, legs, chest, arms)

Table 14-4	(continued)	

CORE SPA PROGRAM FOR A MASSAGE CLINIC	LARGER SPA PROGRAM FOR A MASSAGE CLINIC	LARGER SPA PROGRAM FOR A MASSAGE CLINIC WITH AN ESTHETICIAN AND NAIL TECHNICIAN ON STAFF
	Workday Escape Package	**Manicures**
	Citrus salt glow	Spa manicure
	Aromatherapy massage	French manicure
	Foot spa treatment for tired feet	Gentleman's manicure
		Nail repair and nail art
		Hand hennas
		Pedicures
		Spa pedicure
		French pedicure
		Foot hennas
		Ultimate foot treatment (pedicure, reflexology session, foot mask, paraffin dip, nail art, or henna)
		Pregnancy Package for Moms to Be
		Flowers ritual
		Pregnancy massage
		Signature facial
		Prom Party Package
		Teen facial
		Mini manicure and pedicure
		30-minute aromatherapy massage

for each to make it simple for clients to choose what they want. In this case, one body wrap might focus on detoxification, the second on relaxation, and the third on decreasing muscle soreness.

The therapists at the clinic need to be trained in each of the services and have an appropriate level of knowledge or skill for the treatments they are delivering. In the ayurvedic package described above, the therapist took a special interest in ayurveda and was highly knowledgeable about the body treatments she offered; this is the ideal. At a minimum, the clinic's therapists need to be able to describe the therapeutic benefits of the treatment to the clients and have some background on the products that are being used. For clinics or individuals that do not have the resources to do extensive training, it is advisable to start with a small core menu until each staff member becomes proficient. Only after the clinic owner is sure that all the therapists have mastered the core menu should new treatments be added. These should be added as "specials" one at a time to make sure that the therapists are confident before moving onto a new treatment. Be careful about advertising a service until it has been mastered by the staff members who will deliver it.

A client is often attracted to a treatment because of the way is it described. For this reason, the treatment description must be clear (clients need to know what they are getting) and yet evocative. Strong sensory language captures clients' imaginations and elicits an emotional response. The menu writer should want the client to smell, taste, and feel the treatment just by reading the description. "Uplifting grapefruit body polish" sounds much more exciting than "body polish." "Swiss herbs cocoon" sounds more appealing than "wrap." Ideally, the spa philosophy will shine through in the style in which the promotional descriptions are written. Some spas are very traditional or sophisticated; others are spiritual or even funky and lighthearted. Writing that matches the overall philosophy and style of

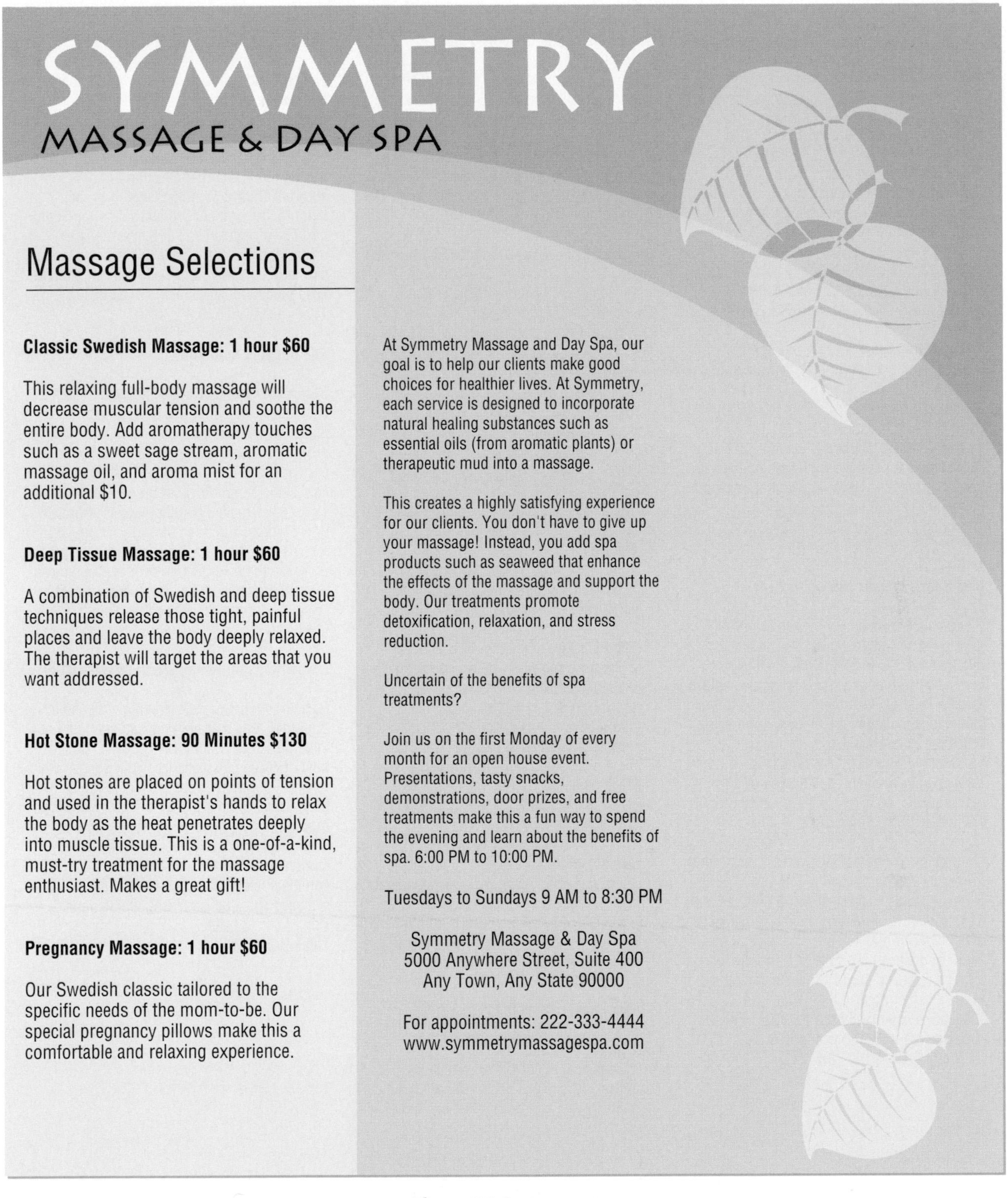

SYMMETRY
MASSAGE & DAY SPA

Massage Selections

Classic Swedish Massage: 1 hour $60

This relaxing full-body massage will decrease muscular tension and soothe the entire body. Add aromatherapy touches such as a sweet sage stream, aromatic massage oil, and aroma mist for an additional $10.

Deep Tissue Massage: 1 hour $60

A combination of Swedish and deep tissue techniques release those tight, painful places and leave the body deeply relaxed. The therapist will target the areas that you want addressed.

Hot Stone Massage: 90 Minutes $130

Hot stones are placed on points of tension and used in the therapist's hands to relax the body as the heat penetrates deeply into muscle tissue. This is a one-of-a-kind, must-try treatment for the massage enthusiast. Makes a great gift!

Pregnancy Massage: 1 hour $60

Our Swedish classic tailored to the specific needs of the mom-to-be. Our special pregnancy pillows make this a comfortable and relaxing experience.

At Symmetry Massage and Day Spa, our goal is to help our clients make good choices for healthier lives. At Symmetry, each service is designed to incorporate natural healing substances such as essential oils (from aromatic plants) or therapeutic mud into a massage.

This creates a highly satisfying experience for our clients. You don't have to give up your massage! Instead, you add spa products such as seaweed that enhance the effects of the massage and support the body. Our treatments promote detoxification, relaxation, and stress reduction.

Uncertain of the benefits of spa treatments?

Join us on the first Monday of every month for an open house event. Presentations, tasty snacks, demonstrations, door prizes, and free treatments make this a fun way to spend the evening and learn about the benefits of spa. 6:00 PM to 10:00 PM.

Tuesdays to Sundays 9 AM to 8:30 PM

Symmetry Massage & Day Spa
5000 Anywhere Street, Suite 400
Any Town, Any State 90000

For appointments: 222-333-4444
www.symmetrymassagespa.com

Figure 14-4 Spa menu.

the spa works best. In a lighthearted description of a seaweed wrap, the treatment might be named the Mermaid Shimmer and start with the line: "Feeling scaly, waterlogged, and listless?" A more sophisticated interpretation might be: "Release yourself to the skin smoothing and body slimming benefits of pure marine algae." In the example below, a seaweed wrap is describe two different ways. In the first description, most of the sensory language has been left out. In the second description, strong sensory language has been included.

Spa Selections

Aromatherapy Salt Glows: 1 hour $80

A salt glow is a revitalizing treatment that stimulates circulation and relaxes and tones muscle tissue while smoothing the skin. Clients have three choices:

1. The Zen Glow infuses spicy ginger with the soothing scents of mandarin and lemongrass. Think CALMING!

2. The Citrus Glow is fresh and uplifting with the scents of grapefruit, lime, lemon, and sweet orange intertwined in a constantly changing aroma melody. Think REFRESHING!

3. The Victorian Garden Glow surrounds the client with the soothing fragrance of an herb garden. Lavender, rosemary, thyme, rose, and just a hint of nutmeg invoke a warm afternoon in the sun. Think RELAXING!

Mud Sport!: 1 hour $85

If you have a sore back or if your workouts have been slowed down by muscle tension, this treatment is for you. Your back is massaged with deep tissue techniques before a warm layer of Parafango* is applied to stimulate circulation and relax sore muscles. While the Parafango works its magic, the backs of your legs are massaged. To end the service, your neck and shoulders are massaged.
Think GOODBYE BACK PAIN!

*Parafango is a combination of a special mud from Italy and paraffin with different melting points. It holds heat for up to 60 minutes and locks moisture at the skin's surface. Because of its superior heat retention abilities, it has been used since the 1950s in Germany for arthritis pain and chronic muscle conditions. At the client's request, the parafango application can be focused for special needs such as sore hamstrings or calves.

Aroma Relief: 90 Minutes $110

This classic aromatherapy massage begins with a consultation and a blend of essential oils created especially for you. The oils are applied in a full-body relaxation massage with enhancers such as rosemary face steam and paraffin dip. You keep your special blend for use at home in a soothing aromatherapy bath or shower. Think MUCH-NEEDED REPRIEVE!

Reflexology Foot Spa Treatments: 1 hr - $80

Reflexology is based on the belief that there are points on the feet, hands, and ears that correspond to all the areas of the body. By activating these points, full-body relaxation is achieved. In each of the treatments described below, the feet are soaked, smoothed with an exfoliation cream, massaged, treated to a series of reflexology techniques, masked to facilitate detoxification, and finished with lotion or powder. Clients have three choices:

1. The Tired Feet Tingle refreshes your feet with a sea salt soak, peppermint exfoliation, kelp mask, and reflexology point work targeting the reflex points associated with mental burnout and exhaustion. Think REVITALIZATION!

2. The Pain-Away Treatment focuses on eliminating foot pain. Your feet are soaked in Epson salt and eucalyptus oil before a bracing rosemary loofah scrub. The massage and reflexology session uses the healing properties of bay laurel and sweet birch oils before thick, warm Moor* mud is slathered on your feet to decrease inflammation and pain. Think LET'S GO DANCING!

3. The Sole Soother is soft and gentle. Lavender, ylang ylang, basil, mandarin, and rose oils caress your feet and allow your body to deeply relax. A paraffin treatment for your hands completes this delightful indulgence. Think TRANQUILITY!

*Moor mud is a high moor peat from Austria that is used in Europe for foot pain, arthritis, and skin and respiratory disorders. It is thick and black with superior heat retention qualities and proven anti-inflammatory action.

The Buff and Bronze: 75 minutes- $90

The buff and bronze is a relaxing treatment that leaves you looking like you just returned from a tropical vacation. Tanned skin has never been so good for you! Your body is buffed, smoothed with moisture creams, and treated to an expert application of auto-bronzant (automatic tanning product). In 3 hours, the product produces a rich, golden tan. The products used at Symmetry are professional quality and look natural. Home care products are available in our gift shop to keep the tan looking fresh. Think BETTER THAN A DAY AT THE BEACH!

Sea Boost: 1 hour $90

Seaweed is a unique product that stimulates circulation and lymphatic flow, boosts immunity, stimulates metabolism, and promotes detoxification. In this treatment, the body receives a dry brush exfoliaton aimed at increasing lymph flow before a warm layer of seaweed is applied and the body is wrapped. While wrapped in this relaxing cocoon, your feet are massaged. A Swedish massage with rich sea creams ends this service. Clients can request the application of a cellulite cream to target areas for body slimming. Think ELEGANCE!

Swiss Herbs Slimming Wrap: 90 mins $100

Relax in our sauna before being wrapped in fragrant linens that have soaked in an herbal infusion. As your body detoxifies, a cooling mist of citrus oils revitalizes your senses and relaxes your mind. Your body is removed from the wrap and treated to an invigorating grapefruit and juniper berry loofah scrub. This cools your body but continues to stimulate circulation and lymphatic flow. To complete this service, a firming cream with seaweed and aloe is massaged into your skin.
Think RADIANCE!

Symmetry
Massage & Day Spa

Figure 14-4 *(continued)*

Seaweed Wrap: After a relaxing foot bath, our specially trained therapist will apply seaweed to your body. Your body will then be wrapped and your feet massaged. The seaweed is then rinsed from your body, and a moisturizer is applied to rehydrate your skin.

Sea Dream: Begin your journey to the sea with a relaxing foot bath of warm salt water and ocean stones. Your body is revitalized with fresh, nourishing seaweeds harvested in the pure waters off the coast of Brittany. Rest, cocooned in warmth, while ocean sounds release everyday worries and your feet receive a pain-relieving reflexology foot massage. Your session ends in a warm aqua shower with skin softening ocean tonic body wash and fragrant moisture balm. Body, mind, and spirit are restored to balance by this inviting "day at the beach."

Although both of these descriptions clearly define what treatment steps the client will experience, the second description sounds inviting and special.

After the menu of services has been developed, the clinic owner or therapist may decide to write an operations manual.

THE OPERATIONS MANUAL

An **operations manual** is really a policies and procedures guide. It provides written support for staff and management so that an appropriate standard is set for the smooth operation of the business, the delivery of treatments, and for customer service. A basic operations manual might contain the following elements:

1. **Job descriptions:** The parameters of each person's job are described to clarify duties and responsibilities.
2. **Master forms:** A master copy of important forms such as the health intake, treatment record, client information form, and spa menu is kept within easy access for quick referral.
3. **Contact list:** A current list of employees and their contact details. It is also helpful to list which services each therapist is trained to deliver.
4. **Employee policies:** Policies on dress code, lateness, sick leave, and shift changes are listed in this section of the operations manual.
5. **Treatment guide:** A treatment guide can be included as part of the operations manual, or it can be a separate document. It lists the equipment needed to perform the treatment, the products that will be used, indications and contraindications for the treatment, the treatment steps, and any retail opportunities that have been identified by the treatment designer. If a therapist has not delivered one of the treatments for some time, this helps to remind him or her of the treatment steps.
6. **Order list:** This is an inventory sheet on which therapists can document that supplies of a particular product are running low and need to be reordered.
7. **Quick reference for reception staff:** It is helpful for reception staff to have a quick summary of the key information on each treatment and the retail items available. The reference might include a promotional description for each treatment, the benefits of the treatment, and specific booking notes for the treatment (e.g., client should plan to wear disposable undergarments or bring an old swimsuit because of the level of exposure required to provide this treatment). The reference might also include information about retail items.

8. **Daily cleaning checklist:** The operations manual should contain a checklist of the cleanup and housekeeping duties to ensure that the facility remains clean and professional at all times.
9. **Opening and closing procedures:** A checklist of the steps involved in opening up the business and closing it each day is useful. This should include a list of equipment that needs to be turned on at the start of the day, such as wax pots, table warmers, and stones for the stone massage. These items also need to be turned off at night to prevent fires.
10. **Maintenance log:** The maintenance log is a running list of maintenance needs. Each employee is encouraged to note what they see or encounter during the course of a day (e.g., in treatment room 3, the cabinet door on the far right does not close completely) to help management sort out these problems quickly.

Just like any aspect of a business, the operations manual needs to be updated and reevaluated on a yearly basis. Some business owners make copies of the operations manual and ask employees to sign that they have read and understood its contents. This ensures that everyone has the same understanding of how the owner would like the business to run.

BUDGET CONSIDERATIONS

Adding spa treatments requires new equipment, back bar and retail products, and additional marketing materials such as the spa menu. The choice of equipment and products should be based on the target market and the amount of money available to invest in the launch of the spa program. During the treatment design process (see Chapter 13), spa products were chosen for each step of the treatment. The cost of delivering each treatment was also worked out, and the price for the treatment was calculated. This information can now be used to assess how realistic the budget is and allows spa owners or therapists to project when they can expect to pay off their spa program launch.

To begin the budgeting process, list the new equipment and products that are needed for the launch of the spa program. This is the "startup budget," or the total cost to launch the spa program, deliver all of the treatments a predicted number of times, and train staff (when appropriate). Some expenses such as the hot towel heating unit, the soda coolers, the product mixing bowls, and the paraffin warmer only need to be purchased once. Other items are consumables, so they will run out at some point (e.g., spa products) or need to be replaced as they wear out (e.g., terry robes, towels). As part of the startup budget, owners or therapists determine how many spa treatments they will have to deliver in order to cover their costs. Table 14-5 lists some areas to consider during the budgeting process.

As part of the budget, the cost of offering the spa program for a whole year needs to be projected. Determine the cost of offering each treatment and then project how many

Table 14-5	Budget Considerations
SPA PROGRAM LAUNCH	**OTHER PRODUCTS BASED ON TREATMENTS**

SPA PROGRAM LAUNCH	OTHER PRODUCTS BASED ON TREATMENTS
1. **New Equipment**	3. **Retail Items**
Hot towel heating unit	4. **Promotional Items**
Soda coolers (one for each treatment room)	Business cards
Product warmers	Menu of services
Paraffin dip	Newsletters or promotional flyers
Washable wool blanket	Open house to launch the spa program
Thermal space blanket	5. **Staff training**
Hot wrap sheets	Training on treatments
Plastic or Mylar body wrap roll	Training on sales of retail items
Client heating devices	Training for receptionists
Terry robes	6. **Regular Expenses**
Terry wraps	Checking account and bank fees
Disposable or washable slippers	Rent, mortgage payment, or lease payment
Disposable undergarments	Office expenses
Bath towels	Linens and laundry
Hand towels	Insurance
Mixing bowls	Electricity and water
Shelving to store product	Telephone and phone book ad
Disposable implements	Cleaning and sanitation products
2. **Back Bar Products**	Continuing education
Cleansing products	Professional fees
Exfoliation products	Furniture and fixtures
Toning products	Staff salaries
Treatment products (e.g., fango, seaweed)	Bathroom supplies
Finishing products	Amenities (e.g., tea, bottled water)
Essential oil kit	
Massage oil	
Massage cream	

treatments will be delivered each month. Calculate the costs of reprinting the menu of services, marketing plans, staff trainings, purchase of new equipment, and the addition of new services as the menu expands.

Budgeting requires a lot of work and a lot of thought, but it helps small business owners know how they are doing and where they need to improve. It allows them to set benchmarks for their employees and themselves. With clear goals in place, the team is more likely to stay focused and provide excellent customer service.

RETAIL SALES

The spa industry makes a percentage of its income by retailing home care products to clients (Table 14-6). Regardless of the size of the business, **retail sales** should be factored into the business plan, budget, and expectation of staff. A dedicated retail area is a must, even if it is small. It should be visually exciting and positioned in such a way that clients see it when they walk through the door. To keep returning clients interested, the business may want to change the color, décor, and some of the products seasonally for fall, winter, spring, and summer promotions. Important retail selling times are Valentine's Day, Mother's Day, Father's Day, Christmas, and New Year's. The retail area must be spotlessly clean and well organized. Testers for products should be available so that clients who come early to their appointment can try out different products. Skin care lines should be grouped according to skin type, and information brochures should be available to provide a background on the products.

The **price point** of each individual product needs to be considered in relation to the target market of the business. For example, a young woman with two small children at home will probably not buy a $45 night cream. With a family budget to think about, the night cream is unlikely to be a priority. A moderately priced skin care trio of cleanser, toner, and moisturizer would make more sense. If the business targets professional women over 40 whose children are probably grown up, the night cream may be a viable retail option.

Some businesses buy retail items wholesale from their spa supplier or from businesses that create retail items especially for the spa industry. If the owner or therapist can afford to buy private-label items, this improves the image of the business and has the advantage that the back bar and retail items are often coordinated. When a product line is purchased from a spa supplier, a product representative often comes to provide training for the staff. Staff training is very important. If the staff members do not know a product, they are unlikely to be enthusiastic about it. The job of the therapist is to show clients the retail products, highlight special product ingredients, point out that this is the same product as what was used in the treatment, and describe the benefits of long-term use at home. Many therapists resist selling retail items, even when they are given a commission. The main reason for this is that they simply have no understanding of sales techniques, and they feel pushy when they try to sell items. Some businesses invest in a dedicated retail sales specialist. These individuals are experts in the spa's products, and their job is to identify solutions to clients' concerns with retail items. They initiate the sale, present appropriate products, and close the sale. In some high-pressure selling situations, the spa may expect one dollar of retail product to be sold for every dollar of service sold.

The business should set up some sort of system for tracking retail inventory. Retail items that sell best should be highlighted. Retail items that sit and collect dust should be cleared in a special promotion and discontinued to make space for other more viable products. If an item is not selling, first check the price point. It may simply be priced inappropriately for the target market. Computerized inventory tracking systems can be purchased for larger businesses. A smaller business may want to set up a simple system such as a running list of items that are sold, the employee who initiated the sale, and the client who purchased the product. A physical inventory needs to be conducted on a regular basis to check written records against stock.

A compensation plan for therapists and staff members is important if the business hopes to generate good sales of retail items. Compensation rates can range from 8% to 22% and are commonly around 10%. Sometimes two individuals are responsible for the sale. The therapist may initiate the

Table 14-6	Retail Items Often Sold at Spas		
Aromatherapy diffusers	Exfoliation gloves	Lip balms
Bath cushions	Face cleansers for skin type	Loofah mitts
Bath oils	Face toners for skin type	Natural hair care products
Bath salts	Facial masks	Nutritional supplements
Bath soaks	Fingernail files	Peppermint foot lotion
Body lotion	Flower remedies	Sea sponges
Body scrubs	Foot masks	Shower gels
Books	Foot soaking aids	Skin bleaching cream
Callus file	Gift baskets	Soap
Candles	Hand lotion	Sore muscle balm
Clay masks	Herb filled dream pillows	Spa bath robes
Cosmetics	Herb sachets for bath	Spa towels
Cuticle oil and nail polish	Home manicure kit	Specialized face creams
Essential oil blends	Home pedicure kit	T-shirts
Essential oils	Incense and incense burners	Wrinkle cream

sale during the treatment and then pass the client onto the receptionist or a sales specialist. In this case, a system will need to be organized in which the two individuals share the commission on the sale. Incentive programs can also be adopted to encourage sales of retail items. For example, the clinic may give the therapist with the top retail sales each month a gift certificate for dinner out at a restaurant or a free service at the spa.

As a spa owner or therapist, it is in your best interest to identify retail sales opportunities and to consider them as part of the treatment. The treatment designer can build retail opportunities into the transitions so that they flow from the treatment itself and are not jarring for the client. Building retail items into the design of the treatment is discussed in Chapter 13.

MARKETING ACTIVITIES

Marketing refers to all of the things that a business or individual does to attract new clients and retain their existing clients. The marketing activities that the business undertakes will be directly related to the work the owner or therapist did in defining the spa philosophy. In that process, the owner or therapist characterized the position in the industry and identified the client groups he or she wanted to reach (target market) with the spa program. The owner or therapist speculated on the target market's perceived health care needs and specialty focus and used this information to guide the choices made in treatment design and the adoption of new services. At this point, the owner or therapist knows who the target clients are and feels certain that the menu of services will be attractive to these clients. The next step is to create a marketing plan that includes activities in promotion, advertising, publicity, customer relations, and potential client education.

Promotional Activities

Promotional activities are actions that are taken to increase visibility in the marketplace and attract the attention of potential clients. These activities may include holding an open house, providing a free workshop, sponsoring an event to benefit the community, renting a booth at a community event or health expo, sending out information newsletters, offering free foot treatments at a local walkathon, mailing flyers that include a special offer to current and potential clients, providing personalized gift items, and providing referral programs. For example, when pregnant women are the target market, a clinic might create a flyer offering a discounted pregnancy spa package available on Saturdays. This flyer should be posted where pregnant women are most likely to see it (e.g., Lamaze classes, fitness centers, health food stores, obstetricians' offices, midwifery centers, maternity clothes shops). Ideally, the flyer would include an education section that alerts pregnant women to the benefits of the treatments included in the package. The infor-

mation provided should not only address the client's needs (e.g., lower back pain, stretch marks that could be prevented, tired feet, low energy) but should also aim to allay any potential concerns they may have (e.g., dangers to the baby, staying in one position for too long).

Printed materials factor prominently in promotion. These items include business cards, brochures, the menu, educational packets, letterheads, envelopes, newsletters, and direct mail pieces. If possible, these pieces should contain a logo and have a similar look and a consistent color scheme so that they blend together well and promote business recognition. These materials reflect the clinic's image, so they should be printed on high-quality paper and designed professionally whenever possible.

Advertising

Advertising is different than promotion because it requires direct payment in order to gain public notice. The most common types of advertising used by health care professionals are the classified ad, the display ad, and phone book ad. Identify where to place the advertisements and then contact the publication for a media kit. The kit will contain the rates for different ads, deadlines for placing ads, and art development information. Statistics show that an advertisement will need to be seen at least three times before it is noticed. It may need to be seen at least seven times before the reader decides to take action. Therefore, it is advisable to place a smaller ad that will run more often than to place a larger ad that will run once. Ads seem to work best when they contain a strong visual image and clearly define the benefits and incentives.

Publicity

Publicity is media exposure that usually arises from an event held at the business. Publicity might arise from an interview, news coverage of participation in a community event, or a feature story about the business or a particular service. For example, a local magazine might have a "tips for better living" section. Try sending in a press release outlining the benefits of reflexology for stress reduction. If the magazine is interested in this "new" approach to stress reduction, they will contact the owner or therapist about the treatment. They may then highlight the treatment in their magazine with a short story about the clinic or therapist. Research the media outlets in the area. Identify those that target the same client markets or that focus on health-related topics.

A press release draws the attention of a media representative to a newsworthy event (Fig. 14-5). The press release is generally one page in length and lists the business name, address, phone number, and contact person in the top left-hand corner of the page. The release date (usually "For Immediate Release") is placed in the top right-hand corner of the page. A headline summarizes the content of the release

For Immediate Release

REDUCE WORK-RELATED STRESS WITH REFLEXOLOGY

Contact:
Melissa Massage

400 Any Street #1
Any Town, Any State
10000

Ph: 255-555-5252
Fax: 252-222-5555

info@bodyinbalance.com
www.bodyinbalance.com

Massage
Aromatherapy
Body Treatments
Reflexology

A balanced
body is achieved
when time is made
for self-care

Take off your shoes and relax! That's how easy it is to reduce work week stress at the Body in Balance massage clinic and spa. The clinic has designed a selection of unique foot spa treatments that target foot pain and stress through reflexology.

Reflexology is a holistic treatment that works on the theory that points on the feet, hands, and ears correspond to all areas of the body. Through stimulation of these points, the body is able to rest, relax, and recover from the pressures of everyday life.

Body in Balance offers a full menu of massage, body treatments, aromatherapy services, and reflexology. Melissa Massage, the owner, is an American Board Certified Reflexologist. She personally designed each of the seven reflexology foot spa treatments offered at the spa.

Athletes will enjoy the Pain-Away Treatment, which uses therapeutic Moor mud from Austria. This special healing mud has been used in Europe to treat joint pain and inflammation. Also popular is the Sedona Clay Ritual, which utilizes the powerful red clays of Sedona, Arizona, together with juniper and sage essential oils.

Melissa notes that "anyone bashful about getting undressed for a spa treatment should try reflexology. Reflexology is a great way to unwind from a stressful work week, and it's literally as easy as taking off your shoes."

To contact a Body in Balance and find out more about reflexology and foot spa treatments, call 255-555-5252.

Figure 14-5 Sample press release.

and is placed in the middle of the page in bold capital letters. The body of the release should contain short, concise paragraphs with the most important information described at the top. The final paragraph should indicate the action the reader is meant to take as a result of the story (book an appointment, attend the event, conduct an interview, and so on). A press release is sent out each time the business participates in a community event, offers a free information workshop, donates its services in support of a charitable cause, introduces a new treatment, or provides an important service to a particular client group (e.g., free fitness checkup on Mondays for seniors).

Client Relations

Client relations refers to what the business does to keep their existing clients and build client loyalty. Most massage therapists truly care about their clients and enjoy building a strong relationship as a partner in good health. This natural tendency of therapists to relate positively to their client is the foundation of good customer relations. The business must also keep good client records; use high-quality products; make realistic claims for their services; provide a safe, comfortable, and sanitary environment; be prompt and reliable; refer to other health professionals when appropriate; return calls quickly; and treat clients warmly and respectfully, even if a particular client is perceived as "difficult." Successful clinics and spas usually go well beyond these foundation activities. They develop action plans to focus in on the particular needs and wants of their target market, and they pamper their clients from the moment they walk through the door. In Chapter 13, client management is discussed in relationship to client retention, and pampering activities are discussed in greater detail.

It is a good idea to set up procedures to maintain contact with clients between scheduled sessions. These activities might include checkup calls the day after the treatment, birthday cards, newsletters, anniversary cards (for the anniversary of the first time the client attended the clinic), and thank you notes for referrals. On special occasions (birthdays, anniversaries), the card can include a small gift in the form of a free treatment (free paraffin dip, free mini facial, 30-minute massage) or product (bath soak salts, lip balm) on the client's next visit. Referral programs are usually organized in the same way. Every time the client refers a friend or family member, the client receives a small gift or discount on the next service. An annual open house event for clients and their guests is a nice way to thank clients for their loyalty. The event might include hors d'oeuvres, seated massage, paraffin dips, a gift of bath salts, and a free spa package as a door prize.

Client Education

Educating people about spa and massage is essential to the growth of the industry. Often clients are confused about the word "spa." They may even think it refers just to a hot tub. Concentrate any education efforts on the target market (or markets) as much as possible. The education plan may include activities such as speaking at the meeting of a support group for a specific condition (e.g., fibromyalgia) or to particular groups (e.g., seniors, pregnant women). Presentations at fitness clubs, health food stores, sporting events, community events, and coffee shops raise the awareness of the general public to the benefits of spa and massage.

Newsletters are an effective way to maintain contact with current clients while also educating potential clients about the business and its services. Newsletters are used to encourage clients to come back and try a new service, use a special offer to bring back clients who have not visited for some time, promote products, build credibility for the business, and give clients information that can improve the quality of their lives. The style, color, and design of the newsletter should match the other printed materials used by the business. Predesigned information brochures and newsletters for health care providers are available from many companies. Using predesigned materials requires less thought and effort but does not feel as personal as a

specially created piece. Many desktop publishing programs come with predesigned templates that allow the writer to simply click and type in their specific information. With a little practice, even a beginner can create attractive materials.

Open house events are another method of reaching new clients. These events might include a presentation on the clinic and its spa program; a display that allows attendees to feel, smell, and try out spa products; and demonstrations of treatments. It is important to have a receptionist ready to book appointments on the spot instead of waiting for clients to call in after the event.

It is helpful to plan a marketing schedule that gives detail on daily, weekly, and monthly marketing activities. Time moves fast, and opportunities to promote the business come and go if a clear schedule is not maintained. Even a small business with a correspondingly small marketing budget should plan to spend 6 to 8 hours a week on short- or long-term marketing activities.

Summary

Before looking for a job at an established spa or adding spa treatments to a private practice or massage clinic, it is helpful to write a spa philosophy statement. The process of writing a spa philosophy statement helps therapists determine their beliefs about health, wellness, and beauty. It also helps them to identify the type of client that they most want to work with and the physical environment in which they want to practice.

Therapists who want to work at an established spa will use their spa philosophy statement to identify good spa matches in the spa industry. They will research their spa of choice, write a cover letter and resume, pursue an interview, and then negotiate an acceptable employment package. Some therapists get additional training or experience and pursue other careers in spa such as the spa product representative, spa educator, spa consultant, or spa director.

Some therapists choose to add spa treatments to their private practice or massage clinic. The treatments that they design for their spa program should fit in with their personal spa philosophy. The owner or therapist will create a menu of services and an operations manual to guide their staff. They will also plan marketing activities to support the launch of their spa program. The sale of retail items is an important aspect of the new business.

There are many opportunities for massage therapists in the spa industry. All therapists will find that self-assessment, good planning, continuing education, and a commitment to exploring new ideas and services will lead to a successful and fulfilling career in spa.

REFERENCES

1. The FDA Manual on Cosmetic Labeling. Available at http://www.cf-san.fda.gov/~dms/cos-labl.html
2. Miller ET: *Salon Ovations: Day Spa Operations.* Albany, NY: Milady Publishing, 1996.
3. Sohnen-Moe C: *Business Mastery: A Guide for Creating a Fulfilling, Thriving, Business and Keeping it Successful*, 3rd ed. Tuscon, AZ: Sohnen-Moe Associates, 1997.
4. The ISPA 2003 Spa Goer Study. Available at http://www.experienceispa.com/learn/resources.html

REVIEW QUESTIONS

Multiple Choice

1. A personal spa philosophy is best described as
_____.
   a. An individual's fundamental beliefs about health, beauty, and wellness
   b. The client groups that a therapist would most like to work with
   c. The type of physical environment in which a therapist would like to work
   d. All of the above

2. Back bar refers to _____.
   a. Drinks served in the treatment room
   b. Behind the scenes at the spa
   c. Large-size professional product containers that are used for the treatment
   d. Products sold to clients in the gift shop

3. The target market refers to
_____.
   a. All the activities the business undertakes to attract new clients
   b. All the activities the business undertakes to keep their current clients
   c. The specific groups of clients on whom the business focuses its promotional efforts
   d. All of the above

4. An individual looking for a spa job should:
   a. Send a cover letter and resume to the person in charge of hiring.
   b. Research the spa and understand its philosophy, treatments, and product lines before the interview.
   c. Be prepared to demonstrate massage and spa skills at the interview.
   d. All of the above

5. A spa director is:
   a. An individual who designs spa treatments
   b. An individual who is responsible for running a spa and making sure it is profitable
   c. An individual who answers the telephone and books clients
   d. An individual who plans marketing campaigns

True or False

6. _____ Demographic indicators and lifestyle indicators can be used to determine the spa's target market.

7. _____ Massage is the most popular treatment offered at spas, and spas are the main employer of massage therapists in the United States.

8. _____ Retail sales should not be encouraged at spas. Spas are places to relax, not shop.

9. _____ A spa consultant is the person who delivers the spa treatment to the client.

10. _____ Spa treatments require more setup and cleanup time than massage, but the therapist can charge more money for the same amount of treatment time.

APPENDIX A

Essential Oils and Their Botanical Names*

COMMON NAME	BOTANICAL NAME AND AUTHORITY
Allspice	*Pimenta dioica* (L.) Merr.
Amyris	*Amyris balsamifera* L.
Angelica	*Angelica archangelica* L.
Balsam fir	*Abies balsamea* (L.) Miller
Basil eugenol	*Ocimum gratissimum* L.
Basil reunion (exotic)	*Ocimum basilicum* L.
Basil sweet	***Ocimum basilicum* L.**
Basil tyymol	*Ocimum gratissimum* L.
Bay laurel	*Laurus nobilis* L.
Benzoin	*Styrax benzoin* Dryander
Bergamot	*Citrus x bergamia* Rissoe Poit
Black pepper	*Piper nigrum* L.
Cabbage rose	*Rosa x centifolia* L.
Cade	*Juniperus oxycedrus* L.
Cajeput (or cajuput)	*Melaleuca cajuputi* Powell
Caraway	*Carum carvi* L.
Cardamom (or cardomon)	*Elettaria cardamomum* (L.) Maton
Carrot seed	*Daucus carota* L.
Cassia	*Cinnamomum aromaticum* Nees
Cassie	*Acacia farnesiana* (L.) Willd.
Catnip	*Nepeta cataria* L.
Cedar texas	*Juniperus ashei* Buchholz
Cedar virginian	*Juniperus virginiana* L.

COMMON NAME	BOTANICAL NAME AND AUTHORITY
Cedarwood atlas	***Cedrus atlantica* (Endl.) Carr.**
Chamomile German	***Matricaria recutita* (L.) Rauschert**
Chamomile maroc	*Chamaemelum multicaulis*
Chamomile Roman	***Chamaemelum nobile* (L.) All.**
Cinnamon	*Cinnamomum verum* J. Presl.
Clary sage	***Salvia sclarea* L.**
Clove bud	*Syzygium aromaticum* (L.) Merr. & Perry
Copaiba balsam	*Copaifera officinalis* (Jacq.) L.
Coriander	*Coriandrum sativum* L.
Cypress	*Cupressus sempervirens* L.
Dill	*Anethum graveolens* L.
Elemi	*Canarium luzonicum* (Blume) A. Gray
Eucalyptus bluegum	*Eucalyptus globulus* Labill.
Eucalyptus dives	*Eucalyptus dives* Schauer
Eucalyptus lemon	*Eucalyptus citriodora* Hook
Eucalyptus smithii	*Eucalyptus smithii* R.T. Baker
Eucalyptus radiata	***Eucalyptus radiata* Labill.**
Fennel sweet	*Foeniculum vulgare* Miller var. *dulce* Battand & Trabut
Fir needle silver	*Abies alba* Miller
Frankincense	*Boswellia carteri* Birdw.
Galbanum	*Ferula gummosa* Boiss.

*Oils that are in bold are the preferred species for use in aromatherapy or are the oils referred to in this text under that particular common name.

COMMON NAME	BOTANICAL NAME AND AUTHORITY	COMMON NAME	BOTANICAL NAME AND AUTHORITY
Geranium	*Pelargonium graveolens* L'Hérit.	Orange blossom (niroli)	*Citrus x aurantium* L. "amara"
Ginger	*Zingiber officinale* Roscoe	Orange pettigrain	*Citrus x aurantium* L. "amara"
Grapefruit	*Citrus x paradisi* Macfady	Orange sweet	*Citrus sinensis* (L.) Osbeck
Helichrysum	*Helichrysum italicum* (Roth) G.Don.f.	Origanum	*Origanum heracleoticum* Benth.
Hyssop	*Hyssopus officinalis* L.	Palmarosa	*Cymbopogon martinii* (Roxb.) W. Watson
Jasmin	***Jasminum officinale* L. form grandiflorum (L.) Kobuski**	Patchouli	*Pogostemon cablin* (Blanco) Benth.
Jasmin	*Jasminum sambac* (L.) Aiton	Pennyroyal	*Mentha pulegium* L.
Juniper	*Juniperus communis* L.	Peru balsam	*Myroxylon balsamum var. pereirae* (Royle) Harms
Lavandin	*Lavandula x intermedia* Emeric ex Lois.	Pine dwarf	*Pinus mugo* Turra.
Lavender spike	*Lavandula latifolia* Medik	Pine longleaf	*Pinus palustris* Miller
Lavender English or true	***Lavandula angustifolia* Miller**	**Pine Scots**	***Pinus sylvestris* L.**
Lemon	*Citrus x limon* (L.) Osb.	Ravensara	*Cryptocarya aromatica (Becc.) Costerm* (old name *Ravensara aromatica* Sonn.)
Lemongrass East Indian	*Cymbopogon flexuosus* (Steudel) W. Watson	Rock rose	*Cistus ladanifer* L.
Lemongrass West Indian	***Cymbopogon citratus* (DC) Stapf**	**Rose**	***Rosa x damascena* Miller**
Lime	*Citrus x aurantiifolia* (Christm.) Swingle	Rosemary	*Rosmarinus officinalis* L.
Linden	*Tilia x europaea* L. (old name or *T. x vulgaris*)	Rosewood	*Aniba rosaeodora* Duke
Litsea	*Litsea cubeba* (Lour.) Pers.	Sage common	*Salvia officinalis* L.
Mandarin	*Citrus reticulata* Blanco	**Sage Spanish**	***Salvia lavandulifolia* Vahl**
Marjoram Spanish	*Thymus mastichina* L.	Sandalwood	*Santalum album* L.
Marjoram sweet	***Origanum majorana* L.**	Savory summer	*Satureja hortensis* L.
Melissa lemon balm	*Melissa officinalis* L.	Savory winter	*Satureja montana* L.
Mimosa	*Acacia dealbata* Link	Spikenard	*Nardostachys grandiflora* DC
Mint cornmint	*Mentha arvensis* L.	**Spruce Canadian**	***Picea mariana* (Miller) Britton**
Mint peppermint	*Mentha x piperita* L.	Spruce hemlock	*Tsuga canadensis* (L.) Carrière
Mint spearmint	*Mentha spicata* L.	Sweet birch	*Betula lenta* L.
Myrrh	*Commiphora myrrha* (Nees) Engl.	Tagetes	*Tagetes minuta* L.
Myrtle	*Myrtus communis* L.	Tarragon	*Artemisia dracunculus* L.
Niaouli	*Melaleuca quinquenervia* (Cav.) S.T. Blake	Tea tree	*Melaleuca alternifolia* Cheel.
Nutmeg	*Myristica fragrans* Houtt.	Thuja white cedar	*Thuja occidentalis* L.
Orange bitter	*Citrus x aurantium* L. "amara"	**Thyme sweet (linalol type)**	***Thymus vulgaris* L.**

COMMON NAME	BOTANICAL NAME AND AUTHORITY	COMMON NAME	BOTANICAL NAME AND AUTHORITY
Thyme Moroccan	*Thymus saturejoides* Coss. & Balansa	West Indian bay	*Pimenta racemosa* (Miller) J. Moore
Tolu balsam	*Myroxylon balsamum* (L.) Harms	Wintergreen	*Gaultheria procumbens* L.
Turmeric	*Curcuma longa* L.	Yarrow	*Achillea millefolium* L.
Vanilla	*Vanilla planifolia* Andr.	Ylang ylang	*Cananga odorata* (Lam.) Hook.f. and Thomson
Vetiver	*Vetiveria zizanioides* (L.) Nash		
Violet	*Viola odorata* L.		

Resources

This list represents a small selection of suppliers, associations, and courses. Spa Bodywork does not endorse any particular product or company.

GENERAL EQUIPMENT AND SUPPLIES

American Salon and Spa
888-230-2040
http://www.americansalonandspa.com

Bio Jouvance
http://www.biojouvance.com

Bouvier Hydrotherapy
http://www.bouvier-hydro.qc.ca

Equipment for Salons
http://www.equipmentforsalons.com

Heat Inc. Spa Kur Therapy Development
800-473-4328
http://www.h-e-a-t.com

International Beauty and Barber Equipment
800-824-7007
http://www.ibbe.net

New Life Systems
800-852-3082
http://www.newlifesystems.com

Skin for Life Salon and Spa Products
866-312-7546
http://www.skinforlife.com

Touch America
800-678-6824
http://www.touchamerica.com

Universal Companies, Inc.
800-558-5571
http://www.universalcompanies.com

Many others: Try the search terms "salon and spa equipment," "spa equipment and supplies," or "hydrotherapy equipment."

SKIN CARE LINES

Aveda
800-644-4831
http://www.aveda.com

Bidwell Botanicals
888-360-3398
http://www.bidwellbotanicals.com

Bioelements
http://www.bioelements.com

Decleor
http://www.decleor.com

Dr. Hauschka Skin Care, Inc.
800-247-9907
http://www.drhauschka.com

Phytomer
http://www.phytomer.com

Skinceuticals
800-811-1660
http://www.skinceuticals.com

Spa Skin
http://www.spaskin.com

MD Formulations
http://www.mdformulations.com

Many others: Try the search terms "spa skin care," "skin spa," or "professional skin care."

SPECIALIZED PRODUCTS AND TRAINING

Abano Terme Bath and Beauty
http://www.abanousa.com

African Shea Butter Company
http://www.africansheabuttercompany.com

The American Institute of Aromatherapy and Herbal Studies
http://www.aromatherapyinst.com

Argiletz Clays
http://www.argiletz.com

Aroma—the People Aromatherapy (products made with therapeutic grade essential oils for the massage therapist)
253-238-6375
http://www.aromathepeople.com

Australia's Earth Beauty Clays and Minerals
http://www.australiasearth.com.au

Dead Sea Cosmetics Company
http://www.deadsea-cosmetics.com

Elizabeth Van Buren Aromatherapy (aromatherapy, natural products, bases, carriers, and trainings)
800-710-7759
http://www.evb-aromatherapy.com

Essential Aura (aromatherapy, natural products, bases and carriers)
250-758-9464
http://www.essentialaura.com

Essential Wholesale (oils, butters, clay, seaweed)
http://www.essentialwholesale.com

Golden Moor, Moor Mud Products
613-764-6667
http://www.goldenmoor.com

Fragrant Earth Aromatherapy
http://www.fragrant-earth.co.uk

The Institute of Integrative Aromatherapy (aromatherapy training)
http://www.aroma-rn.com

Mana Essentials (aromatherapy and products for spas)
http://www.manaessentials.com

Moor Spa Moor Mud Products
http://www.moorspa.co.uk

Natures Body Beautiful Clay
http://www.naturesbodybeautiful.com

The Northwest Center for Herbal and Aromatic Studies
http://www.theida.com

Northwest Essence Aromatherapy
253-884-5600
http://www.northwestessence.com

Original Swiss Aromatics (aromatherapy and trainings)
415-479-9120
http://www.originalswissaromatics.com

Pascalite Clay
http://www.pascaliteclay.com

Premier Dead Sea Company (Dead Sea products, salts and mud)
http://www.premierdeadsea.com

Purely Shea (shea butter)
http://www.purelyshea.com

Repechage Beauty from the Sea (seaweed products)
http://www.repechage.com

R.J. Buckle Associates (aromatherapy training)
http://www.rjbuckle.com

Salt Works (Dead Sea and other spa and bath salts)
http://www.saltworks.us

Samara Botane (aromatherapy, natural products, and trainings)
800-782-4532
http://www.wingedseed.com

San Francisco Bath Salt Company
http://www.sfbscompany.com

Shea Butter Hut
http://www.sheabutterhut.com

SMB Essentials (seaweed powders and more)
http://www.smbessentials.com

Spectrix Lab Essential Oil Analysis (to have essential oils tested for purity)
Larry Jones
831-427-9336
http://www.spectrixlab.com or larry@spectrixlab.com

Thalgo Marine Beauty (seaweed products)
http://www.thalgo.co.uk

Torf Spa Organic Moor Mud
877-811-1008
http://www.torfspa.com

Tsenden Aromatherapy (aromatherapy training)
http://www.spabodywork.com

Well Naturally Products (seaweed powder, clay powder, bulk lotions)
http://www.wellnaturally.com

Many Others: Try the search terms "aromatherapy," "essential oils," "aromatherapy training," "aromatherapy certification," or "essential oil analysis."

STONE MASSAGE

Aromatic Body Stone Therapy (hot stone workshops and equipment)
http://www.spabodywork.com

European Stone Massage (hot stone workshops and equipment)
http://www.europeanstonemassage.com

Stone Temple Institute (hot stone workshops and equipment)
http://www.healingstonemassage.com

Many Others: Try the search term "stone massage."

AYURVEDA

American Institute of Vedic Studies (ayurveda studies)
http://www.vedanet.com

The Ayurveda Company (products)
http://www.bytheplanet.com

Ayurveda Inspired Spa (ayurveda inspired spa treatment training)
http://www.spabodywork.com

The Ayurveda Institute (ayurveda studies)
http://www.ayurveda.com

Banyan Botanicals (ayurveda products)
http://www.banyanbotanicals.com

Diamond Way Ayurveda (ayurveda trainings and equipment)
http://www.diamondwayayurveda.com

Kerala Ayurvedic Pharmacy (products directly from India)
http://www.kapleyayurveda.com

Light on Ayurveda Education Foundation (information on instructors and schools)
http://www.loaj.com

Maharisha Ayurveda (products, studies)
http://www.mapi.com

Many Others: Try the search term "ayurveda studies," "ayurveda training," or "ayurveda products and supplies."

REFLEXOLOGY

American Reflexology Certification Board (ARCB)
303-933-6921
http://www.arcb.net

The International Institute of Reflexology
727-343-4811
http://www.reflexology-usa.net

SPA BUSINESS SITES

Med Spa Solutions (spa consulting, products)
http://www.medspasolutions.com

Plus One (spa design and management)
http://www.plusone.com

Preston, Inc. (spa consulting)
http://www.prestoninc.net

Spa Elegance (a resource site for the spa business or therapist)
http://www.spaelegance.com

Spa Equip (equipment, consulting, products)
http://www.spaequip.com

Spa Trade (a resource site for the spa business or therapist)
http://www.spatrade.com

Many Others: Try the search terms "spa consulting," "spa management," or "spa business."

SPA ASSOCIATIONS

Day Spa Association
http://www.dayspaassociation.com

The International Medical Spa Association
http://www.medicalspaassociaton.org

International Spa Association
http://www.experienceispa.com

SEARCH FOR SPAS

About Spas
http://www.spa.about.com

Spa Finder
http://www.spafinder.com

The Spas Directory
http://www.thespasdirectory.com

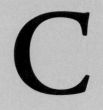

Ready-to-Copy Forms

SPA HEALTH IINFORMATION

Patient Name _____ Date _____

Address _____ State _____ Zip _____

Phone _____ Occupation _____

Emergency Contact _____ Phone _____

Primary Health Care Provider

Name _____ Phone _____

Address _____ State _____ Zip _____

Current Health Information

Please list all conditions currently monitored by a health care provider

_____

_____

 Please list the medications you took today (include pain relievers and herbal remedies).

_____

_____

Please list the medications you took in the past 3 months.

_____

_____

Please list and briefly explain (including dates and the treatment received) the following:

Surgeries _____

_____

Accidents _____

_____

Major Illnesses _____

_____

Tobacco Use: ○ Current ○ Past Comments _____

Alcohol Use: ○ Current ○ Past Comments _____

Drug Use: ○ Current ○ Past Comments _____

Are you currently menstruating?   ○ Yes   ○ No

Have you received a spa treatment before?   ○ Yes   ○ No

If yes, what types of spa treatments have you received? _____

Current and Previous Conditions

Please check all current and previous conditions and give a brief explanation, if appropriate, in the comments section at the end of this form.

Current	Past		Current	Past	
○	○	Headache	○	○	Heart disease
○	○	Pain	○	○	Blood clots
○	○	Sleep disorders	○	○	Stroke
○	○	Fatigue	○	○	Lymphedema
○	○	Infections	○	○	High blood pressure
○	○	Fever	○	○	Low blood pressure
○	○	Sinus condition	○	○	Poor circulation
○	○	Skin conditions	○	○	Swollen ankles
○	○	Athlete's foot	○	○	Varicose veins
○	○	Warts	○	○	Asthma
○	○	Skin sensitivities	○	○	Bowel dysfunction
○	○	Sunburn	○	○	Bladder dysfunction
○	○	Burns	○	○	Abdominal pain
○	○	Bruises	○	○	Thyroid dysfunction
○	○	Aversions to scents	○	○	Diabetes
○	○	Aversion to oils	○	○	Pregnancy
○	○	Allergies	○	○	Cancer
○	○	Sensitivity to detergents	○	○	Fibrotic cysts
○	○	Aversion to heat	○	○	Pacemaker
○	○	Aversion to cold	○	○	Phlebitis
○	○	Claustrophobia	○	○	Raynaud's syndrome
○	○	Rheumatoid arthritis			
○	○	Osteoarthritis			
○	○	Spinal problems			
○	○	Disc problems			
○	○	Lupus			
○	○	Tendonitis, bursitis			
○	○	Fibromyalgia			
○	○	Dizziness, ringing in ears			
○	○	Mental confusion			
○	○	Numbness, tingling			
○	○	Neuritis			
○	○	Neuralgia			
○	○	Sciatica, shooting pain			
○	○	Depression			
○	○	Anxiety, panic attacks			

Other Conditions:

_____
_____
_____
_____
_____

Comments:

_____
_____
_____
_____
_____

Therapist's Name: _____
Signature: _____
Date: _____

SPA TREATMENT RECORD

Client Name: _____   Phone: _____

Date: Treatment Received:	Therapist:	Comments:	Retail Items Purchased:

Date: Treatment Received:	Therapist:	Comments:	Retail Items Purchased:

Date: Treatment Received:	Therapist:	Comments:	Retail Items Purchased:

Date: Treatment Received:	Therapist:	Comments:	Retail Items Purchased:

Date: Treatment Received:	Therapist:	Comments:	Retail Items Purchased:

Date: Treatment Received:	Therapist:	Comments:	Retail Items Purchased:

TREATMENT DESIGN FORM

TREATMENT NAME:		
THE SPA'S OVERALL CONCEPT	THE SPA'S PRIMARY STRENGTH	THE TREATMENT INSPIRATION
THE TREATMENT CONCEPT	PROMOTIONAL DESCRIPTION	
TREATMENT GOALS	INDICATIONS	CONTRAINDICATIONS
CORE TREATMENTS	ENHANCERS/EXTRAS	RETAIL OPPORTUNITIES
TEXTURAL ELEMENTS		
SMELL-SCAPE	MUSIC/SOUND	VISUAL ELEMENTS
SUPPLIES AND EQUIPMENT		
PRODUCT CHOICES		SPECIAL EQUIPMENT

TREATMENT/TRANSITION/CLIENT MANAGEMENT STEPS	NOTES

COMMENTS

Dosha Questionnaire

Client Name: _____ **Date:** _____

	Section One: Prakriti
	Directions: Choose the answer that describes you the most accurately. No answer may fit perfectly, so simply make the best possible choice with the answers provided. Place a V, P, or K in the box to the left.
	My size at birth was small. (V) My size at birth was average. (P) My size at birth was large. (K)
	I am thin and either short or very tall. (V) I am of medium height and body. (P) I am tall and sturdy or short and stocky. (K)
	I have difficulty gaining weight. (V) I gain or lose weight easily. (P) I tend to gain weight easily. (K)
	I have long, tapering fingers and toes. (V) I have fingers and toes of medium length. (P) I have square hands and shorter fingers and toes. (K)
	I have knobby, prominent joints. (V) I have well-proportioned joints. (P) I have large, well-formed joints. (K)
	I have a delicate chin and small forehead. (V) I have a moderate chin and a medium forehead that has a tendency toward lines and folds. (P) I have a large jaw and large forehead. (K)
	I have uneven or buck teeth that are sensitive to either hot or cold. (V) I have even teeth of medium or small size that tend to yellow. (P) I have large, white, even teeth. (K)
	My lips are thin and narrow. (V) My mouth is of medium size. (P) My lips are full. (K)
	My skin is dry, rough, and cold to touch. (V) My skin is fair, soft, and warm to touch. (P) My skin is pale, cold, clammy, and tends to be oily. (K)
	My hair is fine, coarse, brittle, and fine to medium in texture. (V) My hair is fine, fair, or reddish. (P) My hair is thick, oily, lustrous, and wavy. (K)
	My neck is thin, very long, or very short. (V) My neck is of regular proportion. (P) My neck is solid and strong. (K)
	My eyes are small, narrow, or shrunken, and my eye color is dull. (V) My eyes are of average size and are light colored. (P) My eyes are large and lustrous. (K)
	The shape of my face is long and angular. (V) The shape of my face is heart shaped, and I have a pointed chin. (P) The shape of my face is rounded and full. (K)

	My tongue tends to be dry with a thin, gray coating. (V) My tongue tends to have a yellowish or orange coating. (P) My tongue tends to be swollen with a thick, white coating. (K)
	I have a high tolerance to heat and enjoy hot weather. (V) I have a low tolerance to heat and enjoy moderate to cool weather. (P) I have a high tolerance to heat and prefer hot, dry, and windy weather. (K)
	My normal body temperature is cool, and I tend to have cold hands and feet. (V) My normal body temperature is warm, and I often feel too warm or hot. (P) My normal body temperature is cold. (K)
	My sleep is light and fitful. (V) My sleep is sound but sometimes disturbed. (P) I enjoy deep, prolonged sleep. (K)
	I have short bursts of energy, but my endurance is low, and I run out of steam easily. (V) I have moderate energy, moderate endurance, and good reserves. (P) I have good endurance and large reserves of energy. (K)
	In heat, I perspire minimally. (V) In heat, I perspire profusely. (P) In heat, I get clammy, but I don't perspire freely. (K)
	I am always doing different things. I have a tendency to fidget. (V) My activity level is focused and moderate. (P) I can be sluggish and even lazy. (K)
	I have a lot of ideas that I have difficulty putting into action. I have a restless imagination. (V) I am organized, efficient, intelligent, and tend toward perfectionism. (P) I am steady, calm, and not easily disturbed but do not like to be rushed. (K)
	I am good at remembering recent events but have a poor long-term memory. (V) I have a good memory. (P) I absorb information slowly, but once I do absorb it, I have an excellent long-term memory. (K)
	I am creative and expressive. I often change my beliefs. (V) I am goal-oriented, ambitious, and have strong convictions that govern my behavior. (P) I am contented and calm. I have steady, deeply held beliefs that I will not change easily. (K)
	I have difficulty making decisions and change my mind often. (V) I make rapid decisions and believe that they are good. (P) I take a long time to make a decision but stick to the choices I make. (K)
	I dislike routine and need a lot of change. (V) I enjoy planning and organizing my life. (P) I like routine and don't like it when things change. (K)
	When stressed, I become fearful, anxious, and insecure. (V) When stressed, I become confrontational, aggressive, judgmental, and hot tempered. (P) When stressed, I have a tendency to withdraw. Sometimes I am greedy and possessive. (K)
	I am a free spirit. I don't carefully plan my life but go with the flow. (V) I am an achiever, and I am ambitious. I carefully plan each step of my life. (P) I feel safe, steady, and calm in my life. I would prefer it if things remain as they are. (K)
	On a good day, I am secure, grounded, and settled. (V) On a good day, I am confident, warm, brilliant, and witty. (P) On a good day, I am warm-hearted, loving, and active. (K)
	On a bad day, I am cold, distant, and insecure. (V) On a bad day, I am jealous and controlling. (P) On a bad day, I am possessive, lackadaisical, and clinging. (K)

	I know a lot of people, but I have few close friends. (V) I have a few good friendships. I seem to make enemies without meaning to. (P) I have many loyal and close friendships. (K)
	I spend the money I have impulsively and easily. (V) I plan how I will spend my money. (P) I spend money reluctantly, and I like to save. (K)

Totals: Place the total number of Vs under vata, the total number of Ps under pitta, and the total number of Ks under kapha in the spaces provided.

_____Vata   _____ Pitta   _____ Kapha

	Section Two: Vikrti—Indications of Imbalance
	Directions: Choose the answer that describes you the most accurately and place a V, P, or K in the box at the left. If none of these descriptions fit place an NA in the box to the left.
	Recently, my skin has been very dry, or I have dry patches. (V) Recently, I have had heat rashes and spots. (P) Recently, my skin has been oilier than usual. (K)
	Recently, my hair has been dry and brittle, and I have split ends. (V) My hair seems to be thinning or graying more rapidly than usual. (P) My hair has been excessively oily lately. (K)
	I feel underweight and can't seem to gain weight even though I am trying. (V) I keep gaining and losing the same 10 pounds. (P) I'm overweight, and I am having difficulty losing weight. (K)
	Lately, I feel cold a lot. (V) These days, I often feel hot and irritated. (P) Lately, I've been feeling cold and dull. (K)
	I keep waking up and have difficulty getting back to sleep. (V) I have difficulty getting to sleep, but once asleep, I sleep soundly. (P) I am sleeping excessively (9 to 10 hours a night), and I don't want to get up. (K)
	I feel exhausted, restless, and nervous. (V) I feel tense and tired but determined to get the job done. (P) I feel lethargic and have low energy, and I have difficulty taking on new tasks. (K)
	Lately, I feel indecisive, chaotic, and forgetful, and I have difficulty focusing and concentrating. (V) Lately, I feel like I am judgmental of others, overly ambitious, and often negative. (P) Lately, I feel uninspired and resistant to change, and I'm having difficulty retaining information. (K)
	I feel tearful and anxious. (V) I feel angry, aggressive, and confrontational. (P) I feel like I want to hide away from the world. (K)

Totals: Place the total number of Vs under vata, the total number of Ps under pitta, and the total number of Ks under kapha in the spaces provided.

_____Vata _____ Pitta _____ Kapha

Therapist's Comments: _____

_____

_____

_____

_____

_____

Answers to Chapter Review Questions

CHAPTER 1

1. D
2. C
3. C
4. B
5. D
6. Kur
7. Cold water cure
8. Kneipp
9. Radon
10. Female

CHAPTER 2

1. C
2. B
3. D
4. Bar, Liquid
5. Full body
6. Detoxification
7. Disposable
8. 159, 99
9. B
10. B

CHAPTER 3

1. D
2. A
3. B
4. C
5. False
6. True
7. True
8. False
9. True
10. False

CHAPTER 4

1. D
2. A
3. B
4. D
5. C
6. Temperature
7. Length
8. Larger
9. Reflexive
10. Homeostasis

CHAPTER 5

1. A
2. A
3. B
4. A
5. C
6. Distillation
7. 1 to 2 years, 6 months
8. Quenching
9. Climate conditions, soil conditions, extraction method, harvesting method, storage method, shipping method
10. Headache, Nausea, Slight sore throat

CHAPTER 6

1. C
2. B
3. C
4. A
5. Sunburn, shaved skin, condition where the skin is broken
6. Table
7. "Leathery"
8. Physician
9. Esthetician

CHAPTER 7

1. A
2. B
3. A
4. B
5. D
6. C
7. A
8. E
9. B
10. D

CHAPTER 8

1. C
2. A
3. B
4. D
5. A
6. X
7. A
8. X
9. A
10. A

CHAPTER 9

1. D
2. D
3. A
4. C
5. D
6. D
7. 20 to 30
8. 100, Wide
9. White
10. Matured

CHAPTER 10

1. D
2. B
3. C
4. C
5. B
6. B
7. A
8. C
9. E
10. D

CHAPTER 11

1. D
2. A
3. A

4. A
5. B
6. Five elements
7. Vigorous
8. Heavy, cold, slimy
9. Hot
10. Vata

CHAPTER 12

1. D
2. D

3. C
4. D
5. D
6. High-risk pregnancy, Rheumatoid arthritis, High blood pressure
7. Muscle soreness, stress, to promote relaxation
8. Shoes
9. Skin
10. Skin irritation

CHAPTER 13

1. D
2. A
3. C
4. D
5. B
6. B
7. C
8. D
9. E
10. A

CHAPTER 14

1. D
2. C
3. C
4. D
5. B
6. True
7. True
8. False
9. False
10. True

Glossary

Abhyanga: Massage with oil provided by one, two, or more therapists.

Algae: Algae occur in all marine and terrestrial ecosystems of the world wherever there is water. The terms *algae* and *seaweed* are often used interchangeably, which causes some confusion. Seaweeds are algae that have a particular growth form, but the term *algae* also includes a wide range of other terrestrial and aquatic organisms with different evolutionary histories.

Alginate: A substance found in seaweed that has therapeutic properties for skin and body and is often used as a thickening agent in cosmetic preparations.

Antiseptic: An agent that prevents or arrests the growth of microorganisms.

Arch: The bones in the foot are actually arranged to form three strong arches (medial longitudinal arch, lateral longitudinal arch, and transverse arch) that are commonly referred to as the arch of the foot. The arch provides the foot with the strength to support the body while remaining flexible and mobile.

Aromatherapy: The use of essential oils for healing.

Atomizer: A device that breaks down a watery product into a fine mist for spraying onto the body.

Aura mist: An aromatherapy body mist that is used only at the very end of the treatment. It is misted in a high arch over the client from the head to the toes. It should be scented with an aroma that contrasts with the treatment products and fills the treatment room with a refreshing scent.

Ayurveda: The traditional natural medicine system of India dating back more than 5000 years.

Back bar: Spa products often come in two sizes. The larger size is called the back bar and is used by the therapist during the treatment. It is not sold to clients and is not subject to the same labeling requirements as products sold to the public. The smaller size is sold in the retail area for clients to use for home care. It must meet the Food and Drug Administration's labeling requirements for cosmetics.[1]

Barrier function: The ability of the skin to prevent penetration by microorganisms and chemicals that might otherwise damage tissues or enter the circulation. The skin also reduces water loss.

Basalt: A type of igneous rock formed from the solidification of molten magma. Because magma cools quickly on the earth's surface, it generally has microscopic crystals and a smooth texture. Basalt holds heat better than many other rock types, and ocean or river basalt has a smooth surface, so it is one of the best types of stone for stone massage.

Callus: A small area of thickened skin that is caused by continued friction or pressure. The epidermis becomes more active in response to mild, repetitive irritation. This causes a localized increase in the thickened tissue at the surface of the skin.

Claustrophobia: The fear of being enclosed in narrow spaces.

Clay: A variable group of fine-grained natural materials that is usually "plastic" when moist and are mainly mineral in composition.

Cryogenic products: A product that cools the body area to which it is applied.

Cryotherapy: The therapeutic application of cold temperatures.

Cuticle: A fold of skin that partly covers the border of the nail. In a pedicure (or manicure of the hands), the cuticle is pushed back so the surface of the nail appears cleaner and smoother.

Dihydroxyacetone (DHA): The component in autotanning products that causes the skin cells to change color and appear tanned.

Disinfectant: A chemical that destroys harmful microorganisms; usually used on inanimate objects such as floors, walls, and countertops.

Dissolving exfoliants: Dissolving exfoliants are composed of alpha-hydroxy acids (AHAs) and beta-hydroxy acids (BHAs). AHAs include glycolic, citric, lactic, and malic acids. The most widely used BHA in cosmetics is salicylic acid or its related substances, sodium salicylate and willow extract.

Dorsiflexion: Bending the top of the foot (the dorsal surface) toward the shin.

Doshas: One of three subtle energies (vata, pitta, kapha) that hold together two of the five elements.

Dry room: A treatment room in which there is no shower or hydrotherapy equipment. Instead, hot towels are used to remove products from the client's body or clients take showers in a different area.

Emollient: A substance that softens the skin by slowing the evaporation of water.

Emulsion: A mixture of two or more liquids in which one is present as microscopic droplets distributed throughout the other.

Enzymatic exfoliation: Exfoliation that relies on biological action rather than physical abrasion. This type of exfoliation is applied to the skin and then rinsed off. The enzymes used dissolve keratin in the skin, thereby removing dead cells and supporting the natural process of exfoliation. Papain from papaya is an example of one of these enzymes.

Essential oils: Volatile plant oils extracted from certain aromatic plants that have both physiological and psychological effects on the human body.

Esthetician: This word is a variant of the word *aesthetician*, which is derived from *aesthetic*, a branch of philosophy dealing with the nature of beauty. Estheticians are beauty specialists with around 300 to 750 hours of training. Their scope of practice includes skin care, hair removal, and makeup application.

Exfoliation: A process by which dead skin cells are removed to improve the skin texture and appearance. Benefits include increased circulation and lymph flow, increased immunity, and relaxation.

Fango: The Italian word for mud; the term is used loosely to describe products that include mud, peat, and clay.

Father Sebastian Kneipp: A Bavarian priest who streamlined Priessnitz's treatments and combined herbal treatments with water cures.

Fixed oils: Vegetable oils that are nonvolatile such as sweet almond or sunflower. Essential oils readily dissolve into fixed oils, so fixed oils are often used as carriers for essential oils.

Fomentek: A type of water bottle that is designed to lie flat on the massage table.

Functional group: A reactive oxygen or nitrogen-containing unit of a chemical compound.

Galvanic current machine: A machine used by estheticians in facial treatments. It has two different uses depending on the polarity of the current that is used. When the working electrode is the negative pole, it is used with a disincrustation solution to soften blocked sebum in pores. When it is set on the opposite polarity (positive pole is the working electrode), it is used to soothe the skin and encourage the absorption of a water-soluble treatment product.

Hamam: An Islamic bath characterized by a vaulted ceiling and a raised, heated marble platform called a *hararat*, which is used for massage or exfoliation.

Herbal infusions: Herbs steeped in water to produce an infusion. Sheets, bath towels, or hand towels are soaked in herbal infusions and applied to the body for therapeutic purposes.

High-frequency machine: Machine that generates a rapidly oscillating electrical current that is transmitted through glass electrodes. The current produces heat in the skin, which stimulates circulation. It also produces ozone, which acts as a germicide to kill bacteria.

Homeostasis: The body's ability to maintain a relatively constant internal environment despite changing external conditions.

Hunting reaction: Alternating cycles of vasoconstriction and vasodilatation in response to cold.

Hydrotherapy: The use of water in one of its three forms (liquid, solid, or vapor) at specific temperatures for therapeutic purposes.

Interferons: Proteins secreted by some cells that protect them (and other cells) from viral infection.

Kapha: A dosha that is a combination of earth and water.

The Kur system: A German medical system that includes spa treatments as part of a wider system for health and wellness. Kur treatments are medically prescribed and paid for by the national health care system.

Lamina groove: Located between the spinous and transverse processes of the thoracic and lumbar vertebrae, the lamina groove is a vertical depression filled with the fibers of the transversospinalis (multifidi, rotators, semispinalis) and erector spinae (spinalis, longissimus, iliocostalis) muscles.

Learned-odor response: A response that occurs when an odor is paired with a person, place, or thing and a memory link is formed.

Limbic system: The oldest part of the brain where olfactory signals activate smell-related responses.

Luxury spa: A spa with exceptional accommodations, a full range of treatments, the latest advances in spa technology, a full array of wet-room equipment, and well-trained staff.

Marketing: The activities that a business carries out to attract new clients and keep existing clients.

Mechanical effect: The effect on the body of water that is pressurized in sprays, whirlpools, or through jets.

Mechanical exfoliation: A physical process in which the body is rubbed with an abrasive product or with a coarse handheld item such as a loofah.

Menu: A spa menu is like a menu at a restaurant. It lists all of the services that a client could "order" when visiting.

Minerals: Naturally occurring substances that play a crucial role in the body's metabolic processes. They are required by the body to function properly.

Moor mud: A low-moor peat from the Neydharting Moor in Austria that is well known for its anti-inflammatory effects. It is regularly mined and shipped to the United States for spa treatments.

Mucilage: A gelatinous substance found in plants and animals that is extracted for cosmetic purposes from plants such as seaweeds. It is composed of protein and polysaccharides and is used to give cosmetics a creamy substance and to moisturize and protect the skin.

Mud: Soft, wet earth that is mainly mineral in composition (derived from rock) with some percentage of organic matter (matter derived from plant breakdown).

Nail technician: A certified or licensed practitioner who provides care of the nails or applies, repairs, or decorates gel nails or acrylic nails.

Olfactory response: Olfaction is the sense of smell. An olfactory response includes the mental, emotional, or spiritual changes that may be elicited by an aroma.

Operations manual: A policy and procedure guide for the spa staff. It lists important information such as contact phone numbers, dress code, and opening and closing procedures.

Oxidation: A reaction that occurs when the chemicals in essential oils interact with the oxygen that is present in the air. This results in degradation of the oil.

Parafango: A product composed of paraffin and mud. It is mainly used to apply heat to body parts.

Peat: Partially carbonized organic tissue formed by decomposition in water of various plants but mainly mosses of the genus *Sphagnum*.

Pedicure: A treatment in which the foot is soaked, calluses are reduced, the nails are trimmed and filed, the cuticles are pushed back and trimmed, and the nails are buffed or polish is applied to the nails. Nail care is provided only by certified nail technicians or cosmetologists (depending on the laws of the particular state).

Pin and stretch techniques: Techniques in which the muscle is first shortened, then "pinned" at its origin, insertion, or muscle belly, before being lengthened. The effect of this technique is to reset proprioception and lengthen chronically shortened muscles.

Pitta: A dosha that is a combination of fire and water.

Plantar flexion: Bending the bottom of the foot (plantar surface) downward (as in pointing the toes).

Polysaccharides: A class of long-chain sugars composed of monosaccharides that are often used in skin care as antioxidants and water-binding agents.

Poultice: Usually a cloth filled with heated herbs, clay, or a medicated product spread on a cloth and applied to wounds or an injury.

Prakriti: The constitution or inherent characteristics of a person, including his or her physical type, mental type, and emotional type.

Price point: The price the public will pay for a retail item. The business must choose how much of a markup they will add to retail items. This markup becomes the price point.

Proprioception: Proprioception is the kinesthetic sense in which sensory receptors receive information about rate of movement, contraction, tension, position, and stretch of tissue. This information is processed in the central nervous system, which sends motor impulses back to muscle, causing it to contract, relax, restore, or change position.

Quenching: Process that occurs when the action of one compound in an essential oil is suppressed by another compound, thereby making the oil safer for use.

Radon: A naturally occurring atmospheric gas that is radioactive and is released as uranium in rock and soil breaks down. It is used in trace amounts in Europe for the treatment of arthritis and asthma.

Reflexology: A holistic therapy that is based on the belief that specific points on the hands, ears, and feet correspond to specific areas of the body, including the organs and glands.

Retail sales: The spa or clinic may choose to buy spa-related items or skin care products at wholesale prices from distributors. They then mark up these items (average: 40% to 50%) and sell them to the public. This provides the spa or clinic with an additional income stream.

Sanitation protocol: The spa or clinic's procedure for keeping the facility clean and disinfected during operation.

Seaweed: Multicellular marine-based algae that fall into one of three main groups: green algae (*Chlorophycota* spp.), brown algae (*Phaeophycota* spp.), and red algae (*Rhodophyta* spp.).

Shirodhara: The application of a thin stream of oil to the forehead to reduce vata disorders and bring calm to the mind and body.

Signature spa treatment: A special treatment that is only offered by one spa. It is designed to highlight the spa's unique features and particular strengths.

Silicone: One of the elements present in seaweed that binds water to the skin and gives a silky feel when added to cosmetics.

Spa: A commercial establishment that provides health and wellness treatments.

Spa philosophy: The fundamental beliefs that an individual or business holds about health, wellness, and beauty. The spa philosophy might also include a consideration of the clients that the therapist would like to work with and the environment where he or she wants to practice.

Spa program: Collectively, all of the different services that are offered at a spa.

Spa therapy: A general term for a wide range of spa treatment methods or techniques used by various professionals in different settings to support health and wellness.

Spa treatment: A general term for a treatment that uses water, specialized products, and various techniques to bring about relaxation, address a specific pathology, or support overall health and wellness.

Sphagnum: A genus of mosses that grows only in wet acid areas where their remains are compacted over time (sometimes with other plants) to form peat.

Stratum corneum: The outermost layer of the epidermis of the skin that provides the skin with its barrier function.

Sulfur: A chemical element that is an important constituent of many proteins and is often found in thermal pools and in some therapeutic muds. Sulfur is believed to reduce oxidative stress on the body and is used to treat arthritis, sore muscles, skin diseases, and other conditions.

Swiss shower: A shower stall that has pipes in all four corners with 8 to 16 water heads coming off each pipe.

Synergy: When the whole is greater than the sum of its parts and those parts are mutually enhancing.

Taila: Medicated massage oil that is made by cooking herbs into a fatty base such as sesame or coconut oil.

Target market: The client group or groups on which the business focuses much of its marketing campaign. Target markets are defined by demographic and lifestyle indicators. The business designs its spa treatments and other services to meet the needs of the target market.

Terme: Thermal bath. From the Greek *therme* meaning heat, and *thermai* meaning of or related to hot springs.

Textural elements: The word "texture" describes the varied sensations the therapist creates during the treatment by paying attention to what the client sees, hears, smells, tastes, and feels.

Thalassotherapy: The use of marine environments and sea products, including seawater, sea mud, seaweed, and seafood, for healing and wellness.

Thermal mud: Mud that comes from the areas around hot springs. It can be applied at the site while still hot from the spring water, or it can be extracted and heated for later application elsewhere.

Thermotherapy: The therapeutic application of heat

Treatment concept: An abstract idea that helps both to organize the different parts of a treatment and to send a specific message to the client.

Ubtan: An herbal paste used to support detoxification and smooth the skin. It is applied externally to the body.

Universal Precautions: The policy of the Centers for Disease Control on blood and body fluids, which are potentially infectious sources of human immunodeficiency virus (HIV), hepatitis B virus (HBV), and other bloodborne pathogens.

Ultraviolet A (UVA) rays: Sometimes refered to as "aging rays," these rays from the sun penetrate deeper into the skin than ultraviolet B rays and cause photosensitivity reactions.

Ultraviolet B (UVB) rays: Also known as "burning rays," these rays from the sun are the primary rays associated with skin damage and cancer from the sun.

Vasoconstriction: When the lumen of a blood vessel is contracted, reducing the diameter of vessel and decreasing blood flow to a region of the body.

Vasodilatation: When the lumen of a blood vessel is relaxed, increasing the diameter of the vessel and increasing the blood flow to a region of the body.

Vata: A dosha that is a combination of space and air.

Vichy shower: A horizontal rod with holes or water heads that rain water from above a wet table down onto clients.

Vikrti: An individual's diet, environment, work stress, mental or emotional trauma, relationships, or physical injury may cause their prakriti (dosha constitution) to become unbalanced. The unbalanced state is referred to as a vikrti state.

Vincent Priessnitz: An Austrian farmer who became famous for the cold water cure, which consisted of drinking large amounts of cold water, and applications of cold water by packing, immersions, and douches.

Volatility: The rate at which a compound turns from a liquid to a gas at room temperature (i.e., when it evaporates).

Wet room: A treatment room that contains specialized hydrotherapy equipment such as showers that remove spa products from clients' bodies, hydrotherapy tubs, and Scotch hoses.

Index

Page numbers followed by f denote figures; those followed by t denote tables.